Essentials
of
Psychotherapy

Essentials
of
Psychotherapy

Edited by

Samuel M. Stein
Rex Haigh
Jennifer Stein

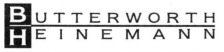

OXFORD AUCKLAND BOSTON JOHANNESBURG MELBOURNE NEW DELHI

Butterworth-Heinemann
Linacre House, Jordan Hill, Oxford OX2 8DP
225 Wildman Avenue, Woburn, MA 01801-2041
A division of Reed Educational and Professional Publishing Ltd

A member of the Reed Elsevier plc group

First published 1999

© Reed Educational and Professional Publishing Ltd 1999

British Library Cataloguing in Publication Data
A catalogue record for this book is available from the British Library

Library of Congress Cataloguing in Publication Data
A catalogue record for this book is available from the Library of Congress

ISBN 0 7506 2655 0

Typeset by Latimer Trend & Company Ltd, Plymouth
Printed and bound in Great Britain by Biddles Ltd, Guildford and King's Lynn

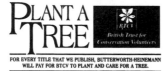

As so much is yet unknown the student is recommended to carry out research in his own way, and if he must read instead of making observations let him read descriptions by many different writers, not looking to one or another as the purveyor of the truth.

Donald Winnicott, *The Child, the Family and the Outside World*, 1964

Contents

Contributors

Gwen Adshead MBBS, MRCPsych, MA Medical Law and Ethics
Consultant Psychotherapist and Honorary Senior Lecturer in Forensic
Psychotherapy, Broadmoor Hospital, Berkshire

Michael van Beinum BSc, MBChB, MPhil, MRCPsych, SAPP
Consultant in Child and Adolescent Psychiatry, Glasgow

Fiona Blyth RMN, MSc
Certified Transactional Analyst and Senior Adult Psychotherapist, West
Berkshire Psychotherapy Service

Philip M. Brown MBChB, MRCPsych
Consultant Psychotherapist, Guild Community Healthcare Trust, Preston,
Lancashire

Gerry Byrne BA, RMN, MA Psychoanalytic Observational Studies
Clinical Nurse Specialist in Child and Adolescent Psychiatry, Park
Hospital for Children, Oxford

Philip Davison BSc, MBChB, MRCPsych
Consultant Psychiatrist, Littlemore Hospital, Oxford

Chess Denman MBBS, MRCPsych
Associate Professional Consultant Psychotherapist, Addenbrookes
Hospital, Cambridge; Member, Society of Analytical Psychology

Chris Evans MRCPsych, MembInstG
Consultant (Research and Development), Tavistock and Portman NHS
Trust, London

Terri Eynon MBChB, MRCPsych
Senior Registrar in Psychotherapy, Humberstone Grange Clinic, Leicester
Mental Health Services NHS Trust

Rex Haigh MA, BMBCh, MRCGP, MRCPsych, MembInstGA
Consultant Psychotherapist, Winterbourne Therapeutic Community,
Reading, Berkshire

James Herdman MA, MBBChir, MRCGP, MRCPsych
Consultant Community Psychiatrist, Thames/Coromandel, New Zealand

Alice Levinson MBBS, MRCPsych
Senior Registrar in Psychotherapy, Cassel Hospital, London and Parkside
Clinic, London

Kate Lockwood MBBS, MRCPsych
Senior Registrar in Psychotherapy, Tavistock Clinic, London and Forest
House Psychotherapy Clinic, London

Gill McGauley BSc, MBBS, MRCPsych
Consultant and Senior Lecturer in Forensic Psychotherapy, Broadmoor
Hospital Authority, Berkshire, and St George's Hospital Medical School,
London

Matthew Patrick MBBS, BSc Hons, MRCPsych
Associate Member of the British Psycho-Analytical Society; Consultant
Psychotherapist, Tavistock Clinic, London; Lecturer in Developmental
Psychopathology, University College London

Jennifer Stein BSc, PhD, MBBCh, MRCPsych
Consultant Psychiatrist in Psychotherapy, Rockingham Forest NHS Trust,
Kettering, Northamptonshire

Samuel M. Stein BA Criminology, MBBCh, MRCPsych
Consultant Child, Adolescent and Family Psychiatrist, South Bedfordshire
Community Health Care Trust, Luton and Dunstable

Steve Thwaites BSc, RMN, Dip in Family Therapy
Clinical Nurse Manager, Highfield Family and Adolescent Unit,
Warneford Hospital, Oxford

Foreword

Dame Fiona Caldicott

This book sets out to delineate the 'essentials of psychotherapy', not an easy task. The editors are successful in describing a field, constituted by many approaches, which largely derive from a small number of theoretical positions. There are therefore many overlaps and differences of emphasis, as well as radical variations between 'schools'.

It is also significant that all three of the editors have trained and also work in the National Health Service in the United Kingdom. The application of such important and potentially beneficial clinical approaches in a health system funded from taxation, and in which treatment is 'free at the point of delivery' has not been straightforward.

The pressure in recent years to demonstrate 'cost effectiveness' of psychotherapeutic treatment has not been espoused as readily in the UK as in some other countries such as Finland. This, as managers have tried to contain costs, has meant that in many parts of the service, patients with psychological and psychiatric symptoms and their advocates, including general practitioners, have perceived that the only service available to them is based on physical treatments.

The challenge to this position has shown the power of the 'consumer'. Pressure to provide a full range of effective approaches has led to a comprehensive review of both the research evidence and the literature concerning efficacy, and finally a widespread expectation that many of the psychotherapeutic approaches described in this book will be made available to patients on the NHS.

While this has been happening, students, trainees and some of the other groups at whom this book is targeted have wanted a text, which guides them through the complexities of the different treatment approaches, suitable for individual patients seeking help.

The chapters are clearly written and cover each approach in a consistent and comprehensive way. For those seeking more advanced texts, a guide to further reading is provided at the end of each.

So this book provides both an introduction to the field of psychotherapy, and also a platform for the reader who wishes to explore some parts of it in more depth. I thoroughly commend it.

Introduction

Rex Haigh, Jennifer Stein and Samuel M. Stein

About this book

There is no single book which draws together all the major psychotherapeutic approaches, and presents them in a common format from which factual information can be quickly obtained and comparisons made. In *Essentials of Psychotherapy* we aim to do just that, using a straightforward and accessible style which may be more associated with lecture notes and revision aids than it is with most psychotherapy texts. We have established a standard set of headings for each chapter, have included bullet lists where helpful, and made use of diagrams and tables to replace or simplify text.

The overall style tries to approximate to introductory lectures for trainees in the subject who are not specializing in psychotherapy, but need to have a working knowledge of it. At times this has clearly limited our contributors' creativity and the exploration of novel ideas, but it has ensured that the essentials are highlighted without being clouded by complexity or controversy. Instead, the reader is guided towards the many psychotherapy books that cover these areas in greater depth and sophistication through the recommended Further Reading and the references provided at the end of each chapter.

Essentials of Psychotherapy was initially aimed to meet the needs of medical students and junior doctors whose training required a broad understanding of psychotherapy. However, psychotherapy is a thoroughly multiprofessional discipline, and many other trainees will also find it useful – either for examinations, or simply for broadening their understanding of this component of mental health. Trainees specializing in one modality of psychotherapy should find the book helpful in providing a working knowledge of the whole field.

This book is also designed to help those clinicians who need to refer patients for psychotherapy. Clear guidance is provided to help determine which therapeutic approaches might be most valuable for particular patients. Psychotherapists who have trained in one approach are often unaware of how their practice compares with, or fits alongside, other psychotherapies. *Essentials of Psychotherapy* will enable them to compare and contrast different theoretical models and clinical techniques, and to generate greater understanding and cooperation between neighbouring schools of therapy.

Administrative and managerial staff involved in commissioning services may have a limited understanding of psychotherapy. This may lead to specific approaches being inappropriately applied to a wide spectrum of patients. *Essentials of Psychotherapy* will enable such staff to differentiate between the rumours and myths about psychotherapy and the facts, encouraging a more careful evaluation of what patients need and how best to deliver it.

Readers without a clinical background who are interested in the development of ideas, or the place of psychotherapy in the caring professions, should find the information set out in a clear way, without the use of complex jargon, and from which a broad understanding can be gained. This will help them to be informed participants in the widespread public debate about the place of psychotherapy.

Essentials of Psychotherapy may also assist prospective psychotherapy patients in deciding whether psychotherapy is likely to help them, and which approach might suit them best. Whilst much of psychotherapy can only be fully understood by experiencing it, there is a growing culture of openness about what psychotherapists actually do. This book also attempts to dispel some of the unhelpful ideas that have led to psychotherapy being perceived as a mysterious practice, away from public gaze or scrutiny.

The authors

All the authors are qualified mental health professionals working in the National Health Service. They are either involved in, or have recently completed, specialist training in psychotherapy. This has ensured that they are familiar with contemporary ideas and modern practice. It has allowed them to distil the essential ingredients of the different approaches without being affected by the personal notions and clinical biases that often influence the experienced practitioner. Whilst this guidance may be extremely valuable in developing specialized and sophisticated practice, it may confuse trainees who are still struggling to grasp the basics of psychotherapy.

The authors have all worked in centres of excellence where research, debate and the development of innovative ideas are encouraged. They have been actively involved in the evolution and shaping of clinical practice and the theory underpinning it. This enables them to communicate current practice with authority, and with a good understanding of recent research and trends. They are also all involved in teaching and training, and are keen to convey their knowledge and enthusiasm for the subject to a wider audience.

The structure of the book

Essentials of Psychotherapy aims to provide an introduction to a broad range of different psychotherapies. Most chapters are about one therapeutic approach, and they are presented in a way that they stand by themselves, but can be compared directly and easily with others.

The general categories covered are the analytic therapies, modifications of these analytic therapies, the influence of cognitive and systemic models, and therapies that involve more than one person. Several chapters directly address the application of therapeutic principles to specific patient groups.

Critical appraisal of psychotherapy is also essential, and the establishment of a robust evidence base for it is drawn together in a separate chapter on *Psychotherapy Research*.

Classical Psychoanalytic theories dating from the early twentieth century are *Freudian Psychoanalysis* (the modern form generally being called 'Contemporary Freudian') and *Jungian Psychotherapy* (often called 'analytical psychology'). The distinct psychoanalytic approaches which later emerged were *Kleinian Psychoanalysis* and the *Independent British School*. *Other Psychoanalytic Developments* included the work of Bion, Kohut, Lacan, Kernberg and Matte Blanco. *Child Psychotherapy* also has a background in psychoanalysis, but has since developed a body of distinct theory and practice.

These therapeutic techniques were then modified and applied to more general clinical work. *Psychoanalytic Psychotherapy* tends towards the classical analytic stance, but is applied in settings where the most intensive approach is not possible or desirable. *Brief Focal Psychotherapy* covers the use of analytic principles in a time-limited format with specific therapeutic goals. The *Conversational Model* has its origins in Jungian analysis but has also been adapted to meet the needs of a more general and diverse patient group. *Humanistic Therapies* cover various different specific treatment methods which have evolved in parallel to, but mostly separate from, the psychoanalytic schools.

Group Therapy, *Family Therapy* and *Therapeutic Community* approaches have evolved in close relationship to psychoanalysis, but they also draw on other theoretical traditions such as systems theory and social psychiatry. *Cognitive Behavioural Therapy* (CBT) comes from a non-analytic tradition, based on theories of learning and information processing. *Cognitive Analytic Therapy* (CAT) has been specifically constructed from these different roots, combining cognitive and analytic approaches.

Forensic Psychotherapy is an evolving discipline with a growing theoretical foundation and method of clinical practice, for particular populations in a specific setting. Likewise, *Psychotherapy in General Practice* makes use of particular dynamic techniques in providing holistic care and emphasizing the doctor–patient relationship.

The structure of each chapter

Historical perspective places each approach in context alongside related therapies. It describes the development of the therapy, including important names, dates and the process by which it evolved.

Principles of theory and practice gives a concise description of the theories that underlie each form of therapy, and the way in which the theory is applied in the clinical setting. This section explains what the therapy is and how it works. It also describes the aims of therapy, where it is relevant and how it differs from other therapies.

Which patient and why? gives an account of who is helped by each therapy. It explains the indications for therapy, contraindications to therapy and the assessment procedure by which patients are selected.

Which therapist and why? covers the necessary background for therapists, the training they need to receive, some details about how this is administered, and the maintenance of safe professional practice and ethical standards through adequate supervision.

Therapeutic setting includes all the practical issues and contextual factors which have an impact on the delivery of therapy, such as rooms, payment and institutional dynamics. Special therapeutic requirements and the advantages of particular settings are considered.

Clinical examples aim to demonstrate how the theoretical issues come to bear on the therapeutic work, and make clear what actually happens in the treatment process.

Problems in therapy include the pitfalls inherent in a particular approach, the mistakes and errors that are commonly made, and misconceptions that may exist.

Evaluation of therapy examines relevant research, considers financial implications, discusses therapeutic efficacy and draws together the evidence base available for each therapy.

Alternatives to therapy gives an account of why this form of therapy may be the first choice, what other options may be suitable, and the interaction and compatibility with other treatments.

Further Reading lists the key books or papers which explain the material of the chapter in more depth and sophistication, whereas the *Bibliography* lists the authors cited and quoted in the text and those who have generally made an original contribution to the development of that approach. Some works may appear in both sections.

One discipline and many: comparing and contrasting

To those unfamiliar with the profession, psychotherapy often looks like a bewildering field with numerous subdivisions, overlaps and splits. Novices may even find it difficult to decide whether psychotherpy is one discipline or many. The editors of this book take the view that it is one discipline *and* many. The chapters are all independently written, to a common structure, and there are many cross-references between therapies. The following discussion presents an overview of all the approaches covered, and uses some of the sections which are standard throughout the book to illuminate the 'headlines' of each different therapy.

Historical perspective: the evolution of psychotherapy

Freud is always seen as the father of psychoanalysis, although the influence of his writings varies considerably between different approaches. Many alternatives to classical psychoanalysis were conceived in rebellion against the dominance of his theories, as all the subsequent psychotherapeutic schools wanted to modify at least part of his model. Some schools, such as behaviourism, were established in almost direct opposition to Freud's thinking and ideas.

The work of Freud and Jung, and the approaches directly related to their teachings, date from the beginning of the twentieth century. Kleinian analysis, the Independent British School of psychoanalysis, group therapy and therapeutic community approaches all emerged in a fairly specific form in the middle of the century. Brief focal therapy, psychodynamic psychotherapy and later analytic developments developed gradually in the second half of the twentieth century. The youngest therapies described in this book are cognitive analytic therapy, cognitive behavioural therapy, family therapy and the Conversational Model of therapy.

Principles of theory and practice

Intrapsychic and interpersonal approaches

A distinction which may be useful for distinguishing the theoretical foundations of the wide range of psychotherapies described in this book is between intrapsychic and interpersonal theories. These are sometimes more simply called 'one-body', 'two-body', 'three-body' and 'multi-body' psychologies. This typology provides a simple framework in which one can begin to comprehend both the similarities and the differences between the various psychotherapeutic approaches.

A *one-body* psychology is primarily concerned with the individual. Relationships with others, and the wider social context, are seen as secondary to the individual's needs and development. In therapy, the focus is therefore on making changes to the individual only; the relationship with the therapist or interactions with other people are not considered as important. Freud's earliest theoretical principles were of this nature, but as soon as transference was described the idea of the patient as an isolated entity was no longer tenable. No modern psychotherapeutic theory now holds this one-body position, although it is the basis for pharmacotherapy and physical treatments of mental conditions. Recent developments in analytic theory are now, to a greater or lesser extent, *relational*.

Similarly, early behavioural theories viewed the individual as a *tabula rasa* (or blank slate) on which learning was imprinted. This learning could then be modified by behaviour therapy. However, behaviour therapists soon realized that this view was too simplistic, and both theory and practice were modified. The importance of a sound working alliance was deemed fundamental as most *antecedent–behaviour–consequence* (ABC) constructions have an irreducible social context. More recently, longer-term cognitive behavioural therapies have examined the patient's relationship with the therapist as part of a schema-focused approach.

The distinction between *two-* and *three-body psychologies* depends upon whether diadic relationships are of central importance (therapist–patient, patient–other, infant–parent), or whether the experience of triadic relationships is paramount (e.g. oedipal theory). In two-body psychologies, the self is actively involved in all the relationships. In contrast, three-body psychologies may also involve the self as a separate observer who is peripheral to the relationship between two other people. Most individual analytic theories fall into the three-body psychology category, although some approaches are closer to a two-body psychology as the focus is primarily on early diadic, pre-oedipal relationships.

Multi-body psychology implies that the whole network of relationships around an individual, which includes the individual, is the predominant determinant of problems and the target of therapy. This is the predominant theory behind group therapy, family therapy and therapeutic community approaches. Elements of work in these therapies will include one-, two- and three-body psychologies but the overriding principle will be that of an individual understood within the context of a web of relationships.

Use of the 'unconscious'

The principles of cognitive behavioural therapy generally exclude the concept of processes and functions which exist outside of conscious awareness. Many family therapists also do not make use of the unconscious, largely because it is felt to be tangential to their work. Cognitive analytic therapy acknowledges its presence and uses it in relation to transference issues, but it does not hold unconscious functioning as a central theoretical principle. Group therapy and therapeutic communities require an understanding of unconscious processes, but also use other concepts as the foundation of their work.

The analytically derived therapies (psychodynamic psychotherapy, brief focal therapy, the Conversational Model) actively use the idea of a dynamic unconscious, particularly in working with the transference, and this makes it a very important element of the theory. The psychoanalyses rely upon it absolutely, and it is the construct against which all clinical material is evaluated. In the analysis of the transference and countertransference, it is the guiding principle by which therapeutic techniques are used and progress is measured.

Research work showing the power of 'non-specific therapeutic factors' suggests that important unconscious work is done in all therapies, even those that do not acknowledge it. It is likely that the experience of a therapeutic relationship exerts a considerable proportion of its impact through unconscious mechanisms such as the provision of safe attachment and a sense of containment. To this extent, one can conceive that all therapies use unconscious mechanisms.

Ways in which the therapist is used

Cognitive behavioural (CBT), cognitive analytic (CAT), family, humanistic and brief focal treatments are structured therapies. In CBT, the therapist conducts the therapy by setting tasks for the patient and working to an agenda. CAT is also highly structured, with specific tasks to be undertaken by the therapist at certain points in the therapy. In family therapy, the therapist concentrates on strategic, structural or systemic approaches. Humanistic therapies differ in the way in which they are structured: for example, psychodrama is explicitly and closely directed by the therapist, and transactional analysis often uses visual aids to share the theory with patients. Brief focal therapy is structured by its limited duration, and the particular themes on which it concentrates.

The analytic therapies are open in their structure, following the principle of free association. In psychoanalysis and its derivatives, there is no agenda and patients are not directed or given any instructions beyond an explanation of the framework of therapy. Group psychotherapy operates similarly, and therapeutic communities generally use a mixture of directive and non-directive techniques. One of the main tools of psychoanalytic therapies is interpretation, which is a considered statement from the therapist about what is happening in the therapy. The way in which interpretations are delivered, and their content, differs between therapies and between practitioners. Some are deliberately tentative (such as the Conversational Model), some are more authoritative and, in groups and therapeutic communities, fellow-patients often make the interpretations.

The extent to which therapists can be spontaneous in their interaction with patients varies with the approach used and their level of experience. Analytic therapists generally maintain a level of therapeutic opacity to help elicit the transference, achieved through abstinence of any personal disclosures to the patient. In CBT such considerations are not relevant, and therapists may be more open. In family therapy, personal disclosures are neither encouraged nor discouraged but could be used as part of the therapeutic material if appropriate. In the humanistic therapies, the open experience of a real relationship between patient and therapist is seen as an important ingredient in itself, so these relationships are generally more spontaneous and less opaque.

Aims of therapy
Analytically based therapies do not have a focal aim. Their intention is wide-ranging personality change, and the material used has no predetermined agenda. The same is true of group therapy and therapeutic communities, except for groups which are set up for a specific purpose. Examples include assertiveness training, anger management and groups for survivors of abuse.

Brief focal psychotherapy works psychodynamically with a definitive focus in mind. Cognitive analytic therapy sets and modifies its own targets as part of the structure of therapy. Cognitive behavioural therapy has an agreed focus and normally works to a predetermined agenda. Psychodynamic psychotherapy and the Conversational Model are more exploratory in nature, and do not work to specific targets or foci.

Family therapies vary in their attention to declared aims and targets, depending on which specific approach is used. Some of the humanistic and experiential therapies will explicitly seek targets and specific areas to work on as an integral part of the sessions. This is particularly true of transactional analysis, Gestalt and psychodrama. Others, such as art therapy and Rogerian therapy, do not necessarily attempt to be directive in this way.

Which patient and why: aetiology and psychiatric diagnosis

The aetiology of conditions which psychotherapy aims to treat is seen differently within the different models. The analytic approaches generally regard problems as ultimately arising from deficiencies in early emotional development, brought about by environmental failure and a variable degree of innate characterological make-up. Thus trauma, abuse, neglect, deprivation and loss have enduring impact with psychological symptoms and mental illness as sequelae which can be ameliorated by appropriate therapeutic intervention. Group and therapeutic community approaches attach a high level of importance to the way in which these phenomena are caused, repeated and treated in the context of a network of relationships. Cognitive behavioural approaches are based on faulty learning, and the associated erroneous cognitions which arise around this. Systemic therapy is atheoretical about the aetiology of disturbance, and aims to bring about change by altering the configuration of the surrounding system.

Analytically based psychotherapies aim for personality change, and are thus often suitable for treatment of personality disorders. The patients frequently present with lifelong relationship problems, dysfunctional help-seeking behaviour (including self-harm and multiple psychiatric admissions) and miscellaneous neurotic and somatic symptoms. Some forms of cognitive behavioural treatment are also useful in treatment of these patients, particularly if a target can be agreed or if the patient is unwilling to embark on an analytic therapy.

Neurotic and affective disorders are treatable by the whole range of psychotherapies. Suitability for a specific type of therapy needs to be determined by careful individual assessment. Organic and psychotic conditions can often be alleviated and ameliorated by approaches informed by psychotherapy, but are not usually amenable to definitive treatment by psychotherapy.

Therapeutic setting

Practical and organizational requirements
Analysis is generally carried out in independent clinics set up for this purpose, or in private practice. The general principle of a quiet, comfortable and undisturbed room is sufficient for the task. Most psychoanalysts generally use a couch so that patients can lie down rather than sit face-to-face, whereas other analytically oriented therapists may or may not use a couch. Analysts working at home need to be careful about selection of patients, attempting to screen out the more disturbed individuals who could pose physical danger or excessive dependency. Organizationally, analysts require little more than sources of referral, availability of supervision and administrative systems for making appointments and charging fees.

All other forms of individual psychotherapy are carried out in a variety of settings: psychiatric hospitals, specialist units, private clinics, therapists' homes, GP surgeries, day hospitals and community mental health centres. Again, the minimum practical requirement is a quiet, comfortable and undisturbed room which is reliably available for the sessions. Cognitive analytic, cognitive behavioural and some of the humanistic therapies will need stationery and equipment for the sessions as they involve discussion of written material and preparation of charts, diaries and contracts. Other 'props' such as cushions and items of furniture are particularly used in Gestalt and psychodrama. Art and creative therapies need materials, water and facilities for storage and clearing up. Child psychotherapy also has particular practical needs, notably specially designed toys and play equipment. As with analysis, patients should not be seen in settings where their potential disturbance cannot be safely contained. The place of these therapies in the context of other services will vary from individual therapists practising with no external contacts except referrals and supervision, to therapy as a small part of a large and complex organization or system.

Family therapy has specific practical requirements, and often needs specifically designed rooms. This includes play equipment, furniture for children of all ages and video facilities for live supervision. The live supervision demands that more than one therapist is available. It therefore normally needs to take place as part of an organization of sufficient size to provide those facilities.

Group therapy requires a room of sufficient size to accommodate a group, and chairs which are comfortable enough for them to sit on for the duration of the sessions. Suitable referrals need to be received at a sufficient rate to establish and maintain a viable group or groups, which can make group therapy easier to practise in an organization than as an independant therapist. Psychodrama, Gestalt, art and other special types of therapy groups all need specific equipment and facilities.

Therapeutic communities require a 'home', with several interconnected spaces for the different activities they are engaged in. This will include a minimum of kitchen, dining room, sitting room, therapy rooms and an administrative office. Residential therapeutic communities will also need bedrooms and bathrooms. By definition, these requirements comprise a specialist unit which could be part of a larger building or organization. Several staff arc needed for a therapeutic community, and they need to be part of an organization which is usually larger than the therapeutic community itself. Examples include psychiatric services, charitable foundations and housing associations. Training, supervision and support need to be in place for therapeutic community staff. Therapeutic communities usually treat moderate to high levels of disturbance, so liaison and good relations with other relevant agencies is required to ensure safety and maintain referral routes, both into and out of the community.

Length and frequency of therapy
Psychoanalysis is, by definition, a lengthy treatment. All the analytic schools would see an analysis as lasting longer than two years, and quite possibly for five years or more. An analysis will often start with once- or twice-weekly appointments, and then build up to four or five sessions per week.

Psychodynamic psychotherapy is somewhat shorter, most commonly between one and three years' duration. Frequency of sessions is once, twice or three times weekly. Brief focal psychotherapy is much shorter, with a set number of sessions which are usually weekly from the outset of therapy. Between six and twenty sessions would be standard practice. Cognitive analytic therapy (CAT) usually comprises of sixteen weekly sessions, although variations are being introduced. The Conversational Model is flexible, usually with weekly appointments for between six and eighteen months. Cognitive behavioural therapy (CBT) also varies, but is generally shorter than analytically based approaches. Appointments are also usually weekly, and a typical course of CBT would be eight to sixteen sessions. Schema-focused cognitive work is often of one year's duration or longer.

Family therapy sessions tend to be longer than other therapies, often lasting up to two hours. They take place less frequently, and monthly or variably spaced appointments are most common. The duration of therapy varies from a small number of sessions to several years.

Group therapy is most commonly held weekly, typically with ninety minute sessions continuing for more than one year, but seldom for longer than three. Group analysis or group analytic psychotherapy is twice-weekly, typically lasting bewteen three to five years, although membership of such a group may continue for considerably longer for some. Groups set up with a specific focus are often of much shorter duration, between eight and twenty weekly sessions.

Therapeutic communities can be set up to be a very intensive form of therapy and may involve residential treatment for several years. A more usual pattern is for treatment to have a maximum period set, often between one and two years.

Availability and cost

Psychoanalysis is an expensive treatment, although patients who are willing to be seen by trainees under supervision can receive analysis with considerably reduced fees. It is only available privately, and predominantly in large cities.

Psychoanalytic psychotherapy and the other open-ended analytic derivatives are available privately or through the National Health Service (NHS). Availability in the NHS is variable, with some areas well provided and no service whatsoever in other districts. The cost is rather less than psychoanalysis, as it requires fewer weekly sessions. Referrals in the NHS are commonly for those patients who have long histories of mental health problems and who have not responded to simpler methods of treatment.

Time-limited treatments (CAT, CBT, brief focal therapy) of brief duration are also available in the private and public sectors. Total treatment cost will be lower as the duration for which therapy is being funded is less. CBT is better supported in the NHS than analytic based therapies, often by psychology departments as a part of mental health services. However, its provision is very variable between different areas.

Group psychotherapy is also practised privately and within the NHS. It is well supported in some NHS areas, although unavailable elsewhere. Its cost is less than individual therapy, although its open-ended nature can make it more expensive than brief individual treatments.

Humanistic therapies are not generally available as definitive treatments in the Health Service, although they are used as part of an integrated approach in some areas. They are widely available in the private sector, and cost will be similar to other open-ended therapies.

Family therapy is used most commonly as part of NHS child and adolescent services, and is quite widely available as such. It is also available privately, and for adults and couples. As the sessions are usually separated by several weeks, it is lower in cost than other therapies. Child psychotherapy is also practised within and outside the NHS, with uneven coverage across the country. Costs will be similar to other individual treatments.

Therapeutic communities which operate as definitive psychotherapy treatments are not available privately, and there is very limited provision overall. Some therapeutic communities are closely allied to general psychiatric services, and others are established as part of specialist psychotherapy services. They can be either residential or day units.

Forensic psychotherapy is generally only available in the health service or criminal justice system. Provision is very variable, and considerably below what should be considered optimal.

Other features

The common threads and divergences between different therapies can also be examined using the chapter frameworks: for example, the background of therapists, the way supervision is conducted, what constitutes satisfactory evidence and the sort of problems encountered. These are included in the individual contributions for each therapy. There is a separate chapter covering research and evaluation as this is an area where the authority of competing paradigms needs to be carefully examined.

A field that is both one discipline and many necessarily has coalitions, conflicts and anomalies. For some, they make psychotherapy a field plagued by division, confusion, insubstantiality and even irrelevance. For others, they are an arena in which creative and contradictory ideas compete for attention, in a way that keeps humanity and compassion occupying a central position in mental health care. We hope the contributions to this book, taken together, show that the tolerance and understanding of these differences is the very essence of psychotherapy.

1
Freudian Psychoanalysis

Alice Levinson

Historical perspective

Sigmund Freud was born in 1856 and, from the age of three, was brought up in Vienna. He came from a Jewish family and his father was in the merchant trade. On starting university he enrolled with the medical faculty, but for many years he pursued an interest in science before completing his medical degree. His scientific background, and his fascination in neuroanatomy and neuropathology, permeate his theory of psychoanalysis.

In 1885 Freud observed Charcot, an eminent physician in Paris, using hypnotism for the treatment of hysteria. This technique so impressed Freud that it changed the direction of his career. On his return to Vienna he collaborated with *Joseph Breuer*, a senior Viennese physician who had some prior experience of treating hysteria with hypnosis. Breuer's method was based on the idea that hysteria resulted from a psychic trauma which the patient had forgotten, and that hypnosis brought the memory back to consciousness with a simultaneous resolution of symptoms. Freud and Breuer worked together on the treatment of hysteria, and together published *Studies on Hysteria* in 1895.

As Freud developed his ideas, his and Breuer's professional interest diverged. Breuer took fright towards the end of Anna O's treatment when she developed an erotic transference towards him, whereas Freud went on to investigate transference phenomena further. Freud found hypnosis and the technique of suggestion both difficult to practise and unpredictable, and therefore abandoned it in favour of the pressure technique and later free association. It was, however, Freud and Breuer's combined work on hysteria that was the foundation of psychoanalysis. The central principle of the unconscious, as well as the concepts of repression and free association, developed from this early work.

An important shift occurred in Freud's thinking at this time about the origins of hysteria. He moved away from the seduction and trauma theory, towards the theory that unconscious sexual fantasies underlie hysterical phenomena. Freud changed his theory as a result of knowledge he gained from his own self-analysis of his oedipal fantasies, as well as from his patients. This change caused controversy as critics accused him of changing the theory in response to public pressure not to expose the incidence of sexual abuse occurring in Viennese society. On the other hand, that he was prepared to change his theories in the face of new observations regarding the importance of unconscious sexual phantasies throughout development, demonstrates his integrity as a scientist.

The early history of the psychoanalytic movement

This is a story of personalities – at the centre of which was Freud – and of how ideas developed between the protagonists, causing legendary conflict along the way. The conflicts mostly arose because Freud wanted talented men around him with whom to share his ideas and to take psychoanalysis into the future, but he was very resistant to accommodating other people's new ideas. He defensively protected his theories, probably because he wanted to establish the discipline of psychoanalysis and maintain clarity. It also seems that, because of his personality, he tended to conceive of his students as his disciples or even children, whom he felt should follow and promote his ideas. He was extremely intolerant of anyone who deviated from his teaching, and they were invariably excommunicated from the Psychoanalytic Movement however close Freud's relationship had been with them. Freud also became suspicious that his disciples would succeed him and plagiarize his ideas. In addition to these tensions, there was rivalry amongst the members of the Psychoanalytic Movement to be Freud's favourite colleague. The history is therefore of a series of very intimate and creative relationships, which frequently broke down to be followed by total rejection.

Wilhelm Fliess (1858–1928) was a Berlin physician, introduced to Freud by Breuer. Freud became dependant on Fliess for his close friendship, as it provided Freud with an audience for his ideas at a time when Freud was very isolated. They corresponded by frequent letters, which have been preserved and provide a record of how Freud changed his ideas on the seduction theory. It was over this subject that their relationship fell apart, as Fliess lost confidence in Freud's method. Fliess believed that because Freud changed his ideas, that they could not have been founded on objective evidence and were therefore not scientific. Fliess made significant contributions to psychoanalytic theory before he departed. He was the originator of the concept of the latency stage of infantile sexuality, and of the idea that man has a bisexual constitution. After their falling out, Freud did not acknowledge these ideas as originally belonging to Fliess.

Alfred Adler (1870–1937) was to be one of the main 'defectors' from the Vienna Psychoanalytic Society. He was a socialist and hoped to bring psychoanalysis into the world of the people at large and to improve society alongside education. Adler was preoccupied with social reality and ego processes, which Freud thought undermined the importance of the unconscious. Adler also considered aggression and destructive drives to be a priority in man's aim towards domination and power, and de-emphasized the role of sexuality, which again was opposed to Freud's thinking at that time. Freud was unable to tolerate these deviations from his theories and, even though he had made Adler President of the Vienna Psychoanalytic Society, he then publicly criticized him for violating the principles of psychoanalysis and ejected him from the Society. Adler went on to form his own school.

Wilhelm Stekel (1868–1940) was from the onset more deviant in his interests than other members of the Society, and was therefore never taken very seriously by Freud. He was, however, an original thinker and made an invaluable contribution to psychoanalysis by emphasizing the destructive forces in human nature. He originated the idea of the death wish, which he termed 'thanatos'. Stekel would not relinquish his independent thinking and was therefore rejected by Freud, who later wondered how he could have overlooked non-erotic aggressive and destructive drives, and yet he had not been able to consider them when they were presented to him by Adler and Stekel. Freud went on to develop his own theory of instincts to include a dualistic life and death instinct.

Carl Gustav Jung (1875–1961) was a favourite pupil of Freud, who recognized him to be a very able and creative man. Jung was a Swiss psychiatrist, which was of value to Freud who had received a hostile response from psychiatric institutions and wanted to spread psychoanalysis abroad. Freud appointed him the first President of the International Psychoanalytic Society in order to move the base out of Vienna. Freud could not accept Jung's religious beliefs (as Freud thought the religious needs of man could be understood through psychoanalysis, rather than allowing religion to have a determining influence on psychoanalysis) and felt that Jung's ideas were too closely linked with mysticism. They differed also on their theory of libido; while Freud restricted it to sexual drives Jung thought the term was more usefully applied to a general psychic energy, and that Freud should be more specific about what was sexual. Tension grew between the two men, and Freud became increasingly suspicious that Jung was trying to take the lead in psychoanalysis. He dramatically expressed his fear by two fainting spells when travelling in the company of Jung to the United States to give public lectures. He seemed unable to reflect upon his anxieties about rivalry and his fear that his theories would be taken over, which led to the expulsion of Jung from the Society.

Ernest Jones (1879–1958) was another influential member of the Society at its beginning. He was the first leader of the British Society of Psychoanalysis. He did not have a medical background, and continued Freud's ethos of training non-medical 'lay' analysts, which contrasted with the practice in the United States, where training in analysis was restricted to doctors. He idealized Freud and stayed on good terms with him. He was however responsible for inviting *Melanie Klein* to join the British Society after she had trained in Budapest and Berlin. Klein was later to cause considerable conflict within the Society because her ideas differed significantly from those of Freud and his daughter, Anna.

Sandor Ferenczi (1873–1933) was a leading Budapest analyst. His contribution was to focus on the therapeutic technique. He had a warm nature, which he used in his technique to relax Freud's more austere approach. He felt that it was necessary to meet the patient half-way, and that the therapeutic relationship should be a genuine interpersonal encounter. He advocated shortening the duration of treatment, and emphasized the intercommunication between patient and analyst, suggesting that the benefits of analysis are not achieved by an intellectual reconstruction of past events but by a genuine emotional reliving in the current therapeutic relationship. He also suggested the use of more 'activity' by the analyst, including expressions of human warmth (which led him to kiss his patients at the end of sessions), as he believed his patients had lacked mothering and love in their early lives. Freud tried to tolerate Ferenczi's deviations, having learnt from experience that his intolerance had led to the loss of the Society's most gifted members. However, eventually Freud did reject Ferenczi from the Movement, fearing that his practice could give psychoanalysis a bad name.

Otto Rank (1884–1939) had a very close relationship to Freud, and was to Freud like an adopted son. He is best known for his theory of birth trauma but his more important contribution was his emphasis on the role of the mother, which has had a far-reaching influence on psychoanalysis. It contrasted with – and compensated for – Freud's centralizing the father's role, and laid the ground for Melanie Klein's ideas. Rank collaborated with Ferenczi on *The Development of Psychoanalysis*, which was received with great suspicion by Freud and his followers. The authors suggested more attention should be paid to the analyst–patient interaction in therapy and the current realities of the transference relationship. They suggested that acting out can be put to therapeutic use in creating an emotional reliving of the past rather than just intellectualized knowledge.

Freud also attracted a number of female followers. These included his daughter, *Anna Freud*, whom he personally analysed and *Helene Deutsch*, who is known for her theory of femininity which developed Freud's theories of female sexuality. She discovered, with *Ruth Brunswick*, maternal transference, and suggested that female homosexuality stemmed from a pre-oedipal tie to a mother (as opposed to Freud who had suggested it was caused by a girl's identification with her father). Other female analysts who contributed to the early movement were *Mira Oberholzer, Marie Bonaparte, Eugenia Sokolnicka, Hermine von Hug-Hellmuth* and *Dorothy Burlingham*.

Principles of theory and practice

Freud's theory of psychoanalysis

In 1895, Freud and Breuer jointly derived an understanding of the mechanism of hysterical phenomena. The cause was thought to be due to psychic trauma which was of a nature that could not be consciously dealt with because it involved an irreparable loss or a sexual experience that was consciously unacceptable. It was therefore excluded from consciousness by repression. As a result, an unconscious conflict was induced and, in order to maintain an economic 'principle of constancy', the unconscious energy was discharged through an alternative channel. The unconscious psychic conflict therefore became converted into somatic symptoms. The hysterical conversion syndrome, which included symptoms of paralysis, contractures, pseudo-seizures and disturbances of vision, memory and consciousness (illustrated in the case study of Anna O), could then be understood as a symbolic representation of the unconscious psychic conflict. The thoughts that have been excluded from consciousness are expressed through a somatic medium. The symptoms may be reinforced and maintained by the process of secondary gain, the syndrome providing the patient with a practical solution to their psychic conflicts. This work led on to the development of two distinct but overlapping models of the mind.

The topographical model of the mind

Freud's next major work was *The Interpretation of Dreams* (1900), which he considered his most important work. Although Freud discovered the power of *the unconscious* in his work on hysteria, it is in *The Interpretation of Dreams* that he gives this discovery full expression. He wrote that: 'The unconscious is the true psychic reality: *in its innermost nature it is as much unknown to us as the reality of the external world, and it is incompletely presented by the data of consciousness as is the external world by the communications of our sense organs*' (Freud's italics).

In this work, Freud developed the *topographical model* of the mind. The mind was conceptualized as a mental apparatus, a dynamic system, consisting of unconscious, preconscious and conscious systems. Unconscious excitation and thoughts are discharged outwards towards the more superficial layers of the preconscious and the conscious, but are met by strongly resistant forces excluding unconscious thoughts from consciousness. He proposed that the process of dream production was similar to that of a hysterical symptom, where a conflict between an unconscious wish and conscious ideas results in repression of the unconscious. The dream or symptom becomes formed as an alternative channel for the discharge of energy, and could be understood as a symbolic expression of the conflict.

Dreams

The motivating force of every dream was thought by Freud to be an *unconscious wish*. This unconscious wish developed into 'dream thoughts' which comprised the 'latent dream'. A process of dream censorship then functioned as a critical agency to exclude the unconscious dream thoughts from consciousness. This can be envisaged as a screen between the unconscious and conscious systems which, during waking life, excludes the dream thoughts from consciousness. However the state of sleep reduces the power of this censorship, allowing the dream thoughts to emerge in a disguised form into the preconscious and conscious systems as the 'manifest dream'. Censorship is part of the process of resistance, and further resistance is then responsible for the forgetting of dreams.

Dream-work was the name given by Freud to the process that converted the unconscious latent dream thoughts into the conscious, but disguised, manifest dream. In this process the unconscious dream thoughts become linked with often trivial conscious thoughts. The displacement of a significant unconscious thought onto a superficial and apparently absurd one is brought about by the pressure of censorship. Displacement serves a dual function. It allows the unconscious excitation to be discharged from the unconscious to the preconscious by pairing the serious thoughts with trivial ones, which allows them to pass through censorship. Simultaneously, by disguising the content of the dream thoughts, displacement protects consciousness from an awareness of the unconscious thoughts. This theory of displacement in dream-work highlights a basic principle of Freudian theory – 'that superficial associations are only substitutes by displacement for suppressed deeper ones'

(1900). The technique of free association is derived from this principle: when the patient is asked to abandon conscious reflection and to say whatever comes to mind, the assumption is that the resulting material – which may appear to consist of arbitrary thoughts – is in fact linked to unconscious ideas that have been censored.

Regression is another dynamic process in the formation of dreams, and is responsible for dreams being mostly recorded in visual images. In Freud's topographical model, the dream thoughts regress to the deeper perceptual system where they get transformed into visual images of a hallucinatory quality. In regression 'the fabric of dream thoughts is resolved into its raw material' and it is responsible for allowing the 'logical relations belonging to dream thoughts to disappear during dream activity' (1900).

Condensation is a related process in dream-work, causing an intensification of the ideational content of the dream thoughts. This intensification is required to force a way through to the perceptual system, thereby enhancing dynamic mobility. However, this intensification also serves to further disguise the dream thoughts.

The overall function of dream activity is to preserve sleep and is carried out through these mechanisms. Unconscious excitation is brought under control by means of dream-work which transforms the latent content into the manifest dream. Disguising the dream thoughts reduces the threat to the preconscious and prevents any disturbance of sleep.

Primary process thinking and secondary process thinking

Primary process thinking and *secondary process thinking* are concepts that are derived from the topographical model. Freud attributed primary process thinking to the unconscious system, where the psychic energy is free and mobile. It is characterized by uninhibited and irrational thought processes. This is in contrast to secondary process thinking, attributed to the preconscious system, where the thought processes are rational due to the censorship of unconscious thoughts. Repression functions to inhibit the unconscious thoughts, in order to avoid painful or unpleasurable thoughts entering preconscious awareness.

The pleasure and unpleasure principles

Primary and secondary process thinking are intimately related to the pleasure and unpleasure principles respectively. The *pleasure principle* belongs to the unconscious and seeks immediate gratification of needs and desires. However the infant, as it develops, learns to delay gratification by inhibiting desires. The capacity to delay gratification is conveyed by the *unpleasure principle* which, through repression, operates to inhibit unconscious thoughts and wishes from reaching the preconscious because they would be unpleasurable to consciousness. As described by Freud (1900), 'the fulfilment of infantile wishes would no longer generate an affect of pleasure but of unpleasure; and *it is precisely this transformation of affect which constitutes the essence of what we call repression*' (Freud's italics).

The structural theory of the mind

Freud moved on to consider the mind in terms of the *structural theory*, in which there is a threefold division of the mind into the *ego*, the *id* and the *superego*. This is a development of the Topographical Model which involved just two systems, the repressed unconscious and the repressing conscious. The topographical model can be thought of as persisting in conjunction with the structural model, providing a dynamic scheme involving unconscious and conscious processes. The structural model offered the advantage of redefining the unconscious and conscious systems through the constructs of the id, ego and superego, which provided clarification and a third division. It is helpful for the understanding of psychopathology, and for the conceptualization of the ego and its defence mechanisms.

The id
The id represents the seat of instincts, especially libidinal but also destructive forces, and is the centre of the pleasure principle. The ego is representative of the external world: it receives perceptual information and serves the *reality principle*. A conflict may arise between the pleasure principle (conveying id impulses) and repression (an ego defence) producing neurotic symptoms.

The ego
According to Freud (1923), the ego 'in its relation to the id is like a man on horse-back, who has to hold in check the superior strength of the horse ... Often a rider, if he is not to be parted from his horse, is obliged to guide it where it wants to go; so in the same way the ego is in the habit of transforming the id's will into action as if it were its own.' One of the functions of psychoanalysis was therefore to facilitate ego development and 'enable the ego to achieve a progressive conquest of the id' (1923).

   Freud thought that the ego developed out of object-cathexes, a process of identification and introjection of these objects, and inhibition of instinctual forces. The ego, Freud maintained, 'is first and foremost a bodily ego' (1923), in that it is the centre of perceptual information from the external world and the physical body. Freud also described the ego as 'a frontier creature', that 'is the actual seat of anxiety' because it is threatened from three directions – the external world, the id and the superego. The ego attempts to repress instinctual impulses from the id but, if it fails in this conflict and gratification of the instincts is also impossible, neurosis may develop.

The superego
The superego was thought to develop out of the resolution of the Oedipus complex by the identifications with the two parental objects becoming united as a precipitate in the ego. In so doing, the superego became an unconscious critical agency of authority over the ego. According to Freud: 'From the point of view of instinctual control, of morality, it may be said of the id that it is totally non-moral, of the ego that it strives to be moral, and of the super-ego that it can be super-moral and then become as cruel as only the id can be' (1923).

The ego's dread of the superego is the fear of conscience, castration and ultimately death. As the superego develops from the oedipal complex, the more powerful and unresolved the complex, the stricter the superego will be. A superego that is excessively domineering will produce an unconscious sense of guilt. Freud considered an unconscious sense of guilt as being a motive for criminal behaviour as it may be 'a relief to fasten this unconscious sense of guilt onto something real and immediate' (1923).

Freudian psychoanalysis centres upon the ego, its defence mechanisms and resistance to change. The ego's defences operate to defend the ego from anxieties arising from the id, the superego and external dangers. The ego's defences are also an important source of resistance, which can be understood as anything that the patient does to obstruct the course of the analysis. Freud recognized five types of resistance, which acted to prevent unconscious processes from becoming conscious: repression, transference, repetition–compulsion, superego influences and secondary gain.

Freud in *Mourning and Melancholia* (1917) describes the interaction between the ego and the superego. For example, a harsh superego, with a correspondingly fragile ego, may affect the course of normal mourning and result in *melancholia*. In normal mourning, there is loss of a real object who, although loved, can be given up with subsequent displacement of these feelings onto another object. In melancholia, the original object choice is more narcissistic and cannot, because of the close identification with the ego, be properly related to as a separate person. Ambivalence in the original relationship results in hate being turned back on to the ego: 'There is identification of the ego with the abandoned object. Thus the shadow of the object fell upon the ego' (1917). This is in contrast to the self-preserving function of a healthy ego, and the superego's capacity to reinforce the ego's love for itself.

Freud's theories on sexuality

Freud's theories on sexuality are important, although some have required modification and rejection in the face of more recent discoveries in infant development. Classical Freudian psychoanalysis has been called a *drive psychology* because of the centrality that Freud gave to the libido theory. He criticized Jung 'for watering down the meaning of the concept of libido itself by equating it with psychical instinctual force in general' (1905). Freud believed that the term libido should be restricted only to instinctual sexual impulses because of the importance they play in the development of psychopathology. He considered that neuroses develop due to repression of excessive libidinal forces. He suggested that neuroses are an outlet for abnormal sexuality, and that perversions are an alternative outlet: 'neuroses are, so to say, the negatives of perversions'.

The infant's sexuality was thought to develop by gratification along *erotogenic zones* that progress from oral to anal to genital. Freud suggested that deviations from normal sexual life, from psychoneuroses to perversions, could be explained by inappropriate sexual experiences during childhood. He proposed that inappropriate sexual excitement could cause the infant to become fixed at that stage of sexual development, and that in adult pathology the person regressed to the phase of sexuality in which they had become fixed in infancy. These ideas have been refuted by developmental psychology, in particular the concept of fixation and regression to infantile 'stages' of development.

The Oedipus complex

The Oedipus complex is one of Freud's theories that has become central to psychoanalytic thinking. It provides a scheme for understanding sexual development and its pathology. Freud (1925) described the different routes that boys and girls take in their sexual development. For boys, the mother, who is the primary object, also becomes the first sexual object. The father is therefore experienced as an obstacle to sexual wishes in regard to the mother, producing hostile feelings and a wish to get rid of the father. The resolution of the Oedipus complex, for boys, is achieved by means of the castration complex. When boys recognize that girls lack male genitalia, they associate this observation with a fear of revenge by their father. They consequently fear for their own genitals, which become invested with self-interest. Boys subsequently deal with their rivalrous feelings toward their father by identifying with him. Their sexuality therefore develops through the dismantling of the Oedipus complex. Libidinal love for the mother is relinquished, but retained as an affectionate relationship, together with continuing identification with the father. However, in what is described as the negative Oedipus complex, the boy may have an affectionate feminine attitude to his father and corresponding jealousy towards his mother.

Girls have a different developmental course to navigate as they have to change their object choice from their mother, as primary object, to their father as the first sexual object. According to Freud, this exchange occurs through the castration complex in girls preceding the Oedipal complex. The girl recognizes the absence of male genitalia in herself and her mother, and consequently develops penis envy. She turns toward her father as he possesses this desired object. As libidinal love develops for her father, ambivalent feelings emerge towards her mother. This process is driven, in part, by the girl's anger that she lacks a penis and because the mother stands in the way of sexual desires for the father. The resolution of the Oedipal complex occurs for girls by relinquishing the hope of a sexual relation with their father and replacing her libidinal love for him by other male objects, whilst intensifying her female identification with her mother.

Freud considered people to have a bisexual constitution, consisting of active and passive elements, corresponding with masculine and feminine attitudes. Bisexuality is therefore a complicating element, as the relative strengths of the masculine and feminine dispositions will determine the outcome of the oedipal situation. Freud considered bisexuality – and most pathologies – to be contributed to by both constitutional and environmental factors. A boy's developing male sexuality may be interfered with by the absence of a father, as it leaves him vulnerable to develop an overclose relationship with his mother and he is deprived of a male adult with whom to identify. He may instead identify with his mother, facilitating the development of homosexuality, transvestism or transexualism.

Freud (1925) described a period of *latency* as part of infantile sexuality. It is during this period that sexual inhibitions develop – which include feelings of shame, disgust and morality – and function as a mental force opposing the sexual instincts. During this period an important process develops called sublimation, defined as 'the diversion of sexual instinctual forces from sexual aims and their direction to new ones'. The capacity for *sublimation* is an important development for the individual; and it is also thought to have had a powerful influence on cultural achievements and the civilization of man. This discourse is expanded in *Civilization and its Discontents* (1930), in which Freud developed the idea of sublimation as partof the life instinct, and how it works in opposition to the death instinct.

Contemporary developments of Freudian theory

Since Freud's death in 1939, there have been major developments in Freudian psychoanalysis. His daughter, Anna Freud, contributed significantly to the understanding of the ego and its defence mechanisms (1937). Later developments have also been made by the integration of different psychoanalytic schools of thought – including some Kleinian theories – and in collaboration with developmental psychology.

Mechanisms of defence

Unconscious interactions between the id and the superego are mediated though the ego. Analysis, by working against the ego's defences, lessens the restrictions of the ego in order to make such unconscious processes conscious. Anna Freud (1937) described how the first task for analysts is to recognize the ego's defence mechanisms, and related therapeutic resistance, which should then become the focus of interpretations. To achieve this, the analyst 'takes his stand at a point equidistant from the id, the ego and the superego'. It is only after these defence mechanisms are understood that attention can be turned to the impulses that the ego is defending itself against, and the analysis turns towards the id. The direction of analysis is therefore twofold, alternating between the ego's defence mechanisms and the id impulses.

Ego defence mechanisms (Anna Freud)
- Repression
- Regression
- Reaction formation
- Isolation
- Undoing
- Projection
- Introjection
- Turning against the self
- Reversal
- Splitting
- Denial
- Sublimation
- Identification with the aggressor

Freud and his daughter recognized vertical splitting of the ego into conscious and repressed unconscious parts. Klein (1946) made an immensely important contribution to the theory of psychoanalysis in describing fragmentation of the ego by minute horizontal splitting, with projection and *projective identification* of the split-off parts occurring in the context of infant development. According to Freud, the process of *projection* is a defence mechanism by which feelings and ideas that are intolerable to the ego are projected into the external world. He understood phobias through the process of projection; the external object becoming the receptacle of internal conflicts and anxiety. Projective identification is a further development of the defence mechanism of projection in which aspects of the self are forced into the other person. Contemporary Freudians recognize the process, but Sandler (1988) warns of a conceptual confusion, if processes in the here and now of adult interactions are couched in theories of infant development, and that conceptually it is important to separate the process of projective identification that occurs in infant development and that which operates between adults. These concepts have become integrated into Freudian psychoanalysis and have added to the understanding of borderline psychopathology. The split-off parts of the ego may be projected and identified in the external world – for example, in other people or even in their own body, which is experienced as separate and alien from their psychological self. These aspects may include feelings, thoughts, images and mental capacities. Patients may, for instance, rid themselves of all unpleasant feelings and experience these as belonging to others, or evacuate their capacity to think.

Developmental psychology

Developmental psychology has changed our understanding of infant development (Stern, 1985). Its theories are based on direct observation of infant development prospectively, in experimental conditions. Development is conceived of as emerging along pathways determined by the growth of the infant's psychomotor capacities within the context of relationships with other persons, and which may deviate from the normal developmental line and take other pathways in response to external experiences. The attempt to understand infant development retrospectively, through theories derived from the psychoanalysis of adult pathology, is now considered inappropriate and incorrect. Contemporary Freudian psychoanalysts generally accept these modifications to Freudian theory in the face of new knowledge being received from developmental psychology. In fact, Freud intended that psychoanalysis should progress in this way as he considered it a science. He wrote that he constructed his theories as provisional hypotheses which he intended should be modified or abandoned as necessary in the light of further observations. Theories of memory are also changing and the concept of repression and its relation to infantile amnesia is now being questioned.

Further developments on the Oedipus complex

The Oedipus complex is a conceptual area where historically there was heated debate about the age of the infant. Freud conceived of the oedipal complex as appearing in the young child at the stage of their becoming more interactive with a third person, whereas Klein put it much earlier, in the infant's first year of life. In contemporary Freudian thinking, there has been some valuable convergence of ideas which has allowed the concept of the Oedipus complex to become more symbolic in meaning. Britton *et al.* (1989) have suggested that the resolution of the oedipal conflict involves the acquisition of a 'third area of mental space'. Mourning the loss of an illusionary, all-inclusive relationship with the primary object (e.g. mother or analyst) and accepting that the primary object has relationships with other people that exclude the child or patient, requires a necessary separation from the primary object. This separation and awareness of the third person allows the potential for a third area of mental space – beyond self and primary object – that can be employed to reflect upon self and other in relation to each other. For example, Britton describes how psychotic patients cannot tolerate the analyst having a separate mind which is out of their control. They experience the analyst's separate mind and thinking (which oedipally represents the parental relationship and intercourse) as threatening the fused link that they wish to have with their primary object and which they fight to maintain in the analytic relationship.

Symbol formation

The separation between self and object enables a shift in mental functioning that includes the capacity for *symbol formation* (Segal, 1957). Symbolic function requires the differentiation between the object symbolized and the symbol, which depends upon a mental capacity that can differentiate between the ego and the object. A failure in resolving the oedipal conflict and separation will make the patient unable to differentiate between ego and object, and therefore have a restricted space to symbolically represent mental states. An impaired capacity for the symbolic or abstract representation of mental states will mean that the patient can only think 'concretely' about internal states. These internal states may then be experienced in bodily ways, causing the patient to act physically towards their own bodies or those of others.

Theory of mind

Fonagy integrates these ideas in an attempt to delineate a capacity of mind that reflects upon the mental states of self and others (Fonagy *et al.*, 1991; Fonagy and Target, 1996). He explains how the psychological self develops through the perception of the self in another person's mind. The process occurs in early development through the dyadic relationship of infant and mother, and the analytic relationship may be understood as providing a similar process. A mother who has sufficient capacity for reflective self-function (Fonagy *et al.*, 1997) is able to reflect upon her own as well as her infant's mental states. This will enable her to think about the infant's internal states as separate from her own. At times when the infant is distressed, the mother will be able to respond with understanding and so provide containment. The infant learns through this relationship process that his internal states are tolerable and explicable, and thereby develops a capacity to think about his own mental states, both independently and in relation to his mother. In contrast, a mother who is unable to reflect upon the infant's mind as independent from her own will not be able to provide containment when the infant is distressed. Instead, the mother will echo the infant's state of mind without modification, resulting in an escalation of anxiety. Fonagy (1996) suggests that the adverse consequences of this developmental pathway are severe and can result in borderline psychopathology as the infant fails to develop the capacity 'to feel themselves from within'. They present with a restricted capacity to reflect upon their own mental states and instead need to search for a sense of self from without. This causes the patient to project intolerable unconscious feelings onto the external world, including their own bodies and other people. As a result, they develop a tendency to experience internal mental states physically through action directed at their own bodies or towards others. In psychoanalysis this process may, very slowly, be reversed as the analyst offers a corrective emotional experience within which the patient can begin to reflect upon their own mental states.

The patient–analyst relationship

Another important movement in contemporary theory is the change of focus from the patient alone to the *dyadic relationship of patient and analyst*. There is now a greater emphasis on the transference as an important clinical instrument in the analysis of the unconscious. The concept of 'clinical facts' as being significant components of the patient's psychic reality in the context of the transference relationship is an example of this development (O'Shaughnessy, 1994). Furthermore, the processes of transference, counter-transference, role enactment and projective identification are, according to Sandler *et al.* (1987), closely connected. It is therefore the interaction between the patient and the analyst that is the unit of analysis, and which is of therapeutic potential.

Aims of therapy

The aims of psychoanalysis are directed towards a fundamental intrapsychic reorganization of the personality. They have continued to evolve alongside developments in the theory and remain open to change.

Aims of psychoanalysis
- The acquisition of insight
- The emergence of a capacity to reflect upon mental states
- A developmental shift towards the three-person oedipal position
- The development of symbolic function
- A reduction of primitive defence mechanisms, such as splitting, projection and projective identification which fragment the ego
- Re-owning of lost parts of the self, or reclaiming of split-off alien aspects of the self
- The neutralization and integration of aggression and other instinctual impulses
- Strengthening of the ego
- A sense of safety
- The development of more secure attachment relationships
- Changing the quality of the transference relationship
- Changes to the patient's internal object relations

The *acquisition of insight* was considered by Freud (Freud and Breuer, 1895) to be the central aim of psychoanalysis, in order to transform 'hysterical misery into common unhappiness'. The emergence of insight enables unconscious conflicts to be made conscious, producing a release of damned up libido (the dynamic theory) and the resolution of conflicts between the ego, id and superego (the structural theory). The concept of insight has shifted from thinking about past conflicts and repression to the capacity to think about unconscious processes in the psychoanalytic relationship and states of mind in the *here and now*. There is also a greater emphasis on *affect*: that thinking is accompanied by the appropriate feelings, so that the patient is able to think with feelings and feel with thinking.

A development to the theory of insight is Fonagy's concept of *reflective self-function* (Fonagy, 1996; Fonagy *et al.*, 1997). The emergence of a capacity to reflect upon mental states, including feelings, thoughts and intentions – of the subject's own mind and in relation to other people's minds – is a developmental achievement. An impairment of reflective self-function may develop as a defence strategy, and can gradually be recovered through a long-term relationship with an analyst who takes on the function for the patient until their own has developed.

A developmental shift towards the *three-person oedipal position* allows the patient to experience their mind as separate from the analyst's, and to develop a third internal mental space to reflect upon the relationship. This shift facilitates the emergence of reflective self-function, and the *symbolic representation* of mental states. The patient can move on from the phantasy of a fused relationship, to develop a level of separateness from their object that allows them to be able to be close to another person at the same time as maintaining their autonomy.

A *reduction of primitive defence mechanisms* (such as splitting and fragmentation of the ego, projection and projective identification) is a central aim of psychoanalysis and results in the ego being strengthened. One of the ways this can be achieved is through the *reclaiming of these split-off alien aspects of the self* (Steiner, 1996). This will involve a process of mourning the loss of the illusionary (false) self-identity, followed by a process of integration of the split-off parts of the ego, which were previously experienced as intolerable and thus evacuated. Using this model, the aim can be understood in terms of the integration of the split-off parts of the ego, to develop a more whole, real robust self.

The *neutralization and integration of aggression and other instinctual impulses* is an aim of psychoanalysis that has its origins in Freud's theory that the *ego is strengthened* by the taming of the instincts, 'where there was id there shall be ego' (S. Freud, 1937). The instinctual forces of eros and death, from which love and aggression are derived respectively, need to be neutralized and integrated within the ego.

A *sense of safety* (Sandler, 1987) is a requirement for need satisfaction, and mediates the development of the reality principle out of the pleasure principle. The sense of safety is more than just a reduction of anxiety, 'it is a feeling of well-being, a sort of ego tone' and develops through the mother's capacity to reflect upon the infant's mental state and contain the infant's affect. A basic aim of psychoanalysis is to enhance the ego's sense of safety. The need for a sense of safety can be understood in terms of attachment theory (Bowlby, 1988) and the need for a secure base. In attachment theory, an aim of psychoanalysis is to move towards *more secure forms of attachment*, in terms of internal mental representations and external relationships. The coherence of an individual's narrative about their early attachment experiences has been found to be a good marker of their attachment security. During the course of analysis the patient has the opportunity to reconstruct their narrative, which can become more coherent due to better internal organization.

Changing the quality and nature of the transference relationship is an unconscious process that works over a long period of time, and therefore differentiates the aims and potential benefits of psychoanalysis in contrast to shorter forms of psychodynamic psychotherapy. Through a long-term relationship with an analyst, a patient's transference can change and become more conscious with insight. This should become reflected in the patient's external relationships, allowing them new ways of relating. The nature of the transference will be closely associated with the quality of the patient's *internal objects* (e.g. self, parents, significant others) and their internal relations to each other. Gradually unconscious changes can occur to the patient's internal objects, and they may become more benign, whole and real.

Principles of practice

The analyst employs a number of techniques, including confrontations, reconstructions, interpretations and the use of their countertransference in order to reveal to the patient his or her internal world, including their conflicts and defences, in order to help them progress to healthier levels of psychic functioning – enabling them to make better adaptations to and resolutions of conflicts.

Free association

Psychoanalysis is an intensive talking therapy, involving five sessions per week. It requires the patient to be able to free associate in order to reach unconscious thinking processes, because it is at the unconscious level that the analyst hopes to be able to direct interpretations in an attempt to bring about psychic change. The patient lies on a couch to facilitate this process of communication, and to avoid the interference of face-to-face contact that accompanies social conventions of ordinary conversation. Free association is a way of thinking and talking, so that the patient says whatever comes into his or her mind without conscious reflection, selection or editing. It enables raw feelings and thoughts to emerge, and thereby provides the material for analysis.

At other times during a session, more reflective thinking is required to enable links to be made between feelings and thoughts and between thoughts themselves. It also allows the patient to link the past and the present, to think about the analyst's interpretations and to think about their own state of mind in relation to that of the analyst.

Transference

Transference is a phenomenon in which past experiences – represented by internal object relations – are revived as applying to the analyst in the present. It is an essential psychoanalytic tool as it reveals the patient's internal world to the analyst. Initially Freud (1940) recognized transference as a form of resistance, but soon discovered that positive transference could be a motivating force and that transference was a powerful psychoanalytic technique. Transference enables the analyst to observe the patient's internal object relations as these are transferred onto the analyst. The revived memories include feelings, thoughts, images, attitudes and fantasies which influence the patient's perception and experience of the analyst and their interventions. It is therefore alive in the current relationship with the analyst and can be worked with.

Freud considered transference to be a universal phenomenon that occurred in all human relationships, but also defined it in the more restricted sense of applying to the patient's relationship with the analyst. Sandler *et al.* (1987) explain that transference 'is not *created* by psychoanalysis, but that psychoanalysis merely *reveals* it and guides the psychical processes towards the desired goal'. It may, however, be intensified and revealed by the analyst not sharing personal information with the patient, thereby becoming a ready receptacle for the patient's projections. How the patient then experiences the analyst is an important part of the assessment of the patient's psychic functioning.

Greenson (1965) emphasizes the repetitive and inappropriate quality of transference which 'must be a repetition from the past and it must be inappropriate to the present'. The inappropriateness may be in magnitude as well as quality, for instance a patient may experience a change in the session time as uncaring or as a harsh rejection, and they may experience an interpretation as threatening and persecutory. The degree of transference reactions provides an indication of the level of the patient's personality disturbance.

The interpretation of the transference has become a central technique of analysis in order to reveal to the patient their unconscious feelings, thoughts and beliefs. Internal and external object relations are recreated in the transference with the analyst so that they can be worked on in the 'here and now' situation. The degree to which the analyst works in the transference will depend upon their theoretical background, their own individual style, the patient's level of psychological functioning, the degree of disturbance and the stage of the analysis. Freudian psychoanalysts put less emphasis on working in the transference. Freudian psychoanalysts are more receptive to the patients external reality, to which their interventions may be directed, although this is imbued by their knowledge of the patient through the transference. Freudians are also interested in the patient's history and its reconstruction in analysis, which is again achieved through the transference relationship.

The therapeutic alliance

The therapeutic alliance is an important ingredient of successful treatment. It is the patient's conscious and unconscious cooperation with the process of analysis and is present when a patient accepts the need to deal with internal problems and to undertake analytic work in the face of psychic pain and resistance. It will depend, in part, on the transference relationship. Sandler (1987) describes it as requiring – but being different from – what Greenacre terms 'basic' or 'primary' transference, which is 'derived from the mother–child relationship but expressed in the confidence in the knowledge and integrity of the analyst and the helpfulness of the method'. It needs, however, to be distinguished from transference as it will be affected by many other factors, including the patient's readiness for treatment and their match with a particular analyst. The alliance is a two-way construction between patient and analyst, and the analyst's capacity for empathy, understanding and containment will help towards building an alliance. The development of a therapeutic alliance may be seen as part of the initial stage of treatment and then continuing simultaneously alongside treatment. In the case of more disturbed patients it will take time – and some psychic change may be required – to create the alliance. The alliance is the foundation for treatment and makes therapeutic change possible.

Countertransference

Countertransference is an essential instrument of psychoanalytic technique. It is a Kleinian contribution to contemporary Freudian psychoanalysis, as Freud originally saw countertransference as an impediment to the analyst's work. Countertransference, in its proper and restricted meaning, relates to the analyst's *unconscious* thoughts, feelings, attitudes and phantasies about the patient which are derived in response to the patient's transference and the analyst's own internal object relations – which will reflect the analyst's past relationships and current state of mind. It is sometimes used in a more general sense to include the analyst's conscious feelings about the patient, although this is better termed the analyst's *total response* to the patient. The psychoanalytic training, in particular a personal analysis, allows the analyst to become more aware of countertransference feelings and to be able to reflect upon their total response to the patient. In doing so they can learn a great deal about the patient and use this in the service of the treatment. The psychoanalyst uses their countertransference as an instrument to explore the patient's transference and internal object relations, and to enable them to observe how they themselves are interacting unconsciously with the patient, which allows them to respond appropriately to patients within the clinical session (Heimann, 1950).

Projective identification

The process of projective identification is connected with counter-transference, the analyst's countertransference being a response to the patient's projective identification. Sandler (1988) defines different stages of projective identification: the first stage is at the level of the patient's fantasy, and the second stage involves an effect on the external object, contributing to the analyst's countertransference. Projective identification can therefore be understood as being connected to transference and countertransference processes. Central to projective identification is the mechanism of control of objects: by getting rid of aspects of the self into the other object, the illusion of being in control is gained. It therefore operates as a defence mechanism to reduce anxiety by the expulsion of unwanted aspects of the self into external objects and through the evocation of familiar role interactions. Another process that is closely related to these processes is *role responsiveness* (Sandler, 1976). The patient will unconsciously attempt to make real and actualize their transference fantasies. One way of doing this is to evoke the analyst's countertransference, and thereby nudge the analyst into a role response.

How does Freudian psychoanalysis differ from other therapies?

Freud developed psychoanalysis for the treatment of neuroses, in particular hysteria. There remains an inclination in Freudian thinking to narrow the scope of psychoanalysis to the neurotic end of the spectrum of mental disorders, compared to Kleinian theory which has developed an understanding of more psychotic disturbance. Anna Freud (1954) advised that analysts should concentrate on the treatment of neuroses in order to perfect their technique before attempting to extend it to the treatment of more severe pathology. Limentani (1972) agreed that 'narrowing the scope of psychoanalysis so that it can operate within its natural limits and not least within the limitations of those that practice it' is required.

Freudian psychoanalysis also differs in theory and technique from Kleinian approaches. There is less emphasis on the transference, countertransference and projective identification. The transference is recognized and used to understand the patient, but the analyst directs their interventions more frequently towards the patient's external reality and relationships. This contrasts with Kleinian analysis in which the tendency is to focus on the patient's psychic reality and the transference relationship.

Which patient and why?

Freudian psychoanalysis may be considered as a treatment of choice for a patient who has neurotic problems, which may be accompanied by a degree of character pathology including relationship difficulties. The patient may have had experiences of loss or trauma which have not been fully resolved or integrated into their personalities.

There is no single assessment approach, but a range of practices that vary from a psychiatric type of interview to elicit data about the patient's presenting problems and past history, to a more psychoanalytic approach resembling a psychoanalytic session. There is also a lack of well-defined criteria for analysability, which stems partly from different theoretical models belonging to the different psychoanalytic groups, but also because the creative nature of the psychoanalytic process means that there is a scarcity of empirical facts. *Symptoms*, on their own, provide insufficient information and *psychiatric diagnosis* is also inadequate as a criterion for psychoanalytic suitability (Zetzel, 1968).

During an assessment the analyst may observe the patient's *ego structure*, its function (in terms of reality testing), its defence mechanisms (such as splitting, projection and projective identification), and its capacity for modification (in terms of adaptation). This gives rise to a well-recognized paradox in that patients who have sufficient ego strength to tolerate the analytic process and have a capacity for change – and are therefore considered suitable for analysis – will be least likely to seek treatment (Fairbairn, 1958).

Limentani (1972) draws attention to the distinction between suitability for analysis and analysability. A patient may be assessed as suitable for analytic treatment, but a symptom or an event in the patient's past or present life may not be analysable. For instance, a symptom of sexual perversion may not change, or a traumatic event may be split off and unreachable.

The assessment of analysability in a single session is a challenging task, for which only guidelines can be given. In the National Health Service (NHS) setting, prolonged assessments consisting of a number of appointments are sometimes offered. In private practice a single assessment appointment is more usual. Schachter (1997) advocates the benefit of longer assessments as they allow the possibility of observing whether it is possible to work with the patient on the transference and countertransference dynamics.

The question is how to assess the patient's *capacity to change*. The patient's *motivation*, their *capacity for psychoanalytic insight* and their *capacity to form a therapeutic alliance* are central elements for a successful analysis. Motivation involves more than simply requesting treatment and needs to include a desire for self-understanding. The patient needs to have sufficient psychoanalytic insight to be able to think about themselves in relation to other people and to be able to understand interpretations. However, as the development of insight is an aim of psychoanalysis, at the stage of assessment there only needs to be a rudimentary capacity to be able to make use of the analytic experience. There needs to be some alignment between the analyst's and the patient's understanding of themselves, and the therapist needs to evaluate the potential for a therapeutic relationship to emerge.

Every psychoanalytic encounter involves the *analyst* as well as the *patient*, and it is therefore important to consider the analyst's contribution to the assessment process. Schachter (1997) describes how the transference and countertransference dynamics are instruments that can be used in the assessment, to assist in the process of exploration, as they are during the analysis. The assessor's personal background will affect their counter-transference to a patient, which will influence what type of patient is taken on, as will their theoretical background.

There are few absolute contraindications to Freudian psychoanalysis. However, some relative contraindications include:

- The risks of *suicide* or developing *psychosis* need to be balanced with the risks of withholding treatment.
- *Substance dependence* often results in patients arriving for sessions intoxicated, missing sessions due to the effects of drugs or alcohol, and using substances as a form of resistance to avoid psychic pain.
- Severe *sado-masochistic tendencies* may contribute to a negative therapeutic reaction in which the patient does not have the capacity to take in anything good from a therapeutic relationship.

- *Compulsive liars*, including patients with Munchausen syndrome, may be unable to engage in a truthful exploration of themselves.

Which therapist and why?

Training

In the United Kingdom, training to become a Freudian psychoanalyst is through the British Institute of Psycho-Analysis based in London. There is an admissions procedure to the Institute designed to assess the applicant's capacity to develop as a psychoanalyst, which includes their interest in unconscious mental functioning and their own analysability. The training takes five years and is intensive. Personal analysis is an important part of the training, which includes an infant observation, theoretical and clinical seminars, and the analysis of two training cases seen five times a week with supervision.

The trainee's own analysis is aimed at enabling them to achieve an in-depth understanding of their own unconscious mental functioning, including their conflicts, anxieties and defences. This will help them to practise safely, so that they are able to differentiate what belongs to themselves and what belongs to the patient, to prevent their projecting their difficulties onto the patient. It also increases their understanding of transference and countertransference dynamics. Supervision of cases supplements this training process.

Matching of therapist and patient

Factors belonging to the analyst have to be taken into account, as they will inevitably affect the patient–analyst relationship. At the assessment stage the analyst's impact on the patient should be considered; as well as which therapist variables would be most helpful for the patient. The type of variables to consider are the *age, sex, cultural-racial background* and *level of experience* of the therapist. However it is difficult to predict matching on a list of variables, which is probably best assessed by the therapist's subjective experience at the first consultation. A transference is likely to emerge during the analysis in a similar form independent of the analyst. However, at the early stages of treatment, the patient may be particularly sensitive to characteristics of the analyst and, if an immediate transference develops, this will have far-reaching effects on the treatment.

Therapeutic setting

The analyst is responsible for creating the setting which will allow the patient to free associate. The analyst constructs the psychoanalytic situation in terms of rules, procedures and conditions which provide the matrix for the therapeutic alliance.

The therapeutic setting provides the *frame* for the psycho-analytic relationship. The *room* provides the regular and undisturbed environment, and the *couch* is part of the setting. These elements provide a spatial matrix for the therapeutic relationship (which may mirror the sensory matrix of the mother–infant relationship) and is the medium for non-verbal as well as verbal communication. The sensory matrix of the setting will help provide the holding environment, which is especially important for patients at earlier pre-verbal levels of psychic organization. Patients, especially those who are more disturbed, may be very sensitive to interruptions and changes to the setting.

Time is another boundary element to the setting. Freudian psychoanalysis involves five sessions a week of fifty minutes duration. There are planned breaks for the analyst's holidays that occur at regular intervals. The regularity and constancy of the time supports the holding matrix of the analytic relationship. It becomes internalized by the patient so that the fifty minutes is experienced rhythmically and provides a ritualistic quality to the analysis. If a session is altered by the analyst it will interfere with the rhythm, while unexpected breaks may make the patient feel seriously let down. The patient may also make modifications to the time, arriving late, leaving early or missing sessions, which is observed by the analyst and may offer information about the patient's internal world and defence mechanisms.

The setting varies depending on the context of the service. Freudian psychoanalysis is available only in the private sector, although there are subsidised schemes providing psychoanalysis. National Health psycho-therapy services seldom offer a five sessions per week psychoanalysis but, as a rare resource, three times a week psychoanalytic psychotherapy, constructed along the theory of psychoanalysis, is sometimes available. In the NHS psychotherapy is usually time-limited, whereas in the private sector psychoanalysis can continue with an open end for a number of years. A further difference is the fact that money passes from patient to analyst in private treatment. The payment can be viewed as part of the setting and will become part of the psychoanalytic relationship: constituting an exchange between the couple it alters the dyadic relationship as the patient has to give something to the analyst for their treatment.

If the setting is within a hospital or clinic, the external environment may feel less personal and more institutional, which may affect the relationship and alter the transference. The patient will develop not just a single transference to the therapist, but a more broadly spread transference to the whole institution. They may develop relationships with the receptionist, secretary and the institution, which become incorporated into their transference. The extended transference to the institution can have a containing function for more severely disturbed patients.

Closer links with psychiatric and medical services can be essential in the treatment of certain types of patients, especially severe borderline personality disorders. When working with patients who are liable to have intermittent psychotic breakdowns during the course of psychotherapy it is extremely helpful to have psychiatric back-up for the analytic treatment. Parallel psychiatric care can support the psychotherapy by monitoring the patient's mental state, managing psychotropic medication if it is required and assisting with their social situation. Psychoanalysts working privately can create links with other services, but it will disturb the setting and the relationship that they have with the patient by stepping outside the usual psychoanalytic encounter. It is therefore better handled before the start of treatment.

Clinical example

A patient of Irish origin came to analysis when he was twenty-six years old, wanting help for his problem with relationships which centred around his sexual inhibition. He had difficulty in making and maintaining relationships, which he presented as being due to erectile impotence on his part (for which physical causes had been excluded). His expressed wish was to be able to have a lasting sexual relationship. He talked of his mother domineering and constantly belittling his father, and seemed to identify with his weakened father. His mother was openly resentful about her husband having had better career opportunities than her, without him achieving the success that she wanted of him. At the start of his psychoanalysis, he was considering another relationship and was therefore seeking help for his sexual impotence.

On entering analysis, his style of free association was of interest as the associations seemed to be coherent and easy to follow. As the analyst listened more carefully, over a period of time, she realized that the patient's 'free associations' were in fact not really free but that he defensively organized his thoughts. He also had a tendency to announce the topic that he was going to talk about at the start of each session, and then rigidly kept to that topic for the fifty minutes, tightly controlling the content of the session, again defending himself against thinking about any more distressing or disturbing thoughts which he had repressed. He did mention a social anxiety that people might think him boring, and he also worried about their reaction to his accent. He spoke in a monotone and in a routine style, and as he talked the analyst began to feel drowsy, finding it hard to concentrate on what the patient was saying.

The analyst reflected upon her experience and wondered what aspects of her countertransference were being evoked by the patient. She thought about how the patient had a fear of disappointing people and of disapproval. This was evident in his relationship with his mother, to whom he felt that he had been a disappointment. It was also present in his relationships with girlfriends, with whom he suffered performance anxiety when he attempted sexual intercourse. He feared that if he was not 'super-man', he would fail them and evoke angry disapproval. The analyst observed how this fear and need to appease his objects had emerged in the transference, through the patient's habitual attempts to please her and give her what he thought she wanted. In doing so he was severely restricting his free associations and his real self.

The analyst reflected on herself becoming drowsy when listening to the patient, and realized that the patient had nudged her into a role response. She had responded to and enacted the patient's fantasy and fear that he was boring and inadequate. The analyst had also noticed that she was feeling irritable and experienced an aggressive urge to prod the patient to liven him up. She realized that she was experiencing the resentful and aggressive feelings that the patient had expelled through projective identification, so that the patient was left feeling flat and devoid of feelings while the analyst was feeling irritable.

Much of the analytical work was focused on allowing the patient to own and express his repressed feelings: including anger and resentment towards his mother, in current relationships with girlfriends whom he had felt the need to appease, and in the transference relationship with the analyst. Interpreting his defence against anger enabled the patient to acknowledge his feelings, of which he had previously kept himself unaware.

Over years, progress was observable within the analysis. The pattern of his associations became freer and less inhibited by his defences. His ego was strengthened through reclaiming lost aspects of himself – in particular his libidinal and aggressive instincts. He became a person with a stronger sense of self, rather than just presenting the compliant, passive side of his character. He had at the end of analysis developed a satisfactory sexual relationship with a girlfriend.

Problems in therapy

Problems that may occur in psychoanalysis
- Enactment: acting out and acting in
- Risk of suicide
- Psychotic breakdown
- Impasse
- Negative therapeutic reaction
- Malignant regression
- Countertransference and role responsiveness
- Role enactment by analyst

Enactment
Enactment includes 'acting in' and 'acting out' phenomena, and may occur when a patient feels unable to use verbal communication and therefore resorts to communicating through action. *Acting in* describes actions that patients may make within sessions, such as protracted silence, walking around the room or physical contact. Freud (1940) described *Acting out* as 'the patient acts it before us … instead of reporting it to us'. This refers to any behaviour that relates to the analytical situation, and it can be understood as a form of communication to the analyst. It is ubiquitous to all analyses and may involve arriving late, missing sessions or the patient behaving differently in their external life as a reaction to the analysis. The meaning of the behaviour needs to be understood in the context of the analytic relationship.

Risk of suicide
Suicide is the most threatening acting out behaviour. The patient, in attempting to kill themself, is also destroying the analytic relationship and making a murderous attack on the mind of the analyst. Freud (1917) suggested that suicide may occur when the patient becomes identified with a lost object, and the self and object become fused. In killing themself the patient is also aiming to kill the object who has abandoned them, in revenge for the pain and despair that they have been made to feel. Suicide may be driven by despair, but may also be part of a sado-masochistic way of relating to their objects. In assessing the risk the analyst needs to reflect on how the patient is relating to them, what sort of object they have become in the

patient's mind, and be aware of not identifying with the patient's despair and anger which could lead to enactment. When the analyst believes that there is a serious risk of suicide they need to take action to make the patient safe. If possible, the analyst should encourage the patient to seek further help for themself; but if this is ineffective, the analyst will need to alert other professionals (a general practitioner or psychiatrist) to take over the psychiatric management. The risk of suicide should, if possible, be considered at the assessment so as to arrange back-up psychiatric support at the start of analysis. It can then be brought into place more smoothly with the patient's consent and is less disruptive to the transference relationship. In the case of a suicide attempt occurring, it is important to bring it into the transference relationship (Campbell and Hale, 1991), to be able to work on the patient's murderous attack towards themselves, the analyst and significant others. This may be facilitated by seeing the patient as soon as possible after the attempt.

Psychotic breakdown
Psychotic breakdown may be provoked in a vulnerable patient by external life events or by the psychoanalytic process itself, through the dismantling of the patient's defence mechanisms and the confrontation of psychic pain. In the assessment, the analyst should have in mind the risk of psychosis developing. Patients with a history of major psychotic illness – manic depression, schizophrenia or other delusional disorders – are at risk of relapse, which could be provoked by analysis. Should such a patient be taken into treatment, it is helpful to have back-up psychiatric management instigated at the start.

Therapeutic impasse
An impasse is said to have occurred in analysis when the patient is neither progressing nor retreating. The patient may appear to be rigidly adhering to and complying with treatment, attending punctually, free associating, bringing dreams and responding to interpretations, but this may be a defensive masquerade. The patient may also not be properly motivated to make psychic change, and may be simply using the analysis as a prop. An impasse is liable to develop gradually and it is often difficult to detect. The analyst may become aware that no real change is occurring, and that the compliance is a disguised form of resistance. It is usually created by an unconscious collusion between the patient's psychopathology and that of the analyst. In the situation of an impasse, the analyst needs to look for ways that they may be contributing to the interaction as well as interpreting the resistance on the part of the patient.

Negative therapeutic reaction
A negative therapeutic reaction is an aggressive and destructive response to the analyst and the analysis. It is therefore a form of resistance, and usually presents as a paradoxical reaction to a correct interpretation or after some progress has been achieved. Rosenfeld (1987) describes how negative therapeutic reactions particularly occur in narcissistic patients and are an expression of destructive impulses, derived from the death instinct. There are a number of situations which may give rise to a negative therapeutic

reaction: a patient with narcissistic personality disturbance may wish to be independent of the analyst, and therefore feels the need to make the analyst useless; the patient may be very dependent on the analyst, but react to this feeling with hatred, which is felt and expressed toward themselves and the analyst; the patient may have envious feelings about the analyst's capacity to understand them, which can lead to attacking of that understanding. In the case of a negative therapeutic reaction, the analyst needs to understand and interpret the cause of the resistance, at the same time addressing its destructive nature.

Malignant regression
There is controversy as to the therapeutic value of regression. Some analysts think it necessary for the patient to re-experience early childhood and infantile states in the transference relationship with the analyst, in order that these difficulties can be worked through in a corrective relationship. It may, however, slide into pathological or malignant regression, when it is out of the patient's and analyst's control. Malignant regression may present with excessive dependency and demands on the analyst, and may escalate to acting out behaviour and the need for psychiatric admission.

Countertransference and role responsiveness
A mistake on the part of the analyst is not to recognize or be able to manage their countertransference, in order to use it analytically to help understand the patient. This can lead the analyst to collude with the patient's psychopathology and defences. It may inhibit the analyst making interpretations to avoid triggering psychic pain, it may allow the analyst to become overinvolved with the patient, and it can also leave the analyst open to role enactment. Sandler (1976) describes how a patient unconsciously attempts in their transference to create a role relationship with the analyst that corresponds to their internal object relationships, and the analyst is therefore nudged into a role response. If the analyst does not become aware of their role responsiveness, they may enact the role and the patient's transference becomes actualized within the psychoanalytic setting.

Role enactment
Role enactment occurs when the analyst is unconsciously driven to respond to the patient in ways that are unhelpful or outside the analytic frame. The analyst is responding to and colluding with the patient's conscious and unconscious feelings, thoughts and defences. The patient may project aspects onto the analyst and, through projective identification, the analyst may unintentionally accept these aspects. These aspects may be positive attributes (leading the analyst to identify with an idealized image of themselves), or they may be negative and hostile, which can lead the analyst to respond in a rejecting manner and thereby enact the patient's phantasies.

Misconceptions

One misconception is that psychoanalysis is preoccupied with the subject of sex. Classical Freudian theory was rooted in a *theory of drives* or instincts.

It put the need for a sexual relationship as a primary drive, and the choice of a partner secondary to this drive. When Freud coined the term libido he meant sexual energy, and criticized Jung for broadening the term to include all psychic energy. The emphasis on instinctual drives contrasts classical Freudian theory from object relations theory, which puts the psychological need for relationships as central. Freud in his own time shifted away from the centrality of instincts, and contemporary Freudian theory has evolved to take into account a more person-related psychology.

Another common misunderstanding is the idea that psychoanalysis is preoccupied with the patient's history and early childhood. The analyst mostly concentrates on the *here and now* of the patient's present reality, including both their internal and external reality and how these converge on the psychoanalytic relationship. Freudian psychoanalysis incorporates a developmental theory that early attachment relationships and experiences are internalized as working models of relationships (Bowlby, 1988), which affect the nature of future relationships. The aim is not to excavate the subject's history in the search for trauma as a form of explanation, but the patient's history is used to help understand the patient in the present. In talking about their past the patient is able to reconstruct their narrative, as they become more aware of their own distortions.

Evaluation of therapy

The evaluation of psychoanalysis remains a challenge for the future. Randomized controlled trials are usually considered to be the research method of choice to evaluate treatments. However, such empirical research of psychoanalysis has not yet been undertaken as the subject matter is not readily investigable by these techniques. There are numerous obstacles to performing this type of outcome research for psychoanalysis, including small sample size, the difficulty of long-term follow-up, high attrition rates, lack of an adequate control group, limited generalizability of the results and the coarse-grained nature of the data.

The Menninger Project (Wallerstein, 1986) is a prospective naturalistic study spanning twenty-five years which incorporates measures at assessment, during treatment and at outcome. The sample included forty-two cases of severe personality disturbance, twenty-two who received psychoanalysis and twenty, psychotherapy. By the end of the study only six of the psychoanalytic sample had traditional psychoanalysis, the others having a modified psychoanalytic treatment, making the results less clear. However some important findings emerged: patients with this severe pathology did as well with supportive psychotherapy as they did with psychoanalysis; a positive transference was a good predictive factor for both groups; and the most disturbed cases with an extremely poor prognosis did not do well in either group. The findings generally support an argument against widening the scope of psychoanalysis for more disturbed patients.

An outcome project of psychoanalysis is being conducted at the Anna Freud Centre. It aims to measure change during and after psychoanalysis, multidimensionally, on a number of standardized measures including psychiatric diagnoses, symptomatology, the Adult Attachment Interview (AAI) and the Reflective Self-Function scale (RSF) (both of which are discussed more fully in the dedicated research chapter). It also includes the analysts' evaluations of change by reviewing a random monthly session which is reported verbatim, and using the 'Anna Freud Centre Young Adult Weekly Rating Scale' (Gerber, 1997). This scale, which is completed by the analyst, has been constructed to measure major themes of the psychoanalytic relationship, including the manifest themes, the analyst's understanding of these, the nature of the transference, forms of resistance and the main theme of the analyst's interpretations. The project aims to use innovative methodology that is scientific – using procedures that are open to inspection and replicable – but which investigates meaningful constructs of psychoanalysis.

Single cases studies have, since Freud, been the most widely used method of psychoanalytic study. They have not been respected as a method of research by empirical scientists but do raise ideas that may develop clinical practice, and can act as a springboard for subsequent larger studies. Kernberg (1994) conducted a case study, audio-recording every session of a patient's treatment over a number of years, and demonstrated how changes in the transference can be measured by observing the nature of the patient's responses to the analyst's interpretations. Moran and Fonagy (1987) showed by a case study of an adolescent girl with brittle diabetes that her diabetic control could be used as an external marker of successful psychoanalytic treatment, and that there was a temporal correlation between interpretations of oedipal conflicts and improved diabetic control.

Psychoanalysis is an expensive treatment. It requires five times a week sessions for a number of years with a highly trained therapist. However, the financial implications need to be compared with alternative treatments, and the use of other resources if no treatment is available. In some cases, an alternative treatment to psychoanalysis could be long-term psychoanalytic psychotherapy in an inpatient setting, such as at the Cassel Hospital which is a therapeutic community. The cost of one year of treatment in a specialist in-patient unit is comparable with, and frequently more expensive than, five years of private psychoanalysis as an out-patient. There are now a number of cost-effectiveness studies (e.g. Menzies *et al.*, 1993) showing an overall cost reduction when the cost of the treatment is set against a reduction in the use of other resources (such as psychiatric treatment, the use of accident and emergency services, general practitioner visits, medical and surgical interventions, social services involvement and unemployment benefits). The benefits of psychoanalysis may be slow to achieve, but are thought to be more permanent and long lasting than other forms of psychological treatment.

Alternatives to therapy

A patient may start in psychoanalytic psychotherapy and then for various reasons progress to psychoanalysis. This may occur if a patient has demonstrated during psychotherapy that they can use the psychoanalytic approach and if the therapist feels that they could benefit from more intensive treatment. A therapist may also suggest increasing the number of sessions per week for a patient who finds it difficult to tolerate the gaps between sessions.

Psychoanalysis may be considered after general psychiatry has failed to produce change in a patient with personality disturbance. It may be considered if a patient has the psychological capacities to use psychoanalysis, if they can be contained in the out-patient setting and if they can afford it. If they do not fulfil these requirements, therapeutic community treatment is an alternative for personality disordered patients who have not been helped by general psychiatry. Therapeutic communities have evolved for the treatment of such individuals and are available on the NHS. The environment offers containment for the patient whilst they undergo psychoanalytic psychotherapy; it also offers a group experience with other patients with similar disturbance, and a process of living and working together in a community. They can be residential or day units.

In private psychoanalysis with more disturbed patients, where there is a risk of psychotic breakdown or suicide, it is very important to liaise with the local consultant psychiatrist to arrange back-up psychiatric care. In cases where there is a high risk of acting out through violence or sexual perversion, it may be appropriate to have back-up forensic psychiatric management or links with a forensic psychotherapy service.

Acknowledgements
I would like to thank David Leibel and Joan Schachter for their help with this chapter.

Further reading

Bateman, A. and Holmes, J. (1995) *Introduction to Psychoanalysis: Contemporary Theory and Practice.* London and New York: Routledge.

Freud, A. (1937) *The Ego and the Mechanisms of Defence.* London: Hogarth Press. (Reprinted by Karnac Books, London, 1993.)

Freud, S. (1900) The interpretation of dreams. In: *Standard Edition of the Complete Psychological Works of Sigmund Freud*, vol. 4/5. London: Hogarth Press.

Freud, S. (1916/17) Introductory lectures on psychoanalysis. In: *Standard Edition of the Complete Psychological Works of Sigmund Freud*, vol. 15/16. London: Hogarth Press.

Freud, S. (1901–1922) *Case Histories I: 'Dora' and 'Little Hans'.* The Pelican Freud Library. London: Penguin.

Freud, S. (1909–1920) *Case Histories II: 'Rat Man', 'Schreber', 'Wolf Man', 'A Case of Female Homosexuality'.* The Pelican Freud Library. London: Penguin.

Freud, S. and Breuer, J. (1895) Studies on hysteria. In: *Standard Edition of the Complete Psychological Works of Sigmund Freud*, vol. 2. London: Hogarth Press.

Gay, P. (1988) *Freud: a Life For Our Time.* Dent and Sons: London. (Reprinted by Papermac, London, 1989.)

Jones, E. (1962) *The Life and Work of Sigmund Freud.* London: Hogarth Press.

Roazen, P. (1979) *Freud and His Followers.* London: Peregrine Books.

Rycroft, C. (1995) *A Critical Dictionary of Psychoanalysis.* London: Penguin Books.

Bibliography

Bowlby, J. (1988) *A Secure Base: Clinical Applications of Attachment Theory*. London: Routledge.
Britton, R., Feldman, M. and O'Shaugnessy, E. (1989) *The Oedipus Complex Today*. London: Karnac Books.
Campbell, D. and Hale, R. (1991) Suicidal acts. In: Holmes, J. (ed.), *Textbook of Psychotherapy in Psychiatric Practice*. London: Churchill Livingstone.
Fairbairn, W.R.D. (1958) On the nature and aims of psychoanalytic treatment. *International Journal of Psychoanalysis*, **39**, 374–385.
Fonagy, P. (1996) When cure is inconceivable: the aims of psychoanalysis with borderline patients. Presented at *The Changing Aims of Psychoanalytic Therapy*, University College London, June, 1996.
Fonagy, P. and Target, M. (1996) Playing with reality. I: Theory of mind and the normal development of psychic reality. *International Journal of Psychoanalysis*, **77**, 217–233.
Fonagy, P., Steele, H., Moran, G. *et al.* (1991) The capacity for understanding mental states: the reflective self in parent and child and its significance for security of attachment. *Infant Mental Health Journal*, **13**, 200–217.
Fonagy, P., Steele, M., Steele, H. and Target, M. (1997) *Reflective-Functioning Manual: Version 4.1 for Application to Adult Attachment Interviews*. London: University College London, Psychoanalysis Unit.
Freud, A. (1937) *The Ego and the Mechanisms of Defence*. London: Hogarth Press. (Reprinted by Karnac Books, London, 1993.)
Freud, A. (1954) The widening scope of indications for psychoanalysis. *Journal of American Psychoanalytic Association*, **2**, 607–620.
Freud, S. (1900) The interpretation of dreams. In: *Standard Edition of the Complete Psychological Works of Sigmund Freud*, vol. 4/5. London: Hogarth Press.
Freud, S. (1905) Three essays on the theory of sexuality. In: *Standard Edition of the Complete Psychological Works of Sigmund Freud*, vol. 7. London: Hogarth Press.
Freud, S. (1917) Mourning and melancholia. In: *Standard Edition of the Complete Psychological Works of Sigmund Freud*, vol. 14. London: Hogarth Press.
Freud, S. (1923) The Ego and the Id. In: *Standard Edition of the Complete Psychological Works of Sigmund Freud*, vol. 19. London: Hogarth Press.
Freud, S. (1925) Some psychological consequences of the anatomical distinction between the sexes. In: *Standard Edition of the Complete Psychological Works of Sigmund Freud*, vol. 19. London: Hogarth Press.
Freud, S. (1930) Civilization and its discontents. In: *Standard Edition of the Complete Psychological Works of Sigmund Freud*, vol. 21. London: Hogarth Press.
Freud, S. (1937) Analysis terminable and interminable. In: *Standard Edition of the Complete Psychological Works of Sigmund Freud*, vol. 23. London: Hogarth Press.
Freud, S. (1940) An outline of psychoanalysis. In: *Standard Edition of the Complete Psychological Works of Sigmund Freud*, vol. 23. London: Hogarth Press.
Freud, S. and Breuer, J. (1895) Studies on hysteria. In: *Standard Edition of the Complete Psychological Works of Sigmund Freud*, vol. 2. London: Hogarth Press.
Gerber, A. (1997) 'The Anna Freud Centre Young Adult Weekly Rating Scale'. Unpublished manuscript of PhD in progress, Anna Freud Centre, London.
Greenson, R.R. (1965) The working alliance and the transference neurosis. *Psychoanalytic Quarterly*, **34**, 155–181.
Heimann, P. (1950) On counter-transference. *International Journal of Psychoanalysis*, **31**, 81–84.
Kernberg, O. (1994) Identity diffusion and structural change: research findings. Presented to the *Fourth International Psychoanalytic Association Conference on Psychoanalytic Research*, London, March, 1994.
Klein, M. (1946) Notes on some schizoid mechanisms. *International Journal of Psychoanalysis*, **27**, 99–110.

Limentani, A. (1972) The assessment of analysability: a major hazard in selection for psychoanalysis. *International Journal of Psychoanalysis*, **53**, 351–361.

Menzies, D., Dolan, B. and Norton, K. (1993) Are short term savings worth long term costs? Funding treatment for personality disorders. *Psychiatric Bulletin*, **17**, 517–519.

Moran, G. and Fonagy, P. (1987) Psychoanalysis and diabetic control: a single case study. *British Journal of Medical Psychology*, **60**, 357–372.

O'Shaughnessy, E. (1994) What is a clinical fact? *International Journal of Psychoanalysis*, **75**, 939–947.

Rosenfeld, H. (1987) Narcissistic patients with negative therapeutic reactions. In: *Impasse and Interpretation. Therapeutic and Anti-therapeutic Factors in the Psychoanalytic Treatment of Psychotic, Borderline, and Neurotic Patients*. London: The New Library of Psychoanalysis, pp. 85–105.

Sandler, J. (1976) Countertransference and role-responsiveness. *International Review of Psychoanalysis*, **3**, 43–47.

Sandler, J. (1987) *From Safety to Superego*. London: Karnac Books.

Sandler, J. (1988) The concept of projective identification. In: J. Sandler (ed.), *Projection, Identification, Projective Identification*. London: Karnac Books, pp. 13–26.

Sandler, J., Holder, A. and Kawenoker-Berger, M. (1987) Theoretical and clinical aspects of transference. In: J. Sandler (ed.), *From Safety to Superego*. London: Karnac Books, pp. 264–284.

Schachter, J. (1997) Transference and countertransference dynamics in the assessment process. *Psychoanalytic Psychotherapy*, **11**, 59–71.

Segal, H. (1957) Notes on symbol formation. *International Journal of Psychoanalysis*, **38**, 391–397 (and in *The Work of Hanah Segal*, London: Free Association Books, 1986.)

Steiner, John (1996) The aim of psychoanalysis in theory and practice. *International Journal of Psychoanalysis*, **77**, 1073–1083.

Stern, D. (1985) *The Interpersonal World of the Infant*. New York: Basic Books.

Wallerstein, R. (1986) *Forty-Two Lives in Treatment: a Study of Psychoanalysis and Psychotherapy*. New York: Guilford Press.

Zetzel, E. (1968) The so called good hysteric. *International Journal of Psychoanalysis*, **49**, 256–260.

2

Jungian Psychotherapy

Jennifer Stein

Historical perspective

Jungian psychotherapy originated with the life's work of Carl Gustav Jung (1875–1961). A pastor's son, Jung grew up in rural Switzerland. Much of his early childhood revolved around his struggle to make sense of religious practices, and his father's part in them. This experience ran parallel to his observations of his parents' marriage, which was an unhappy one. While Jung's mother was extroverted and concerned herself with practical, down-to-earth issues, his father was introverted and struggled to live up to his Christian beliefs. Although his parents attempted to appear united, it was evident to Jung, who was a sensitive and intelligent child, that there was a great deal of conflict between them, and that they represented opposite polarities of personality. Jung described his mother as having 'a hearty animal warmth' and being 'a ready listener'. He saw her as being gifted in a creative sense, and felt that she had a deep sense of her own personality, which as he remarked 'struck to the core of my being' (F. Fordham, 1953). Despite this, Jung found comfort from his father who was enlisted into a maternal role when his mother was ill in hospital. The disappearance of his mother for several months when Jung was only three years old seems to have been responsible for an enduring attitude Jung had towards women, seeing them as unreliable.

At the age of eleven Jung went to Basle Gymnasium, where he found his teachers to be unresponsive and unaware of his personal progress and development. School bored him and he felt a sense of loss at being taken away from his playmates in the local school, being placed instead in the 'great world' (Jung, 1963). He began to develop neurotic fainting spells, and was away from school for a period of six months. This allowed him to spend endless happy hours absorbed in his own inner world. Perhaps as a result of his father's concern, however, Jung suddenly came to terms with the need to accept reality. His studies picked up, and he began to have some insight into his earlier unhappiness, recognizing the unexpressed rage and grief which had contributed to his fainting attacks.

Towards the end of his schooling Jung became more aware of his scientific interest and, with his father's support, took up medical studies at Basle University in 1895. In 1900 he went to work at the Burgholzli Mental

Hospital in Zurich as an assistant to Eugen Bleuler, and in this intellectual atmosphere Jung was able to develop his ideas about the psyche. In particular, he became interested in psychotic illness, and in 1907 published *The Psychology of Dementia Praecox*. This book provided the opening for meeting Freud, who invited him to Vienna.

Freud was twenty years older than Jung, and was something of a father-figure to him. The two men developed a close relationship, although their interests were always slightly different. Freud was particularly preoccupied with neurotic illness, while Jung turned to the psychoses, and psychotic aspects of ordinary individuals. Jung diverged from Freud in his wider interests in religion and mythology, and rejected Freud's exclusive concentration on infantile sexuality. Both Jung and Freud accepted the notion of an inherited 'primaeval experience' in the psyche (Freud, 1916/ 1917) but Jung gave it greater prominence in his concept of the collective unconscious. While for Freud the instincts formed the basis of individual experience and unconscious motivation, Jung felt that there was a wider inherited component in the unconscious which related to society and the human race in general.

An interesting parallel finding for Jung was his discovery of a recurring sexual motif in mythology and religion, and he developed this in his work known as 'Psychology of the Unconscious' (1912; *CW*, 7). He proposed that a son's incestuous feelings for his mother were spiritual and were stimulated by searching for a new self through a rebirth experience. Since this idea was at odds with Freud's theories, the two men broke apart. Jung left the psychoanalytic movement and his former friends deserted him, seeing him as a mystic. Moreover, the impact of the outbreak of the First World War stimulated in Jung a number of powerful images of destruction which heightened his sensitivity and increased his interest in psychotic phenomena.

Jung began to explore his own inner experience at this time and was more open to his irrational impulses. He evolved a method of self-analysis, stimulated by his work with psychotic patients in Burgholzli. Jung carefully recorded his fantasies, visions, dreams and thoughts, often painting the images, which he found allowed the emotional content to emerge. He gave himself access to activities more often associated with a child's play, and using stones and bricks he built models of small towns. At the same time he related to his dream figures in an attempt to gain greater awareness of previously hidden, or unconscious, parts of his personality. Freda Fordham (1953) writes, however, that, 'He recognized the material as similar in character to what is produced by the insane, but it was also "the matrix of a mythopoeic imagination which has vanished from our rational age", i.e. is no longer valued'.

In contrast to Freud, Jung conceptualized the libido as a non-specific psychic energy and developed a theoretical perspective which viewed the psyche as a self-regulating, dynamic system. He viewed libido as passing between two opposite poles. The forward movement he called progression (which satisfies the conscious life) and the backward movement he called regression (which satisfies the unconscious). The latter is associated with a state in which the individual feels a need to withdraw and where mental activity is less directed – a kind of '*reculer pour mieux sauter*'.

Jung went on to develop an interest in Eastern religion. He looked on both religion and alchemy as metaphors for individuation, the process of becoming whole, to which Jung felt his psychology aspired. Jung saw the alchemical texts as expressing unconscious fantasies. He wrote, 'The experiences of the alchemists were, in a sense, my experience, and their world was my world ... I had stumbled upon the historical counterpart of my psychology of the unconscious' (F. Fordham, 1953). Jung also travelled widely to lecture and to research his ideas. In Africa he found that he was 'touched [in] every possible sore spot in my own psychology' and found 'the stillness of the eternal beginning, the world as it had always been, in the state of non-being' (F. Fordham, 1953).

Storr (1983) wrote, 'It is characteristic that his autobiography contains next to nothing about his personal relationships. Jung wished to ... shield his family from the glare of an unwelcome publicity. It is also true that the psyche was of over-riding importance to him. "You are only interested in the collective unconscious", said his wife on one occasion' (F. Fordham, 1953). Jung's wife, Anna, also developed an interest in analysis and took patients. She died in 1955 before she could complete her research on the legend of the Grail.

Jung retreated finally to his house at Bollingen, on the shores of the Lake of Zurich. He was unreliable in his reaction to visitors, though often being very friendly and interested in students, and unsophisticated people. He seemed to convey the sense of a great man, and made a significant impact on those who met him. His own observation of himself was that he needed 'other people both more and less than most' (F. Fordham, 1953). He died at the age of eighty-five, in 1961.

Jung did not wish to establish a school of theory but said 'I prefer to call my own approach "Analytical Psychology", by which I mean something like a general concept embracing both psychoanalysis (Freud) and individual psychology (Adler) as well as other endeavours in the field of "complex psychology"' (*CW*, 16). He made a major contribution to the general body of psychoanalytic theory through his attempt to give equal weight to the inner or inherited psychic processes as to the outer environmental ones. Both during his lifetime and following his death several institutions were established to promote Jungian psychotherapy, including the C.G. Jung Institute in Zurich (1940) and the Society of Analytical Psychology in London (1940). Jung published his ideas in many articles and books, including his *Collected Works*. Analytical psychology has been developed more recently by the post-Jungian writers, among them Michael Fordham, Kenneth Lambert, James Hillman and Eric Neumann.

A clear account of the different schools within analytical psychology is given by Samuels (1985). Broadly these may be divided into the Zurich School of Jungian Psychotherapy, which lays greater emphasis on the use of myths, and the London School, which pays more attention to the transference and incorporates a developmental approach which owes much to Klein's writings. Samuels describes three main schools – the classical school, the developmental school and the archetypal school. Exponents of these schools would be Adler, Fordham and Hillman respectively.

Principles of theory and practice

Theoretical principles

Michael Fordham (1978) makes the point that 'in the history of analytical psychology, observations came first and then theoretical constructions'. In his book he gave 'priority to the practice of analytical psychology as an experience'. The following framework was developed by Jung, and subsequent Jungian writers, in order to organize and explain the information which came from clinical practice.

The psyche

Jung conceived of the mind as a psyche in which there are both conscious and unconscious parts. He divided the psyche into the self, the ego, the personal unconscious and the impersonal or collective unconscious.

The self

In Jungian psychology the self is seen as being the centre of the personality. Jung's self differs from the psychoanalytic concept of feelings of self-hood or personal identity which Jung located in the ego and which can be reflected on by the conscious mind. The idea of the self gives rise to a sense of what we mean when we talk about wholeness. In Jungian terms, wholeness is arrived at through balance and the self represents 'the potential for integration of the total personality' (Samuels, 1985). Much of the self is often unconscious and only becomes conscious through the self archetype, with the task of mediating opposites within the psyche and being responsible for the appearance of deeply meaningful symbols which lead to insight and healing.

The self can also appear as images in dreams. A frequent symbol of the self is the divine child, or a treasured object. Jung thought that the mandala symbols – concentrically arranged figures which are commonly found in dreams – were also an expression of the self. As the self becomes more conscious, one-sided attitudes are compensated for and an individual becomes a more balanced personality, coming to terms with who they are, not what they should be.

The ego

In Jungian psychology the ego represents the centre of consciousness, but not the centre of the psyche. Jung saw the ego as a mirror for the unconscious. He postulated that the ego and ego-consciousness have a complementary relationship with the unconscious, 'so that what is known tells us something about what is not' (Samuels, 1985). The ego contains an individual's conscious attitudes and ways of behaving. Since these are learnt primarily through the child's relationship with important others, such as parents, the ego comes to have a close relationship with the personal unconscious and, in particular, the shadow. The ego is seen as being dependent on the whole psyche; this varies between individuals, however, depending on how dominated the person is by their unconscious. Specific functions of the ego are memory, identity and personal continuity. The degree and nature of ego functioning varies with health and maturation. An awareness of the ego, or ego consciousness, is therefore a dynamic process which unfolds over time and may be accelerated by analysis or psychotherapy.

In Jungian writing, ego consciousness is symbolized in a variety of ways. An example may be found in the creation myth (Genesis) and in many other similar accounts of the creation of light from other cultures. The ego can also be equated with the idea of the hero, whose journey in many myths and stories 'signifies a renewal of light and hence a rebirth of consciousness from the darkness' (*CW*, 5). The immature ego is seen as being formed from a coalescence of 'islands of consciousness' (*CW*, 8) which can be viewed as parts of the ego as they arise from the unconscious.

The personal unconscious

The personal unconscious is seen as containing repressed material from an individual's own experience. Since the psychic material which is contained in the personal unconscious is repressed, it does not form part of the ego. The repressed or personal unconscious contains aspects of an individual's personality which are incompatible with their ideals and ethical attitudes. It results from the interaction between that individual and their parents and society. Jungian theory postulates the operation of defences as a means by which this repression is achieved.

Collective unconscious and archetypes

The collective unconscious is seen as being derived from innate, and probably inherited experience. Jung called the organizers of this experience *archetypes*. Archetypes 'express the primitive concepts, needs and aspirations of humanity' (Samuels, 1985). The archetype may be viewed as an innate pattern, which becomes 'clothed in images' (Whitmont, 1964) through the subjective experience with the external world, especially the mother. The archetype therefore represents a potential for personality development, and the archetypal image is a reflection of the form the personality is taking up, as a result of external experience in the world. The formation of images may be influenced by myths, fairy tales and religious images. The experiencing of such images often has an awesome, or powerful impact on an individual, and this has been termed *numinosity*. Archetypal images which have not been modified by personal experience are particularly likely to exhibit themselves in a more dramatic way, and evoke primitive emotions and affect. Although this can be part of normal experience, it is seen particularly well in psychotic phenomena, and in the projections of borderline patients.

The archetypal system can therefore be observed through particular constellations or clusters which tend to separate out in different personalities. Jung wrote, 'It is a well-nigh hopeless undertaking to tear a single archetype out of the living tissue of the psyche; but despite their interwovenness the archetypes do form units of meaning that can be apprehended intuitively' (*CW*, 9). The following archetypal images are commonly observed: the shadow, the anima and animus, the wise old man, the divine child, the great mother and the trickster.

The shadow

The shadow is seen as being closely associated with the personal unconscious. It contains both the personal and the cultural shadow, and represents those aspects of an individual, or a society which have been neglected or repressed. It contains the desires and emotions which are incompatible with social standards or an individual's ideal personality. While some repression is helpful in everyday living, the damming up of strong feelings often results in them becoming overwhelming. 'The shadow', says Jung, 'is a moral problem which challenges the whole ego personality' (M. Fordham, 1957). Through natural developmental processes, parenting tendencies and education, an individual reaches a compromise between himself and what society thinks he ought to be. This leads to the development of a mask, or persona, which hides the shadow behind it. The shadow is often projected on to other people, and can then be observed if the process has been recognized. The process of projection is also a way in which other archetypal images may be seen.

The persona

The persona is a collective phenomenon which appears to be individually developed but, as described above, largely arises out of cultural influences. There is pressure on an individual to incorporate the persona into his or her personality in order to simplify relationships. 'People who neglect the development of the persona tend to be gauche, to offend others, and have difficulty in establishing themselves in the world' (F. Fordham, 1953).

The anima and animus

It is integral to Jungian theory that both feminine and masculine elements are potentially to be found in any individual. Jung said that 'an inherited collective image of woman exists in a man's unconscious with the help of which he apprehends the nature of woman' (CW, 7). Freda Fordham (1953) makes the point that the archetypal feminine image, or anima, is only a general expression of femininity and only becomes available to an individual through real contact with women. The anima is therefore an innate capacity which can lead to the development of a feminine side in men. Such integration also helps a man feel more comfortable with his masculinity.

Men frequently project their anima image on to women who are important to them and become fascinated by it. As Jung wrote, 'Every mother and every beloved is forced to become the carrier and embodiment of this omnipresent and ageless image which corresponds to the deepest reality in a man' (CW, 9). The types of images which are associated with the anima are therefore very varied. There are often two sides represented in these images, the Madonna figure and the Siren, and this results in both the idealization and deprecation of women.

The fascination which is aroused through the projection of a man's anima on to a woman may be understood as his recognition of a previously unconscious part of himself which he needs. Jung therefore referred to the anima as a man's soul. It is often difficult for men to accept the more negative anima image as being part of their own personality and this results in the man being a prisoner to the power of the dragon female image.

The masculine element in women is called the animus. The animus is often associated with the thinking function, and with conscious and directed thought. Although the animus figure often originates with the father, it also tends to be expressed as a group of men. The animus function can be observed in the woman through her own behaviour, for example overcritical and judgemental statements, particularly when related to the work sphere. It may also be projected on to a man, and results in a blinding to the woman of that man's actual personality.

As with a man and his anima, a woman becomes fascinated by the projection of her animus on to a man, and this can explain the tendency some women have to seek close relationships with powerful men. Whereas the anima produces moods in a man, the animus produces opinions and can make women aggressive and prejudiced. On the other hand, the animus can stir up a search for knowledge in women which will help to modify the primitive nature of the animus, and give a woman's personality more balance. Projection of the anima and animus are characteristic of 'states of being in love' and more psychotic delusional states. They may also manifest themselves through an apparent deficiency of the opposite function, for example a man who is possessed by his mother's animus may fail to identify with his own masculinity (see clinical example).

Complex

Jung arrived at his concept of complexes primarily from his work with psychotic patients, using association tests. He observed that certain ideas and affects in an individual have a tendency to cluster together. These clusters, or complexes, may be derived from either the personal or the collective unconscious, or may be a combination of both. The individual is often unaware of the operation of such complexes. Complexes are viewed as being split off from the control of consciousness, having a life of their own. Their origin is often in an emotional shock, which may either be from an early childhood event, or from a more current conflict. Complexes do not necessarily imply a pathological state, however they do indicate that some aspect of the psyche has been unassimilated, and they therefore act as a stimulus to psychic growth much in the way that Winnicott's frustrating good-enough mother does. An example of this process would be the increasing preoccupation a woman might have with her reliance on men. This may be viewed as a father-complex, which becomes integrated into her personality through her greater awareness of a need to identify with women, or a mother figure. The resulting psychic growth leaves a woman with less powerful feelings in relation to men, and a capacity for a more equal relationship with them.

The opposites

In Jungian psychology there is a great awareness of the necessity for the presence of opposites within facets of the personality, and that the balancing of the opposites comes about by a process of self-regulation. A one-sided attitude is frequently accompanied by a set of traits or symptoms which represent the opposite aspect. For example, neurosis is viewed as a one-sided or unbalanced development of the psyche. It is the role of the self to balance the opposing tendencies in what is termed a compensatory process. Compensation comes about through dreams, resistances, slips of the tongue, or other habitual but often unnoticed ways of behaving.

Psychological types

Jung attempted to classify human beings according to their psychological types. He distinguished two main attitudes to life as exemplified by the extroverted type and the introverted. In the extrovert, libido or psychic energy is directed out to the object of interest in the external world. In the introvert, libido is drawn in from the object, to the internal world. While the extroverted type is sociable and feels at ease with himself in the world, the introverted type withdraws, preferring reflection to activity. The two attitudes often stand in conflict to one another, though it is usually the case that the conscious attitude is accompanied by an unconscious opposite attitude. Jung called the latter the inferior function. Jung described four other functions which are used to establish an identity: thinking, sensation, feeling and intuition. These functions differentiate between intellectual and emotional experience. In order to differentiate feeling and thinking Jung wrote, 'When we think, it is in order to judge or to reach a conclusion and when we feel it is in order to attach a proper value to something' (*CW*, 6).

Although the use of typology has perhaps diminished in importance in contemporary Jungian practice, there remains a considerable body of opinion in favour of their use, as discussed by M. Fordham (1978). There are a number of psychological tests which look at typology (Myers, 1962; Wheelright, 1964). The Myers–Briggs Type Indicator (Myers, 1962) incorporates a distinction between judging and perceiving and results in a clarification of sixteen subtypes of personality function.

Alchemical metaphors

Jungian psychotherapy uses a variety of alchemical terms in order to describe aspects of the analytic process. Most of these terms refer to the transference relationship between the patient and the therapist. Jung thought that the alchemical paradigm better described the analytic process than the religious one. In the Christian religion Jung saw the opposites of light and good/darkness and evil as being left in open conflict, whereas alchemy 'is rather like an undercurrent to the Christianity that ruled on the surface. It is to this surface as the dream is to the unconscious and just as the dream compensates the conflicts of the conscious mind, so alchemy endeavours to fill in the gaps left open by the Christian tension of opposites' (*CW*, 12). The following terms have a symbolic relation to Jungian analysis.

Vas: This describes the alchemical vessel in which the base elements were mixed. In analytic terms, the vas represents the holding situation of the analysis. This is described in both Jungian writing and in other psychoanalytic writing as containment.

The **coniunctio:** In alchemical writings this described the coming together of the different elements in the vas, with the production of alchemical gold. The elements were often represented by male and female figures. In Jungian analysis the coniunctio has come to mean the union of opposites, symbolizing the interaction of the analyst and the patient, and the integration of the conflicted aspects of the patient's psyche. The coniunctio, or marriage, also represents the possibility of the emergence of a third, newly found aspect or element. Thus the alchemical metaphor encompasses the creative aspect of the analytic situation.

Transformation: The alchemical process involved the transformation of elements and relied on the transmutability of the components of the process. This image of the possibility of psychological movement is an essential part of the theoretical underpinning of Jungian therapy.

The symbol

In Jungian psychology the symbol is described as 'the best possible description or formulation of a relatively unknown fact, which is nonetheless known to exist or is postulated as living'. 'It is a living thing ... an expression for something that cannot be characterized in any other or better way. The symbol is alive only so long as it is pregnant with meaning' (*CW*, 6). This contrasts with the idea of the sign, which is seen as standing for something which is known about and can be described. In Jungian practice then, the symbol combines both personal and collective elements of the psyche, and the adoption of a symbolic attitude facilitates what is known and what is not known. Patient and analyst together arrive at meaning through the experience of integrating opposite aspects of the personality. Jung postulated that the psyche spontaneously produces symbols when the intellect cannot make sense of an inner or outer situation. A symbol may express conflict which helps unconscious experiences become known about. An image may be both a symbol and a sign: for example the cross for a religious Christian is a symbol of their spiritual life, while for a non-believer, the cross is a sign of Christianity. When a symbol is perceived and recognized it may lead to a feeling of integration and enrichment. This is particularly true of the symbols of the self or of wholeness, such as the child, or mandalas. Such 'peak experiences' have been described as 'joyous shock' and often accompany a discovery of otherness or difference. The developmental parallel to this type of experience is the oedipal resolution, and what Jungian writers term the emergence consciousness.

Individuation

While Jung emphasized individuation as 'a second half of life' process, Michael Fordham, a more recent Jungian writer, postulated that the process of individuation operates from birth. Individuation is seen as a process of realization of the self. It is often the case that once individuals have fulfilled their earlier developmental tasks such as self-education, and family responsibilities, they reach a time when they are thrown back on to themselves, and begin to contemplate the meaning of their life. Such people become more aware of their wider personality, and enter into a deeper relationship with the self. It was this process which Jung was primarily talking about when he coined the term individuation. Fordham widened the use of the term, emphasizing the more unconscious aspects of the development of the personality, which come about from the very beginning through interaction with environmental influences. Fordham's work brought Jungian theory more into line with other developmental theories, and this has had a particular influence on the London School of Analytical Psychology.

Reductive and synthetic processes

Jung regarded Freud's theory and practice as reductive in nature. He particularly wanted to emphasize a more synthetic or expanding approach to the psyche. Individuals will differ in their needs in this respect. Some may be at a stage in analysis or life situation when emphasis on personal material may be more productive, leading to a more reductive therapy which tends to help clarify and summarize experiences. This equates with a more concise narrative style. For others, particularly later in analysis or later in life, an emphasis on more impersonal material leading to an appreciation of symbolic experience and thought may be desirable. This may be helpful where there is a need for the individual to distance himself from personal experience, perhaps because it is too traumatic, or because there is no longer the opportunity to engage with it, as in later life.

While Jung emphasized the need in many people in later life to move towards a greater awareness of the self, particularly as experienced through the collective unconscious, Michael Fordham believed that a child should not be held from experiencing and recognizing very highly charged personal experiences, and primitive feelings, impulses and thoughts emanating from the collective unconscious. A considerable proportion of the London Jungian analysts would now be of the view that 'reductive analysis is in fact a synthetic process, defined as bringing together in a healing way disparate elements in the psyche, and that the distinction as it was first formulated owed more to Jung's need to separate from Freud than from experiences in the consulting room' (Astor, 1995). Other Jungian writers have also emphasized the undesirability of trying to divide the collective and personal unconscious when a clinical perspective is considered (Williams, 1963).

Amplification and active imagination

The process of amplification is the application of myths, fairy tales or other collective 'knowledge' to what the patient presents in the therapy, in order to elucidate or 'make ample' what might only be a rather unformed piece of experience, for example a dream image, a bodily sensation, or a single word. Amplification is linked to active imagination which Jung encouraged and instructed patients in, in order to facilitate the production of symbols. He asked his patients to write down dreams, record associations and to paint, model and draw in order to facilitate the process. This is very different from the more conscious use of fantasy.

There is debate within the Jungian school of psychotherapy about the value of amplification and active imagination, and M. Fordham (1978) believed that its use tended to isolate patients from their everyday life experiences and from the transference. Others believe that the value of amplification is its potential to put individuals in touch with the collective unconscious. Active imagination may be a valuable source of material which reveals cultural and personal history, and the patient's potential for individuation. Fordham (1978) writes that 'perhaps the most interesting feature of active imagination is that it gives a person a respect for the reality of the psyche and can lead on to creative achievement because of this. To gain through direct experience a conception of the psyche as a relatively autonomous and helpful apparatus, which can produce its own ideas, feelings, revelations, and can be related to living, seems to be therapeutic.'

Intuition

Intuition, one of Jung's psychological functions, was described by him as being 'dependent on unconscious processes of a very complex nature'. Because of this peculiarity, he defined intuition as 'perception by the unconscious' (Jung; *CW*, 9). Intuition is facilitated by the process of empathy. A capacity for empathy is widely recognized as an essential quality in any psychotherapist: 'it involves putting oneself in the place of, or inside, another person without losing sight of who one is' (Samuels, 1985). Empathy ensures the best possible attention and observation of the inner world and makes intuition possible.

The problem with intuitive acts and experiences is that they are not amenable to rational investigation. Kohut (in Samuels, 1985), though not a Jungian, puts the case for intuition, which is so central to Jungian psychotherapy. He writes, 'talent and experience combine to allow either the rapid and preconscious gathering of a great number of data and the ability to recognize that they form a meaningful configuration, or the one step recognition of a complex configuration that has been preconsciously assembled'.

This definition of the intuitive process has been further developed in the work of Louis Zinkin (1991). Zinkin, both a Jungian and a group analyst, drew attention to recent child observation work by Stern (1985) and linked it with classical Jungian ideas. Stern's observation of the mother's resonance with the child's needs has much in common with Jung's description of the intuitive function. The intuitive process is also central to the flexibility of analytical technique described in contemporary Jungian therapy by Zinkin (1974) and Fordham (1978).

The dialectical process

Jung saw analysis as a dialectical process involving both an interaction between two persons (patient and the therapist) and an interaction between the conscious and unconscious aspects of the patient's psyche. In Jungian psychology it is not the analyst who is seen as the container, but rather the relationship between the patient and the therapist. The therapist therefore does not analyse from a distance but is himself as much in the analysis as is the patient. Both the patient and the therapist unconsciously influence each other, the encounter between the two personalities being like the mixing of two chemical elements. He wrote that 'in a dialectical procedure ... the doctor must emerge from his anonymity and give an account of himself, just as he expects his patient to do'. Jung believed that the personal qualities of the therapist were of great importance, and that every therapist himself should undergo a thorough analysis. Jung went on to say that, 'The intelligent psychotherapist has known for years that any complicated treatment is an individual, dialectical, process' (*CW*, 16).

Jung believed that the dialectical relationship was based on processes that neither the patient nor the therapist could consciously control, but that it is the therapist's task to be conscious of the part that his unconscious processes may play in his interaction with his patient. Michael Fordham (1957) concluded that the therapist's countertransference is an indicator of the patient's transference, and enables the therapist's ego to analyse and use countertransference information as part of the therapeutic technique. He saw this process as the basis of the dialectical procedure. Zinkin (1974) viewed 'the dialectical procedure [as] essentially conceived as a dialogue in which two people of equal status address one another spontaneously ... [However] Jung's emphasis on the equal status of analyst and analysand (symbolized by their sitting facing each other) has somewhat obscured the fact that each participant has an essentially different role. The increasing use of the couch by analytical psychologists in Great Britain has perhaps reflected a realization that the analyst and patient can have quite different roles without the status or individuality of the participants being in question.'

Transference and countertransference

Jung did not write very much about transference, believing that 'most psychotherapeutic procedures do not involve transference analysis' (M. Fordham, 1957). From his use of word association tests, however, he 'realized that it was quite impossible to exclude the personal equation in any psychological work' (Baynes, 1950). Jung agreed with Freud that what happens between a patient and therapist was 'the alpha and omega of the analytic method' (*CW*, 16), but he saw this transference relationship differently from Freud. Jung paid more attention to the archetypal content of the transference than to the personal content.

Contemporary Jungian analysts differ in their approach to the use of the transference. While there has in the United Kingdom been a trend towards a more psychoanalytic model of the transference, with greater attention to the here and now personal experience with the therapist, the Zurich school and some groups within the United Kingdom remain adherent to the archetypal transference which focuses on the collective unconscious.

Countertransference has been greatly developed by post-Jungian writers. Michael Fordham (1957) makes the point that although the psyches of both the patient and the analyst are involved in a process which neither can control consciously, 'the analysis depends upon the relatively greater experience of the analyst [in this process in order that he] can meet the patient's [needs]'.

Aims of therapy

Jung disagreed with the approach of Freud and Adler in terms of what he called its 'technical rules'. He wrote, 'We must not mind doing tedious but conscientious work on obscure individuals, even though the goal for which we strive seems unattainable. But one goal we can attain, and that is to develop and bring to maturity individual personalities . . . I therefore consider it the prime task of psychotherapy today to pursue with single-mindedness and purpose the goal of individual development, only in the individual can life fulfil this meaning' (*CW*, 16). Jung went on to describe psychotherapy as 'An encounter, a discussion between two psychic goals, in which knowledge is used only as a tool. The goal is transformation . . . no efforts on the part of the doctor can compel this experience.' As Samuels (1985) writes, 'We may conclude that the goal of analysis is mutual transformation. What happens in the treatment may change the analyst, illumine his life, face him with problems and opportunities of which he was cogniscent.' Jung had asserted that unless the analyst felt a personal impact arising out of the analysis, nothing would come of it. The analyst must be affected by what is happening: 'analysis presupposes not only a specific psychological gift but in the very first place a serious concern with the moulding of one's own character' (*CW*, 4).

Gordon (1979) makes a distinction between curing and healing, both of which take place in analysis. 'The former is concerned with ego development and the integration of drives and archetypes. Healing on the other hand is a "process in the service of the whole personality towards ever greater and more complex wholeness".' Samuels (1985) makes the point that analytical psychology has 'tended to work on a growth model rather than a cure model'. There are parallels and aims with the psychoanalytic schools. Gitelsohn (in Samuels, 1985) says the following: 'One of the as yet unsolved problems of psychoanalysis is concerned with the essential nature of the psychoanalytic cure. It is not insight; it is not the recall of infantile memories; it is not catharsis or abreaction; it is not in relation to the analyst. Still, it is all of these in some synthesis which has not yet been possible to formulate explicitly. Somehow, in a successful analysis the patient matures as a total personality.'

Often the patient does not present with these deep-seated aims for therapy. Although Jungian psychotherapy offers the opportunity for a full exploration of the personality, and the adaptation of the individual to their life, general principles of psychodynamic psychotherapy can be used by the Jungian therapist in a more eclectic approach. In such cases it would be the therapist's aim to help the patient identify problem areas in their life and experience transference relationships linked to an understanding of past and present relationships. In this way a broad spectrum of psychiatric problems can be tackled.

Although a patient may present with discrete symptoms, for example depression or relationship difficulties, it is often possible to identify, with such people, a longstanding problem with their sense of ease with themselves and with others. The aim of Jungian therapy, as with all analytic therapies, is to link the more superficial problems with which many patients present with underlying personality characteristics and life experience. Many patients have never had the opportunity, perhaps particularly during their childhood, to feel that they have been understood by significant others or to have their needs met. The establishment of a relationship which allows for these experiences is a broad aim of Jungian psychotherapy. More specifically, a Jungian approach would concentrate on the analysis of the opposites within a person's personality, with the aim of bringing about a fuller awareness of personal characteristics, which can facilitate greater fulfilment in current and future relationships both in work and social spheres.

How does Jungian psychotherapy differ from other therapies?

While it has been said that the process of Jungian analysis depends upon the impact of the patient on the therapist and vice versa, the analytic stance of the therapist helps to guide and contain the process. This is true of all analytic therapies but Jungian psychotherapy differs in the following important ways.

- The therapist and the patient focus on the patient's self. This is equated with a need for coming together or individuation.
- There is a recognition of ego development which helps the individual to separate, to develop a personal identity and an awareness of external achievement.
- The conflict between separation and merging is seen as essential and there is an emphasis on integrating or reconciling these opposites.
- The patient is encouraged to acknowledge both a wish to move on in life, and a desire to go back to their origins. This yearning in therapy can result in regression. A temporary regression is therefore seen as positive, and is similar to Balint's (1968) notion of benign regression.
- From a Jungian perspective, the more psychologically mature a person is, the greater is their capacity for holding together conflicting states or attitudes, and thereby discriminating self from others.
- In more disturbed individuals with early life problems, the therapist may find himself being a carrier for the self of the patient. Through countertransference experience the therapist facilitates the patient forging a link between his ego and his self. The therapist does this by keeping in touch with the patient as a whole person, something which the patient is unable to do for himself.
- The holding or containing function of Jungian psychotherapy is similar to that postulated by Winnicott and Bion. While Bion emphasized the containing role or reverie of the therapist, Jungian psychotherapy places greater weight on the united role of the unconscious of both the patient and the therapist.

- The process of integration of the opposites in the personality involves an individual looking at their shadow side and becoming aware of the collective unconscious through archetypal experiences.
- There is an emphasis on the recognition of images and the use of active imagination and amplification.

Principles of practice

'Psychotherapy is the treatment of the mind, or rather the psyche, by psychological methods' (F. Fordham, 1953). Jung described four stages in psychotherapy which he habitually used.
- *Catharsis*: While there are benefits to cathartic confession, Jung was aware that this process does not work in those people in whom there is a resistance to uncovering unconscious feelings, or where a patient is either over-enmeshed, or out of touch with their therapist. In the latter case, there may be repeated cathartic activity, without relation to the therapist as a person.
- *Elucidation*: Elucidation is thought to coincide with the introduction of the interpretative method by Freud. Elucidation involves interpretation in order that childlike aspects in the adult can be linked both to a retrogressive longing for paradise and also to a creative forward movement in the adult where positive playful qualities may be valued.
- *Education*: Jungian therapy may sometimes incorporate education, in order to help the patients adapt to everyday reality. This aspect of technique derives from the work of Adler. Although it stands in contrast to the usual analytic method, education can be very useful in those patients with a poor capacity for symbolism, either in neurosis or borderline personality functioning.
- *Transformation*: Transformation is a process specifically described by Jung, which requires the analyst to be involved in a dialectical process, and to use what we would now describe as countertransference experiences. Jung wrote, 'You can exert no influence if you are not susceptible to influence. It is futile for the doctor to shield himself from the influence of the patient and to surround himself with a smoke-screen of fatherly and professional authority. By so doing he only denies himself the use of a highly important organ of information ... One of the best known symptoms of this kind is the countertransference evoked by the transference ... Between doctor and patient, therefore, there are imponderable factors which bring about a mutual trans-formation' (*CW*, 16).

Lambert (1974) felt that the analytic endeavour involves a capacity for agape (pronounced 'agapay') in the therapist. Agape, often translated from the Greek as love or charity, also expresses the idea of esteem. Agape may be seen as one aspect of a therapist's analytic stance alongside patience, control of anger and subtlety. A number of writers have discussed the need for the therapist to endure a patient's tendencies to depression, diminishment and self-destruction, and to avoid the temptation to promote premature positiveness and growth. Lambert mentions his own struggle with the instinctual need to retaliate, and Jung was clear that an analyst must be able to risk changing his own personality for the sake of his patient. Jungian psychotherapy promotes the idea of a facilitating analytic stance which allows an individual to explore his difficulties in a non-persecutory environment. In practice both the therapist and the patient are engaged in a process which seeks out meaning, and expands the patient's psyche, through relatedness with the therapist.

Post-Jungian writers have emphasized the necessity for 'not knowing beforehand' (Michael Fordham in Astor, 1995). Fordham recommended the idea of retaining previously gathered data about a patient in some imagined mental filing cabinet. Astor comments that 'while there is nothing wrong with using filing cabinet material in sessions it is preferable that its use is determined by the relation to the patient on that day'.

Zinkin (1974) describes three phases in every analysis:

- Patient and therapist establish a working relationship which is mutually satisfactory.
- The patient experiences an increased sense of separateness with more capacity for an 'as if' situation. This is accompanied by an increasing development of symbolic thinking.
- The patient begins to be able to lend parts of himself to the therapist, in a way which feels that they are not lost, but can be retrieved when necessary.

From a Jungian perspective, the practice of psychotherapy may be best viewed as a circular or spiral, rather than a linear process. Jung (*CW*, 14) described the process of psychotherapy in the following manner: 'The way to the goal seems chaotic and interminable at first, and only gradually do the signs increase that it is leading anywhere. The way is not straight but appears to go round in circles ... We can hardly help feeling that the unconscious process moves spiral-wise round a centre, gradually getting closer while the characteristics of the centre grow more and more distinct.' Zinkin emphasizes that spiral processes require controls, and that the control is the responsibility of the therapist. The therapist must keep the balance between distance and closeness, between separation and entanglement, between emotional response and detached interpretation.

Which patient and why?

The indications for Jungian psychotherapy are very broad. Jungian therapists working within the National Health Service (NHS) may need to modify their Jungian practice in order to provide a broad psychodynamic approach to patient assessment and treatment. Patients suitable for this type of treatment will therefore be similar to those identified as being suitable for other psychoanalytic psychotherapy treatments. A Jungian analysis of four or five sessions each week for a period of several years will be the treatment of choice for those individuals with severe characterological problems such as obsessive compulsive neurosis, borderline personality disorder and long-standing depressive disorder. Many of these patients will have experienced very early failure in attachment to primary caregivers, and a significant number will have experienced infantile trauma such as sexual abuse. In practice this treatment is rarely available in the NHS, although an analytic therapy of twice-weekly frequency for two or three years may be an option for a limited few.

The majority of psychiatric illnesses may be treated with Jungian psychotherapy that has been modified to suit individual patient needs. The therapist retains his Jungian perspective and applies the analytic understanding to less intense (once- or twice-weekly) and shorter (three months to two years) therapies. Contraindications to Jungian psychotherapy would be a lack of psychological-mindedness, and extreme concreteness in thinking, which may be related to intellectual capacity or an aspect of neurotic or psychotic defences. This may also be very predominant in psychosomatic illness. Individuals with acute psychotic illness would be unsuitable for analytic therapy except in a very specialized setting. The active use of alcohol and drugs usually makes an individual unsuitable for this kind of treatment although it is sometimes possible for such people to start therapy with a view to phasing out their substance abuse.

Some patients may present with a personal style which would seem to be best suited to a cognitive behavioural approach. In some of these cases it may be important initially to focus on symptom relief and harness existing cognitive skills. This might be appropriate in severe obsessional disorder or in those with obsessional personality traits who tend to use intellectualization and rationalization to defend themselves against their feelings. It is often the case however, that such patients can benefit from a more exploratory therapy in order to help them gain greater access to their emotional life.

It is important that patients presenting for psychotherapy are actively involved in the search for treatment and have a willingness to work with the therapist. A capacity to engage in the therapeutic process and to form a therapeutic alliance may be gauged from an assessment interview. A patient's response to interpretations during this process is an important indicator of suitability for therapy, although the therapist needs to be sensitive to the possibility that patients often need a period of induction into the method before they can begin to work more therapeutically. The therapist would be looking for signs that the patient has a curiosity about their state of mind, and/or feels compelled to pursue the treatment in order to explore their difficulties because they feel they have no other choice. Jung described one-third of his patients as having 'senselessness and aimlessness of their lives ... In the majority of my cases the resources of the conscious mind are exhausted (or, in ordinary English, they are "stuck"). It is chiefly this fact that forces me to look for hidden possibilities. For I do not know what to say to the patient when he asks me "What do you advise? What shall I do?" I don't know either. I only know one thing: when my conscious mind no longer sees any possible road ahead and consequently gets stuck, my unconscious psyche will react to the unbearable standstill' (*CW*, 16).

Which therapist and why?

There are a number of organizations in the United Kingdom and in other countries which train candidates in Jungian psychotherapy or analytical psychology. There are differences in breadth and depth between the trainings.

Most involve between three and four years of seminars and the taking on of a number of training patients under supervision. A personal analysis is also an ongoing requirement, and most people will undergo between three and five sessions per week for a number of years. Individuals wishing to train come from varied professional backgrounds. While it is not necessary to have a medical qualification, it is a requirement of the training that individuals gain some experience in clinical mental health work.

The selection procedure for training is a rigorous one. There is an attempt to select people who have the capacity to analyse patient material and situations, and to illuminate this with their own experience. A capacity to use countertransference experience, and to refine intuitive capacities, are important characteristics of would-be therapists. Some candidates also find that an interest in mythology and the wider creative arts may give them an insight into analytical psychology.

The therapeutic alliance is a strong determining factor in the success of a therapy and the selection of a therapist for any particular patient is important, depending both on the professional training of the therapist and their own personal characteristics. The theory of Jungian practice provides a broad framework for psychotherapy, although much depends on the way in which the patient and the therapist are able to interact with each other.

Samuels discusses the archetype of the wounded healer, which is seen in post-Jungian theory to represent a split in both the patient and the therapist. He writes: 'If it is the case that all analysts have an inner wound, then to present one-self as "healthy" is to cut off part of one's inner world. Likewise if the patient is only seen as "ill" then he is also cut off from his own inner healer or capacity to heal himself. It is likely therefore that psychological factors play a part in the choice of a career in psychotherapy and in the degree to which any one therapist is able to help a particular patient' (1985).

Therapeutic setting

The therapeutic setting in Jungian psychotherapy is similar to that used in other psychoanalytic psychotherapies. Although Jung's patients did not use a couch, it is increasingly being used particularly within the London School. In contrast to a more formal Freudian approach, the analytical psychologist may sit alongside the patient rather than behind. With the analyst in sight or partially so, the patient may choose whether to engage in eye contact and more direct relating, or to use the proximity of the therapist as an aid to exploring a more inner free associative experience. However, there is much variation amongst Jungian therapists in this aspect of technique and setting.

As with other psychoanalytic therapies, the therapist does not usually give much direct information about herself. This allows greater opportunity for the patient 'to use' the therapist in a way which serves the patient and a transference can be generated which is impinged upon as little as possible by the therapist's own life. Since many therapists work in their own homes, they will of necessity reveal a certain amount of information about themselves and this is often greedily looked for or angrily rejected by patients. Any response can be analysed in terms of what it means to the patient.

Within the NHS, the patient often knows rather less about the therapist and the institution itself plays a part in the therapeutic setting. This is particularly important for borderline patients. Principles of theory and practice in Jungian psychotherapy can be integrated very satisfactorily into the health service setting. More difficult patients may benefit from both the concrete containment of the institution and the inner psychic containment which is created in the therapy itself. Jungian therapists are trained to facilitate patients and therefore can become very flexible in their approach. The therapeutic boundaries may be held within that relationship through a commitment to a therapeutic alliance both by the patient and the therapist. It is, however, the therapist who must be responsible for this. In this way disruptions in the actual physical nature of the setting can be managed.

An appreciation of how Jungian psychotherapy parallels other ways of working aids the process of integration and particularly helps communication between different professionals. As with all psychoanalytic psychotherapies, there is great value within the body of theory in its application to institutional settings, and therefore in facilitating the work of mental health professionals.

Clinical example

James is a twenty-five-year-old architect who referred himself for analytic psychotherapy because of his difficulty in making and keeping relationships, and his subsequent depression which on one occasion led to an overdose. James had previously had counselling but did not find that this helped him, and had a sense of needing a more intense form of help. He underwent two years of Jungian analysis with sessions four times weekly.

At his assessment interview, James was able to make use of the silences which the therapist left for him. While he did not describe persecutory feelings, the assessment did elicit his feelings of aggression, particularly towards women. When the female therapist interpreted this to him, he was both surprised and angry. James did not wish to acknowledge this aspect of himself, which we might term his shadow. James described a family situation which was enmeshed and which offered him a little scope for escape. James was still living at home and felt unable to confront his father in an adult way for fear of upsetting his mother. James enjoyed a 'special' relationship with his mother and felt unable to relate to his father, consequently experiencing disappointment and anger because this left him without a suitable role model.

At the time of starting his analysis, James was aware of his need to move on in his life. This presented him with difficulties, and he was aware that there was a mismatch between his intellectual development and his emotional development. James was aware of his need for personal development in terms of his professional career, however this took him away from his family of origin and isolated him still further from his father. During his analysis, James demonstrated a number of archetypal patterns which contributed to his feeling of 'stuckness'. James's lack of identification with his father was accompanied by an identification with his mother's animus. In other words, James equated his maleness with the masculine element in his mother, and not with his father's masculinity. This left James with no sense of an integrated feminine and masculine identity, and his despising of his father could be seen to be a result of projections of his own aggression which he was unable to integrate. James's sense of the feminine, or his anima, was also threatening for him since it had not been mediated by his real relationship with his father. As a consequence, James had an idealized view both of himself and the world, with unmediated archetypal patterns of relating to others holding sway in his internal world.

James appears to have adapted to this situation by identifying with the hero archetype. This resulted in him despising both the real male adult, with all its failings, and also the child, who was equated with an impotent feminine role. James often saw himself as a helpless child, unable to challenge his parents in an adult way, and thereby to liberate himself. As the hero, James's primary activity was of rescuing others which opposed the part of him which needed to be rescued. There was a denial of the inner aggression or dragon figure within himself, which was projected onto others.

James rarely attended for more than three sessions weekly, and was able after a year of analysis to admit that he found the intensity too frightening. James's fear was connected with getting in touch with his own aggressive impulses, which he found to be intolerable. His aggression was instead acted out in the transference; by his non-attendance, by an affair he had during his analysis and by his difficulty in paying for his sessions. The therapist experienced herself as 'useless' in many of the sessions, and this was later confirmed to be how James felt in his relationships with others. The therapist used her countertransference experience to understand something which James found difficult to put into words. From this, the therapist was able to gain an understanding of James's past, in particular how he had not been able to fully work through his preverbal experiences with others, and how he subsequently had difficulty with oedipal, or three-person relationships.

James's mother had been seen by the family as fragile due to a diagnosis of diabetes, and in the transference James demonstrated his enmeshment with her. His mother, while appearing to offer intimacy, also seems to have undermined his capacity for mastery and control. James reacted to this with a great deal of passive aggression. This aggression was made overt during the analysis and awakened his sense of longing for early infantile experiences, leading him back to a feeling of being in a familiar place which was at the same time new to him. This circular or spiralling process of discovery and rediscovery was both frustrating and rewarding for James. He began to learn that his idealized fantasy of a direct move from his family of origin to a family of his own could not be achieved without change in himself.

Problems in therapy

Problems in therapy may arise when a therapist has not achieved a sufficient degree of flexibility in order to adapt technique to a particular patient or therapeutic setting. It is likely that a Jungian therapist in the NHS would need to have a good working knowledge of a variety of different types of psychotherapy in order to communicate with other professionals and to understand their approach to mental health problems. The essence of Jungian therapy is the flexibility of technique which involves sensitive tailoring from patient to patient, and from moment to moment of depth, confrontation and empathy. It is for this reason that the analytic technique cannot be manualized in the way that other therapies have been. Problems with either particularly difficult patients or inadequately trained therapists are likely to be ameliorated by regular and high quality supervision of the work.

The problems which are attached to other psychoanalytic therapies are also potential sources of trouble in Jungian therapy. These include:

- Acting out behaviour
- Idealization of the therapist
- Erotic transference and countertransference which is missed or avoided
- Negative transference which is not interpreted
- Delusional transference in dangerous patients
- Regression which threatens the therapeutic alliance and is uncontained by the therapy

Evaluation of therapy

Jungian psychotherapy, as with other psychoanalytic therapies, has not been well researched but has relied on individual clinical experience and observation. The use of meta-analysis has been helpful in bringing together a variety of studies, however the studies tend to be brief, non-analytic and do not address typical NHS medium-term analytically oriented therapies. More specifically, in terms of Jungian psychotherapy there have been a number of studies carried out in Manchester (Guthrie, 1991; Guthrie *et al.*, 1993) which have employed a randomized control trial design, and have demonstrated significant improvements using a brief Conversational Model of therapy which is based heavily on Jungian psychotherapy. Barkham and Hobson (1990) researched the use of the Conversational Model in a very brief intervention (two plus one sessions). Hobson, a Jungian analyst and NHS Consultant, was also a founder member of the Society for Psychotherapy Research in the United Kingdom. Other Jungian-trained clinicians are attached to psychotherapy institutions which have looked at psychotherapy from a research or cost-effective perspective and have demonstrated its efficacy (Menzies *et al.*, 1993).

A number of researchers have devised instruments which look at typology or personality type from a Jungian perspective (Myers, 1962; Wheelright, 1964). These studies are in marked contrast to the outcome studies which are currently in vogue but represent an attempt to look more objectively at personality functioning in addition to the way in which this is approached by Jungian therapy. This methodology is particularly relevant to the question of therapist-patient matching which is so crucial in psychotherapy. The University of Essex has recently set up a department funded by the Society of Analytical Psychology and led by experienced Jungian analysts which will train and encourage research into analytical psychology.

Samuels (1985) suggests that those with an interest in research, and 'a desire to update that knowledge [should] go ... where the disagreements are'. Quoting Popper he says, 'We do not know how or where to start an analysis of this world. There is no wisdom to tell us. Even a scientific tradition doesn't tell us. It only tells us where other people started and where they got to.' Samuels therefore makes the point that there is a strong case to be made for basing a quest for knowledge not on consensus, but on conflict. He goes on to say that 'Starting at the beginning is no guarantee of comprehension'. This is a frequent experience of those beginning research into psychotherapy, and many concepts are only understood with time and experience. As William James put it in 1911, 'Ideas become true just so far as they help us get into satisfactory relations with other parts of our experience' (Samuels, 1985). A Jungian viewpoint on evaluation therefore, would be to emphasize the complexity of the patient–therapist relationship, and of the analytic endeavour. While much research, especially the randomized control trial model, relies heavily on a rational approach to the subject matter, many writers, including Storr (1979) have emphasized the art of psychotherapy.

In addition to researching Jungian therapy through the Conversational Model, Hobson applied a critical approach to many Jungian concepts. He suggested that the feeling of numinosity, widely connected with an archetypal image, refers more to the experience of the individual and less to something in the image. This implies that 'The sense of awe becomes a subjective matter for a person and it follows that some will have a propensity for this type of experience' (Samuels, 1985).

As with all psychoanalytic casework, much individual therapy has been described in the literature. Such naturalistic studies have been acknowledged as contributing to a knowledge base (NHS Executive, 1996). However, the handling of the data has not yet become sufficiently operationalized to aid current attempts to evaluate Jungian analysis in a statistical way.

Alternatives to therapy

A decision as to the suitability and/or advantages of psychoanalytic therapy will usually be determined during an assessment. The general criteria which indicate the choice of individual Jungian therapy rather than group analysis or brief therapies are similar to those for other psychoanalytic therapies. Occasionally some patients have a trial of therapy and either decide to end therapy themselves, or come to a decision with their therapist that this particular form of treatment is not helping them. There is very little written on the advantages of one psychoanalytic therapy over another.

Ambivalence on the part of the patient should alert the assessor or therapist to the possibility that this particular patient would benefit from an alternative approach. Psychiatric review should always be borne in mind as a possible requirement in those individuals with severe pathology. It is sometimes the case that patients will opt for a more supportive and symptom-relief oriented treatment. Pharmacological treatment may be used in combination with Jungian psychotherapy, although patients may decide to tail off medication during therapy. In patients with serious mental illness, such as bipolar illness or schizophrenia, this decision would need to be taken in conjunction with both the psychiatrist and psychotherapist. It is also occasionally helpful for people to engage in an individual therapy at the same time as taking part in other forms of therapy such as family therapy.

Samuels (1985) writes of the limits of analytical psychology. He puts the question, 'How fluid can practice be with regard to a particular patient before it becomes professionally responsible to refer them to another analyst or even to another kind of practitioner?' Both Glover and Adler attacked eclecticism, Adler feeling 'that one must accept that we have to make a choice'. He was against internal Jungian diversity and accepted the idea that Jungian psychology might 'lose on the side of understanding physical phenomena, object relations and some actual therapeutic insight'. By contrast, Storr (1979) expressed the idea that eventually psychological schools would become integrated since similarities outweigh differences. Samuels (1985) agrees with this viewpoint if one is talking about a process of cross-fertilization. He nevertheless makes the point that it is 'necessary for the analyst or therapist to work with conviction, even passion. If this is lacking then something may be lost.'

Further reading

Fordham, F. (1953) *An Introduction to Jung's Psychology*. London: Penguin Books.
Samuels, A. (1985) *Jung and the Post-Jungians*. London and New York: Routledge and Kegan Paul.
Storr, A. (1983) *Jung: Selected Writings*. London: Fontana.

Bibliography

Jung's work is conventionally referred to according to the *Collected Works (CW) of C.G. Jung*, volumes 1–19. London: Routledge and Keagan Paul.

Astor, J. (1995) *Michael Fordham. Innovations in Analytical Psychology*. London and New York: Routledge.
Balint, M. (1968) *The Basic Fault. Therapeutic Aspects of Regression*. London: Tavistock.
Barkham, M. and Hobson, R.F. (1990) Exploratory therapy in two-plus-one sessions. II – A single case study. *British Journal of Psychotherapy*, **6**, 89–100.
Baynes, H.G. (1950) Freud versus Jung. In: *Analytical Psychology and the English Mind*. London: Methuen.
Fordham, F. (1953) *An Introduction to Jung's Psychology*. London: Penguin Books.
Fordham, M. (1957) *New Developments in Analytical Psychology*. London: Routledge and Kegan Paul.
Fordham, M. (1978) *Jungian Psychotherapy: a Study in Analytical Psychology*. Chichester: John Wiley.
Freud, S. (1916/1917) *Introductory Lectures on Psychoanalysis*. Reprinted 1973. London: Penguin.
Gordon, R. (1979) Reflections on curing and healing. *Journal of Analytical Psychology*, **24**, 207–219.
Guthrie, E. (1991) Brief psychotherapy with patients with refractory Irritable Bowel Syndrome. *British Journal of Psychotherapy*, **8**, 175–188.
Guthrie, E., Creed, F., Dawson, D. and Tomenson, B. (1993) A randomised controlled trial of psychotherapy in patients with refractory Irritable Bowel Syndrome. *British Journal of Psychiatry*, **163**, 315–321.
Jung, C.G. (1957–79). *Collected Works*. London: Routledge and Kegan Paul.
Jung, C.G. (1963) *Memories, Dreams and Reflections*. London: Collins and Routledge.

Lambert, K. (1974) The personality of the analyst in interpretation and therapy. In: M. Fordham, R. Gordon, J. Hubbock *et al.* (eds), *Technique in Jungian Analysis*. London: Heinemann.

Menzies, D., Dolan, B.M. and Norton, K.R.W. (1993) Are short-term savings worth long-term costs? Funding treatment for personality disorders. *Psychiatric Bulletin*, **17**, 517–519.

Myers, I. (1962) *The Myers–Briggs Type Indicator*. Palo Alto, CA: Consulting Psychologists Press.

NHS Executive (1996) *NHS Psychotherapy Services in England: a Review of Strategic Policy*. Wetherby: Department of Health.

Samuels, A. (1985) *Jung and the Post-Jungians*. London and New York: Routledge and Kegan Paul.

Stern, D.N. (1985) *The Interpersonal World of the Infant*. New York: Basic Books.

Storr, A. (1979) *The Art of Psychotherapy*. London: Heinemann.

Storr, A. (1983) *Jung: Selected Writings*. London: Fontana.

Wheelright, J. (1964) *Jungian Type Survey: the Grey–Wheelright Test Manual*. San Francisco: Society of Jungian Analysts of North California.

Whitmont, E. (1964) Group therapy and analytical psychology. *Journal of Analytical Psychology*, **9**, 1–22.

Williams, M. (1963) The indivisibility of the personal and collective unconscious. In: M. Fordham *et al.* (eds), *Analytical Psychology: a Modern Science*. Reprinted 1973. London: Heinemann.

Zinkin, L. (1974) *Flexibility in Analytic Technique*. In: M. Fordham *et al.* (eds), *Technique in Jungian Analysis*. London: Heinemann.

Zinkin, L. (1991) The Klein connection in the London School: the search for origins. *Journal of Analytical Psychology*, **36**, 37–61.

3
Kleinian Psychoanalysis

Matthew Patrick

Introduction

Many psychoanalysts, psychotherapists and psychiatrists working in Britain and across the world today have been influenced by the work of Melanie Klein. The impact of Klein's thinking has not been limited to the work of a particular group of psychoanalysts working with a single 'house style'. Rather, clinicians from different backgrounds, often nominally attached to different psychoanalytic 'groups', have integrated into their work and thinking various aspects of her technique and theory. Her work has, indeed, been one of the major influences on the development of psychoanalysis in Britain this century. This chapter provides a brief historical perspective on Mrs Klein and her work, and on the work of those who have developed her theoretical and clinical contributions. The chapter also describes some of Klein's and other 'Kleinian' analysts' major contributions to psychoanalytic theory, describing how these are linked with a particular approach to clinical work.

Historical perspective

Melanie Klein (née Reizes) was born in Vienna in 1882, the daughter of a doctor. As a young child she also had a desire to study medicine, but became engaged at the age of seventeen and, in 1903, married Arthur Klein. By all accounts the marriage was not a happy one, and the couple were later divorced. They had three children.

In 1910, Klein and her family moved to Budapest. She did not develop an interest in psychoanalysis until 1914–15, by which time she was in her thirties, when she encountered the writings of Freud. Klein subsequently began an analysis with Sandor Ferenczi and became a member of the Hungarian Psychoanalytic Society. She was a pioneer of child analysis and, early on in her career, developed her distinctive method known as the 'Play Technique' (Klein, 1955). Underlying the 'Play Technique' was Klein's belief that the analysis of young children could be conducted in much the same way as that of adults, except that play with toys was used to supplement verbal free association. In 1921, Klein moved to Berlin at the invitation of Karl Abraham. She eventually persuaded Abraham to take her into analysis but he died just eighteen months after the analysis had begun. In 1926 Klein moved again, this time to England at the invitation of Ernest Jones, a leading figure in the British Psycho-Analytical Society. She remained living and working in London until her death in 1960.

Whereas Klein's work had not received wide support while in Berlin, in London it was more popular. She quickly established herself in the British Psycho-Analytical Society and continued to develop her ideas, drawing on her work with children but increasingly relating this to work with adults. Many of these ideas were challenging and led to disagreements within the Society. This escalated with the arrival, in 1938, of a group of Viennese analysts, including Freud and his daughter, Anna. During a period that came to be known as the Controversial Discussions (1943–44), points of theoretical and clinical difference were argued over and, as a result, three distinct groups were created within the British Psycho-Analytical Society: the Kleinian Group, the Contemporary Freudian Group and the Independent or Middle Group. Unlike psychoanalytical institutions in other countries, however, the British Society did not split in several smaller organizations and still retains a single integrated training structure.

Amongst Klein's early supporters were Susan Isaacs, Paula Heimann and Joan Riviere. These analysts were of particular importance in helping to clarify a number of Klein's ideas at the time of the Controversial Discussions. These included her formulation of the nature of internal objects and the internal world, and the nature and function of unconscious phantasy, a realm in which psychological and physical experience are represented in the mind in terms of human relationships. Later Wilfred Bion, Herbert Rosenfeld and Hanna Segal became key members of the Klein Group, all contributing to the growing body of Kleinian theory. Rosenfeld's work focused particularly on the understanding of psychotic states and the role of narcissism in these disorders (Rosenfeld, 1965). Hanna Segal developed Klein's work in relation to symbol formation, and later in relation to the areas of aesthetics and creativity (Segal, 1986). The work of Bion has been of especial importance in the development of Kleinian theory and practice. He contributed to the psychoanalytic understanding of group processes and psychotic states, and set out a developmental model of the human capacity to think. In addition his work exploring aspects of early human relationships, including his model of 'containment', has had a tremendous influence on subsequent practitioners (see Anderson and Segal, 1992). In more recent years, the work of Betty Joseph has had a particular impact on clinical technique, and on the understanding and use of transference and countertransference in the analytic situation (for example, *Psychic Equilibrium and Psychic Change*, 1989). Other analysts, such as Britton and Feldman, have contributed to the development of psychoanalytic understanding of the Oedipus complex and its role in early development (Britton *et al.*, 1989), while analysts such as Steiner have contributed to our understanding of the complex ways in which defensive systems may be organized into more or less stable 'psychic retreats' (Steiner, 1993).

Principles of theory and practice

Principles of theory

Melanie Klein's work was particularly concerned with describing the earliest infantile conflicts and anxieties, encountered in both children and adults, and with trying to understand the primitive mental processes associated with such anxieties. While her contributions to psychoanalysis cover a wide range, amongst the most important of these are:

- Internal objects and the concept of an internal world
- The primitive mental processes of splitting and projective identification
- The paranoid–schizoid and depressive positions

Bion's development of the concept of containment has also had a great impact on clinical practice

Internal objects and the internal world

When Freud first began writing about psychoanalysis in the 1890s, his intention was to formulate a new and scientific account of the workings of the human mind. Thus he made use of concepts and language from the physical sciences that lent an air of rigour and objectivity to his works. The psychological theory that emerged was couched in terms of energy, its conservation, displacement and discharge. The style of such theorizing, however, contrasts markedly with Freud's clinical case descriptions which are much more human, detailing with great understanding his patient's anxieties, conflicts and wishes. Even in his early theoretical writings Freud was pointing toward a more interpersonal (or 'object relations') model of psychological functioning. In his 1917 paper 'Mourning and Melancholia', Freud suggested that psychotic depression arose when individuals found themselves faced with the loss of a person whom they both loved and hated, a loss which was managed by 'internalizing' the relationship. He argued that a part of the patient identified with the lost person who had now been internalized, and that the patient then directed his hatred towards this part of himself in the relentless disparaging attacks so characteristic of this form of depression. In Freud's terms, the shadow of the object had fallen upon the ego. With the lost figure now installed in the patient's mind, the loss in external reality can be avoided but only at the cost of terrible depression. Freud came to suggest that it was through such processes of identification that young children could come to establish the functions of external figures within their minds.

Klein's work on the nature of internal objects and internal object relations, the representations in the mind of people and of relationships between people, was initially based largely on her work with children. She questioned whether the establishment of internal objects was dependent upon, or necessarily brought about by, the loss of an ambivalently loved object as Freud had suggested. Rather, Klein argued, each infant is capable of relating to figures that are identified as separate from the self at birth, and that introjective processes (those psychological processes involved in taking in to the mind from outside) were active and created internal objects from birth (Hinshelwood, 1991). This position has now found considerable support in the work of infancy researchers such as Daniel Stern (1985). Object relationships are sometimes described in terms of 'part-objects' as opposed to 'objects'. The term part-object is used to describe an object or figure in the mind that is less integrated than a 'whole person'. An example of this might be when a patient (or indeed anyone) feels caught up with a particular aspect of their relationship with another person such that they lose sight of the broader picture, of the complexities of the relationship and of the person with whom they are involved. The patient may, at this point in time, be relating to only one aspect of a person, for example their cruelty. In the patient's mind, this 'part' has come to represent the whole person.

In her work, Klein went on to develop Freud's notion of internal objects into the notion of an internal world. This notion describes the way in which each individual lives within their own version of the world. Their perception of external reality and of interpersonal events might be coloured or even shaped by representations or models that they carry in their own minds. Klein's model of the internal world was fundamentally an interpersonal one, comprising representations of people and of relationships between people, including the self, built up through infancy and childhood. She argued that these internal figures were experienced by the infant, and later in the adult unconscious, as having a degree of autonomy and separateness from the self, although they always existed in relation to a particular representation of the self in the way that one's relationship to a person with a particular defining characteristic, say as your parent, defines your position in relation to that figure as their child.

Klein argued that the earliest internal objects were based largely on the infant's experience of his own bodily sensations and impulses. She argued that the infant, with his primitive capacity to recognize the existence of a relationship between the self and figures distinct from the self, tends to represent his physical experiences in terms of such relationships in his mind. In this way, pain and frustration are felt by him as if they were hostile attacks from a malevolent or 'bad' object in his mind. The infant feels assaulted, not aware of the absence of a good object but rather aware of the presence of a bad object. Pleasant experiences, such as a full stomach, on the other hand, might be experienced by him as deriving from a relationship with a 'good' feeding object, an experience of a relationship with a warm, nourishing and loving object.

In her formulation of the internal world and internal objects, Klein was one of the founders of what is now known as object relations theory, along with Fairbairn, Guntrip and Winnicott.

Primitive mental processes

In her writing, Klein describes a number of what she termed 'primitive mental processes'. Amongst these, the mechanisms of splitting and projective identification are of particular importance (Klein, 1946). One reason for this is that these mechanisms not only function as defences against early anxieties, but are also necessary for the establishment and maintenance of various forms of psychic equilibrium. They may, to a greater or lesser extent, determine the way in which an individual experiences the external world.

Klein argued that the infant struggles to manage intense and conflicting emotions of pleasure and discomfort, love and hate, at times fearing that bad will overwhelm good in his mind. A central task for the infant is then to protect himself and to ensure his survival, and the survival of the objects he loves in his mind.

Splitting refers to the way in which either an object or the self may be divided and then reconstituted within the internal world. In this context the word 'object' might be understood as a representation of 'others' in an individual's mind, while the word 'self' relates to a representation of 'I-ness', or 'that which I am'. When there is splitting of the object, separate representations are constructed in the mind, each carrying particular characteristics from the original representation. In its simplest form, objects may be divided into good or bad. Similarly the self may be divided, for example aggression and hostility may be separated off from more loving tendencies. Klein emphasized that no splitting of an object takes place within the internal world without a corresponding split in the self. When object representations are seen as intrinsically linked to aspects of the self, the nature of the self is in part defined by the nature of the object to which the self is relating.

Splitting in its simpler forms may be used as a defence, by the splitting off of aspects of the self perceived as bad. Under the pressure of primitive anxieties, Klein also described a more profound form of splitting in which the object and self may be fragmented. While such an activity is designed to rid the individual of intolerable experiences, it more usually results in an exacerbation of anxiety and fear as the self then feels threatened by a multitude of persecutory objects.

Within Klein's model, splitting is very often associated with another primitive mental mechanism, that of projective identification. Projective identification describes a process that takes place at a quite unconscious level of the individual's mind, in which, in the internal world, a part of the self with certain attributes and characteristics is 'split off' and then relocated or 'projected into' an object, the object is then experienced as having (identified with) the characteristics of that part of the ego. In this way, the individual may cease to be aware of, say, a state of need or hunger, but may feel themselves to be in the presence of a figure who needs something of them. When taken with the process of introjection, by which external objects are taken in and established in the internal world, one can see how splitting and projective identification are essential to the process of constructing the objects Klein suggested populated the internal world.

Klein and subsequent workers have described a variety of ways in which projective identification may be employed, that is the variety of attitudes that the self may have in relation to the object designated as the recipient for such a form of projection. For example, projective identification may be employed with the intention of communicating certain states of mind to the object, or the intention may simply be to evacuate the self of a particular state of distress or anxiety. In more disturbed states of mind, the intention may be to penetrate and take control of an object in a more aggressive and hostile way. Within a clinical setting, as an analyst or therapist one may feel moved, filled up, or even assaulted by states of mind that make thought impossible.

More recently analysts have described the variety of ways in which these unconscious processes operating on figures in the patient's internal world, such that objects are identified as possessing certain characteristics at a point in time, may in fact be lived out in a real way in exchanges between two people. In the consulting room the experience is that the analyst is either invited to, or is 'nudged into' acting out the role associated with a particular projection (Joseph, 1985). In this way, the patient may actually create an experience in external reality in which the object is identified as possessing certain characteristics, while the patient is free from such characteristics, and indeed is free from all knowledge of what has taken place, as the process is unconscious. So, a very depressed patient may start attending sessions erratically, engendering a state of uncertainty and anxiety in their analyst who may even be worried that the patient has attempted suicide, while the patient upon return describes having felt much better.

The paranoid–schizoid and depressive positions

In her paper 'Notes on Some Schizoid Mechanisms' (1946), Klein described a constellation of anxieties, defences and object relationships that she felt were characteristic of the earliest months of infancy. She argued that, during this period of time, the infant is subjected to anxieties that threaten to overwhelm his immature ego. The infant is a passionate being, struggling to survive, to protect his good internal objects and good relationships. As described earlier, the source of some of these anxieties is related to the infant's experience of his own physical state, for example of discomfort, pain or hunger.

Other anxieties were believed by Klein to be intrinsic, particularly the 'death instinct' as described by Freud in his later work. This concept refers to intense hate and anti-life impulses that Freud and Klein believed to exist alongside love in the unconscious. The infant's first response to such severe primitive anxiety is to project it outwards and away from himself into an object experienced by the infant as separate from the self, to get rid of it. This object, in Klein's writing 'the breast', is then identified as a source of external persecution.

The breast, however, is also identified by the infant as the source of his good experiences, for example of fullness and warmth after a good feed. The infant manages this situation by splitting the breast (in unconscious phantasy) into a good and a bad breast, and by struggling from then on to take in the good breast while keeping the bad breast at bay. In this way, Klein described how a world of part-objects is created, each containing split-off aspects of the infant's experience, goodness and badness, pleasure and pain. This world has nightmarish qualities, everything in it is black or white, good or bad, potentially malevolent or beatific. The characteristic anxiety of this state of mind, called by Klein the paranoid–schizoid position, is that bad objects represent a persecutory threat to the self.

It is important to realize, however, that it would be unlikely now that an analyst would talk to their patient about their experience of good and bad breasts. Instead, an analyst is more likely to concentrate on describing the patient's experience of the analytic relationship, and of their analyst, which may at times be of a helpful, nurturing or comforting figure, while at other times may be of a more persecuting or hostile figure. The analytic encounter is thus one in which the struggle is to understand a very human and personal relationship, and then make use of this in helping the patient to understand the world they find themselves living in, both internal and external.

Klein argued that the paranoid–schizoid position underlay psychotic states. Now, we would perhaps see this kind of mental organization most clearly in borderline patients, in which the propensity to experience others as either ideal or malign is so predominant.

Klein envisaged development over the second three months of life as an integrative process by which the loved and hated, good and bad, objects become aspects of a single, whole object – a person. When the infant comes to realize that his love and hate have been directed at one such integrated whole object, he also becomes aware of feelings of concern for the object, and guilt for the attempts he has made to psychically destroy the object within the internal world. Finally, the infant experiences a strong wish to repair the object, to make reparation. It is this constellation of anxieties and object relationships that Klein termed the depressive position (Klein, 1935, 1940).

In the depressive position, depressive anxiety relates to the damage feared done to the object through attacks by the self. By way of contrast in the paranoid–schizoid position, paranoid anxiety relates to the threat of damage to the self by the object. It is in the move from paranoid–schizoid to depressive positions that the infant's character becomes enriched through a stepwise relinquishment of the old and incorporation of the new. The characters in the infant's internal world become more three-dimensional, relationships are more complex and omnipotence is given up with an acceptance of loss and imperfection in himself and his objects.

While describing the paranoid–schizoid and depressive positions as being a normal part of infant development, Klein argued that throughout adult life the individual moves between these positions in terms of their experience of the world. In this way she suggested that all people have a capacity for more paranoid states of mind, in which they believe that they are under attack from the world around. Any given individual, however, may have a greater or lesser propensity for such states of mind, or a greater or lesser capacity for the more integrated modes of experience associated with the depressive position. This notion of a shifting equilibrium is one that all Kleinian analysts use to orientate themselves to a patient's clinical material and to what it expresses of the patient's relationship to, and experience of, the analyst.

Containment

While considering that constitutional factors and the active role that the infant may play in determining its environment are of great importance, Klein (1946) referred to 'love and understanding of the infant ... as the infant's greatest standby in overcoming states of disintegration and anxieties of a psychotic nature'. Wilfred Bion (1962; 1967) developed this idea into a much more specific hypothesis. Bion suggested that for individuals to develop coherent ways of representing relations between self and other, and for thinking about the contents of their own mind, they need to develop within a particular kind of interpersonal setting.

Bion argued that young infants require a sensitive and emotionally 'containing' caretaker or caretakers, if they are to develop their own capacities to 'contain' and assimilate experiences and feelings. If there is no sensitive caretaker available, then they may be unable to integrate difficult or frightening anxieties, experiences or parts of the self. Such a failure may lead to a retreat to the primitive defences which characterize Klein's paranoid–schizoid position. The infant may then respond by attempting to rid himself of overwhelming feelings through splitting representations of self and other into unrealistic idealized or denigrated figures, with an associated disruption in the experience of self.

Such vigorous defences then lead to an internal world in which all is either ideal or malign, with associated disruptions in the experience of self and external reality. Bion argued that the infant's experience of a relationship with an object who is able to tolerate and make sense of seemingly incomprehensible psychic states then, in time, allows the infant to take in such a containing function. This aids the infant in moving toward the more integrated mode of experience characterized by the depressive position.

Aims of therapy

Freud summarized the aim of psychoanalytic treatment, typically succinctly, as helping a patient to rediscover their capacity for love and work. Winnicott added play to this description. Within the work of Melanie Klein, underlying these aims is the belief that anxiety associated with unconscious phantasies may inhibit such capacities. Where anxiety is too great, the individual may resort to primitive, omnipotent defences including splitting and projective identification. Klein argued that these defensive manoeuvres fundamentally weaken and deplete the personality and inhibit psychological development. The aim then of analytic work, through the interpretation of the transference, is to help the patient to reintegrate such split-off aspects of their personality. In accepting, tolerating and understanding a patient's projections within the analytic situation, the analyst is also offering the patient a 'containing' function that the patient may then, over time, take into themselves. These aspects of the analytic experience may then help the patient to a greater capacity for bearing what Klein described as the depressive position, in which the patient relates to others as 'whole objects', and is able to tolerate the anxieties associated with such a situation.

Another way of framing this might be to say that the aim of an analysis is to help the patient develop enough strength to tolerate encounters with external reality, and with their own internal reality. Thus each patient may have to face both their own loving and hateful feelings, their own creativity and their own destructiveness. The development of such strength may then allow the patient to shift the balance between these internal forces.

Principles of practice

Psychoanalysis is concerned not so much with explaining the present in terms of the past, but rather with exploring the nature of an individual's interpersonal relationships and, through this, with understanding something of the organization of that individual's internal world. The concept of transference is central to this work – the idea that each person's mental representations of interpersonal experience or internal object relations, may determine the perception and patterning of their current relationships. The focus of study within the analytic situation is what is happening between the patient and analyst while it is happening. The idea is that by working in the 'here and now' of the patient–analyst relationship, access is gained to a level of internal organization and functioning that would otherwise remain inaccessible or unobservable. In an analysis, the analyst comes to experience what it is like to be a figure within one of the patient's internal relationships. He or she is ascribed various roles, and is made to feel things and sometimes to do things that have a specificity in relation to a particular patient. It is the analysis of this current encounter between patient and analyst that yields the analytic perspective on the structure and functioning of the mind. Explaining the present in terms of the past is inevitably a more tentative part of psychoanalysis. All of the above, however, is true of most (and not just Kleinian) analytic practice in Britain today.

Many analysts now place a particular emphasis on understanding the transference as a 'total situation' (Joseph, 1985). This total situation includes not just the patient's conscious and unconscious experience of and attitude towards the analyst, but also the analyst's conscious and unconscious experience of, and attitude towards, the patient. Within this context, all associations are considered to relate to the nature of this transference, if not in content then in style of delivery or in their intended function. For example, let us suppose that an analyst makes an interpretation to a patient. The patient pauses for thought and says 'Yes, that feels right'. The patient then has an association, the content of which seems to exemplify and support what the analyst has said. The association seems genuine and moving, and there is a sense that something important has been understood. Now, suppose that the same analyst were making the same interpretation but to a very different patient. This patient is also silent; but then, without commenting directly upon the interpretation, he or she offers an association that seems to move the situation forward, introducing a new and rather different element. The content of this association seems linked with the interpretation and, as this situation is repeated, the analyst believes that the analysis is progressing well. Until, that is, it gradually becomes clear that what superficially appears to be helpful free association, actually serves to allow the patient never to consider anything in a thoughtful way. Instead, the analyst is placed in the position of following after the patient. In time, the patient's sense of superiority over the analyst becomes clearer, as does the patient's certain knowledge that they know just what the analyst will interpret in relation to each new piece of material.

Joseph has described the dangers of interpreting the content of the patient's material, rather than interpreting where you and the patient are in the transference. Implicit in the example above is the notion that the analyst may 'act out' a role on behalf of the patient for some time before it becomes understood. Others have pointed out how aspects of the analyst's 'countertransference' experience, particularly the state of mind engendered in the analyst by the patient, is largely unconscious and is very likely to be acted out (Steiner, 1993). This formulation is very different from the notion of the patient 'making the analyst feel things' at a conscious level, although this certainly can and does also happen. The work of these authors has led to the development of a model of transference and countertransference relationships in which the evolving and involving relationship between analyst and patient may be of great subtlety, operating at many different levels. It may only be observable once it has developed over some period of time and is then being lived out by patient and analyst, as it is by the analyst who follows dutifully after his patient believing that all is well and that the analysis is developing nicely. Interpreting in 'the here and now' of the analyst–patient relationship thus involves taking into account content, form and intended function of an association in relation to what may have preceded it.

Among the ways in which the work of Klein, and those analysts who have developed her ideas, may influence psychoanalytic practice, two deserve particular attention. The first of these relates to the importance of 'negative transference'. In her work with young children, Klein found that phantasies of destructiveness, hostility, aggression and hatred were common. These phantasies were very often associated with powerful anxieties as experienced by the children. Klein later identified similar phantasies in her work with adults. While she believed that every communication between patient and analyst may contain an important balance of positive and negative attitudes, of love and hate, Klein argued that these 'negative' phantasies were those most immediately related to the most pressing forms of anxiety. These observations have led many analysts to believe that the interpretation of 'negative' aspects of the transference, when they are present, is of great importance in alleviating patients' anxieties and in demonstrating that such phantasies are communicable without concretely leading to a destruction of the analyst's mind. The intention of such work is to help the patient to reintegrate split-off aspects of their personality, although such a reintegration may also involve a patient facing the ways in which they contain destructive capacities and qualities as well as more constructive ones.

The last of the influences of Klein and her followers that I will describe here relates to the level at which interpretations are made when addressing a patient's anxiety. Of course an analyst working with a patient over a period of time will make many different sorts of interpretations in many different contexts, some relating to events in the patient's life, some relating to aspects of the analyst–patient relationship, and some linking these two to aspects of the patient's story. However, when addressing unconscious anxiety, some analysts are perhaps more likely to interpret what they consider to be the content of the patient's most pressing anxiety rather than the defences organized against the experience of that anxiety. Some have described this as the difference between an 'onion-peeling' style of work, and analytic work characterized by the making of 'deep' interpretations, deep in the sense that they bypass defensive strategies and address unconscious anxieties in a more direct fashion. As with the interpretation of negative aspects of the transference, the main reason for this style of work is a belief, based on clinical experience, that the direct interpretation of unconscious anxiety is the most effective way to alleviate such anxiety.

How does Kleinian psychoanalysis differ from other therapies?

The model of a drive- and instinct-based psychology relates mostly to Freud's work in the early part of this century, and is very different to the object relations-based psychology that is the dominant theoretical and clinical framework employed by analysts in Britain today. What then are the ways in which the contributions of Mrs Klein and subsequent 'Kleinian' analysts may influence the practice of a particular analyst's clinical work? A part of the answer lies in Klein's contribution to psychoanalytic theory. One example of this would be her formulation of the paranoid–schizoid and depressive positions, a model of two very differing modes of psychological functioning that many analysts make use of in orienting themselves to a patient's material: are the patient's anxieties of a primitive persecutory nature, or are their concerns more linked with a sense of guilt, sadness and a wish to repair damage? There are also, however, a number of facets of an analyst's clinical technique that may be influenced to a greater or lesser extent by the work of Klein and her followers.

Which patient and why?

The factors that make a patient suitable for an analysis of this sort are in many ways no different from those that would make a patient suitable for any psychoanalytic treatment. They include a degree of self-interest, a capacity to tolerate the distress and psychic pain associated with facing truths about oneself and a degree of psychological-mindedness. The indications for a psychoanalytic treatment may include a certain constellation of defences or a character structure which might remain untouched, or indeed be reinforced, by a less frequent or different mode of psychotherapy. Similarly, some highly disturbed patients may be assessed as needing the containment offered by a more frequent therapeutic intervention, especially if the risks of exploring certain aspects of mental functioning may be experienced by the patient, perhaps accurately, as too dangerous, and the risk of breakdown too high. Within a psychoanalytic treatment, such a breakdown may sometimes, to a degree, be controlled or contained within the structure of the treatment. Some individuals may also feel that in addition to a need for treatment, they have a curiosity about the workings of their mind and the structure of their personality, and wish to undertake an endeavour in which these things will be explored in depth.

In addition to patients who may be suitable for a 'Kleinian analysis', the work of Melanie Klein may be helpful and relevant to other patients. Within psychiatric and National Health Service (NHS) settings, Klein's work is of immediate relevance to the treatment of disturbed patients, especially those with diagnoses of severe personality disorders (for example, borderline personality disorder) but also in contributing to the understanding of those with psychotic disorders. Her work is also of immediate relevance to the *management* of such patients in that it offers a framework for understanding the anxieties and states of mind engendered in those individuals or groups who may be struggling to help a disturbed individual. Such an understanding may be a prerequisite to the successful outcome of any psychotherapeutic endeavour, or indeed to the successful outcome of any more general psychiatric interventions, and perhaps particularly those taking place in in-patient settings.

At the same time, Klein's work is also of relevance for the understanding of the more primitive psychopathology that exists in all of us. Indeed we all have a capacity for slipping into an experience of the world that is captured in Klein's description of the paranoid–schizoid position, a world of anxiety and fear, of persecution and nightmarish distress.

Assessment of the suitability of a particular psychotherapeutic or psycho-analytic intervention for a particular patient should involve a dynamic assessment interview, in which some preliminary exploration is undertaken with the patient as to the nature of their difficulties. In such an assessment, some of the factors outlined above would be looked at, including the patient's capacity to make use of interpretative work. The assessment should also include an exploration of the potential harm that a particular intervention might do to a patient, for example in threatening breakdown, but also the potential harmfulness of a patient to their analyst, for example some assessment of potential dangerousness. Milton (1997) has written very thoughtfully and at greater length on the task of psychoanalytic assessment within NHS settings.

Which therapist and why?

The training of psychoanalysts in Britain takes place under the auspices of the British Psycho-Analytical Society, which was founded by Dr Ernest Jones in 1919. Applicants are eligible for consideration if they are medically qualified or undergoing medical training, or if they have a university degree or its equivalent. Non-medical applicants need to demonstrate some relevant clinical experience or professional responsibility for the development or welfare of individuals. The training is not divided by group, but focuses on a thorough grounding in psychoanalytic work through three components: personal analysis, supervised clinical work and theoretical teaching. Nominally, Kleinian analysts are those who have had an analysis with a Kleinian analyst, although clinical work and style does not always fall that neatly into such artificial divides. An analyst from any group may be more or less influenced by the work of analysts nominally attached to other groups. There are other excellent trainings in psychoanalytic psychotherapy, a number of which revolve around three times a week treatments as opposed to four or five, although such therapists may also see patients more frequently.

Therapeutic setting

Klein's work has not just been taken up by one group of analysts within the British Psycho-Analytical Society. Rather, her work has found relevance and application in many different settings, including NHS psychotherapy services offering psychoanalytic psychotherapy and in more general psychiatric settings. The clinical setting for an analysis does not differ according to whether one is a Contemporary Freudian, a Kleinian or a member of the Independent Group. The treatment is conducted on a four or five times weekly basis. The patient has set times for their sessions, and can expect their analyst to be punctual and to provide a consulting room that offers privacy and consistency, free from interruption. Patients lie on a couch with their analyst usually sitting behind them, as opposed to sitting face to face as would typically occur in a once-weekly psychotherapeutic treatment. Beyond the concrete setting, however, the patient might expect to encounter an individual who does not intrude their own life into the encounter, and who is prepared to listen to the patient and not respond in a judgemental way, but who will, rather, try to make sense of the responses evoked in him to formulate interpretations that will help to clarify aspects of the patient's experience.

Clinical example

The features of this style of clinical work can be illustrated with this example taken from a session early on in the analysis of a patient, Miss LK. The example is chosen not only to illustrate a style of work, but also to illustrate how one might think about and conceptualize material after a session, indeed might only be able to after a session, before continuing the work the following day.

Miss LK is twenty-seven years old and has a sister four years her elder. She was referred with complaints of depression, loneliness, lack of self-confidence and a coping facade which she felt was too convincing, preventing others from recognizing how she really felt.

When Miss LK was six, her father left the family home abruptly after an affair. For several reasons the break-up of the family was made particularly painful. Two difficult years followed, during which time Miss LK's mother struggled to bring up the two children alone. There were frequent times at which her mother was apparently overwhelmed by the task, breaking down and crying when feeling that she was unable to control her children. At the end of two years the patient's mother remarried and had another child, and things within the family improved.

When talking about her past, the patient always emphasized her belief that she had survived best. Her mother and sister had been more disturbed, she felt, by her father's departure, and had both needed treatment around the time of his leaving. She also described having sat in the car with her sister on the way to and from her sister's therapy sessions, and the way in which her sister used to punch and tickle her – 'trying to drive her mad'. Miss LK underachieved at school and left aged eighteen with only two O' levels, although clearly very bright. She immediately found a job in a residential care setting, looking after disturbed children. At the time of her referral, she was dominated by feelings of anger and upset at the way in which she was too often left alone to cope with difficult situations at work by uncaring senior staff who should have known that she did not have sufficient experience.

In this brief piece of history one can begin to see the possible ways in which this patient had made use of splitting and projective identification in managing states of distress that she felt she was unable to manage. In relation to the departure of her father, distress and disturbance was located not in the patient, but in her sister and mother. This disturbance, however, after having been split off and relocated in objects external to the patient in her mind, now represented a threat to the patient in that it threatened 'to drive her mad' should it find its way back into her. A similar situation was observable in relation to her work, in that she chooses to look after disturbed children, perhaps because they represented an ideal receptacle for her own distress and disturbance associated with feelings of abandonment.

Two weeks before her first break, Miss LK began her session by telling me about difficulties at work in which she had to deal with hopeless and inadequate staff. She was dismissive and haughty. When I suggested that she felt surrounded by incompetents and always had to shoulder all of the responsibility she rounded on me and witheringly said that she supposed that I was talking about the analytic sessions, well she wasn't, so I could keep my pseudoanalytic interpretations to myself. At this I indeed did feel a bit crushed, thinking that perhaps my intervention had been rather clumsy and forced. The patient then told me about a situation with her boyfriend that had occurred the day before, in which he had been unable to listen to something she had wanted to say because he had things on his mind. In her session, the patient reacted by saying that she felt this was fine. She both understood and felt it was how it should be – he needed his own space. She then told me that, later on the same day, her boyfriend had tried to make amends but that she had felt there was nothing to make amends for, and couldn't understand why he had then been upset with her.

At this point I plucked up my courage and said to the patient that I thought she was saying (I had become a little cautious) that she dealt with rejection in a particular way. Rather than getting angry, 'everything is just OK'. But, in addition, I said that I thought that there was more to it than this. Here, in the session, before a break, she made it clear that our relationship was irrelevant to her, and that when I made 'pseudoanalytical interpretations' I was in fact simply trying to make myself important to her, confirming my inadequacy. As with her boyfriend, I should not think that I was important enough for her to feel anything concerning my impending unavailability.

What I was trying to show the patient in this interpretation was the way in which I now contained an experience of being inadequate, unable to gain and hold her interest, peripheral to her life. I wondered whether this experience also contained an aspect of her feelings concerning her father's departure, if she had been more adequate perhaps father would not have left. I did not suggest to the patient that she felt any of these things, however, because at this point in the session, clearly she did not!

Miss LK responded to my intervention in a curious way. She told me that she had just had an interesting thought, and then repeated to me almost exactly what I had just said to her. In effect, she had appropriated my thoughts and negated the existence of my interpretation completely.

In response, I said that it seemed that something interesting had just happened, pointing out what I felt she had just done. Miss LK looked at me and, rather like a school teacher, started to talk about how provoked her mother had always been by her and her sister's fighting. She remembered her standing in the doorway, hands clenched, her knuckles white. The patient went on to tell me that she knew that her mother hadn't known how to cope, and that this left her feeling very guilty.

It was not until after the session that I began to understand what in fact might have taken place. The patient had been extremely provocative, and yet I had tried to take up her depression concerning the break. When she appropriated my thoughts, negating the existence of my interpretation, I said *to her that this was 'interesting'. In the session, in effect, I had become the one who said that anything she did was OK. Furthermore, on reflection it now seems that what was important at this point was not the patient's depression, but her sense that I was unable to cope with her behaviour and with my anger at her, and so avoided it, reinforcing the patient's feeling that no one could tolerate the violence of her feelings.*

Problems in therapy

There is a common misconception that the work of Melanie Klein involves a sole focus on destructiveness and negative aspects of the personality. In fact, Klein wrote movingly about the importance of more loving feelings within the personality. Within an analysis, it is the balance between such conflicting forces that is the focus of exploration. In some cases, indeed, patients may feel more awkward about the more positive aspects of the transference than the negative. A second common misconception of Klein's work is that any observation by a patient about their analyst or their analysis is based on projection rather than reality. In fact, nothing could be further from the truth. In an analysis, patients have the opportunity to come to know the character of their analyst extremely well, if not at a conscious level, then certainly at an unconscious one. Furthermore, it is now widely accepted that certain roles can be recreated between a patient and analyst, and that an analyst's countertransference may be largely knowable only through observation of how the analyst finds himself functioning in relation to a particular patient, or feels impelled to function. In this regard, patients are often extremely accurate in their observations and may provide very helpful guidance to their analyst as to how he may be acting.

There also seems to be a belief that followers of Melanie Klein accord absolute paramouncy to the internal world, taking little heed of factors in external reality. Once more this is far from the truth. While facts about reality are hard to know with any certainty from material brought to a session as one may be presented with a particular slant on events (and indeed it would be a little surprising if one were not!), contact with reality is considered of great importance. Indeed, one might at times feel a need to interpret a patient's focus on their relationship with their analyst as a turning away from the reality of their life outside of analysis.

The variety of mistakes that analysts may make in their clinical work are beyond the scope of this chapter but one of the commonest areas of difficulty relates to the understanding of the transference. When beginning to work in a dynamic way with patients, it is often hard to get to grips with what or indeed where 'the transference' is. If a patient comes in and talks about how angry they may be with their mother for being unsympathetic and unavailable, it may be tempting to say something along the lines of 'I think that you may be angry with me', assuming that in the patient's mind you represent this maternal figure. This may not, however, be the case.

Perhaps the simplest way of thinking about the transference is to try to ask a number of questions of oneself:

• Who or what am I for this patient at this point in time?
• What is the intended function of the mood created by the patient?

- What is the patient trying to do to me?
- What does the patient feel that I am trying to do to him?
- What situation is being recreated in the room between the patient and myself?

In this way, in the example given above, one can then see that the patient may be relating to his analyst as a sympathetic figure, or may be trying to win the analyst over to his side in a battle with mother. Alternatively, the patient may bring the material in a manner that leaves the analyst feeling unmoved and maybe even irritated. Indeed, the analyst may make an interpretation, only then to notice the slightly critical tone of it. The analyst may then realize that he has enacted the relationship being described by the patient, that the scene is now alive in the session and can potentially be worked on. This is not to say that such enactments on the part of the analyst are advisable, or to be encouraged. If the pressure to act can be noticed without acting, so much the better, but subtle enactments may constitute an unavoidable part of the analytic encounter that needs to be understood.

Evaluation of therapy

In the United Kingdom, psychoanalytic treatments are generally only available in the private sector. A number of means-tested vacancies are, however, available through the London Clinic of Psycho-Analysis as a part of their training activities. In private practice, a patient's fees may depend on the experience and training of the analyst although many analysts will also consider a patient's financial circumstances when negotiating fees. In a number of European countries financial support for psychoanalytic treatments is available from health insurance companies, who calculate that the cost of treatment is less than the costs of other interventions for difficulties that may reoccur over many years.

Much has been written about psychoanalytic treatments and their outcomes over the past hundred years, and this subject is dealt with in other chapters. There is little literature comparing different psychoanalytic approaches beyond descriptions of individual's experiences of them. In addition, there are obvious difficulties in subjecting psychoanalytic treatments to randomized controlled trial designs, although a number of large studies of this type are now being undertaken in different centres around the world. Much of the literature on the efficacy of these interventions is, then, in the form of case studies or series of case studies, or involves research designs that would now be considered less robust than randomized control trials. At the same time, it is worth noting that an increasing body of research is accumulating that looks at the validity of psychoanalytic hypotheses and theory. The overlap between psychoanalytic theory and attachment theory has proved to be a rich source in this regard (e.g. Patrick et al., 1994). The development of new measures from other fields has also made the task of researchers a little easier, and in some ways has made 'conventional' research more interesting to psychoanalysts, although many still regard the psychoanalytic method itself as the research tool par excellence when exploring the nature of an individual's internal world, and the nature of their intersubjective experience.

Alternatives to Kleinian psychoanalysis

There are, of course, many alternatives to a psychoanalytic treatment. There are psychoanalytic psychotherapies offered at frequencies of between one and three times a week, there is group psychotherapy, cognitive behavioural psychotherapy, cognitive analytic psychotherapy and so on. There are day hospitals, in-patient psychotherapy units, drug treatment and other forms of more conventional psychiatric management. In a way, perhaps the question relates more to issues of local resources. If a patient has been assessed as most suitable for a psychoanalytic treatment, but this is not available, then more available local resources need to be considered. Relatively short-term dynamic psychotherapies may be of tremendous benefit, even to very disturbed patients, and there is increasing evidence for the efficacy of cognitive behavioural and cognitive analytic treatments in patients with lifelong characterological difficulties. Indeed, for some very troubled patients there are situations where a less intensive treatment may be more manageable for the patient. When assessing referrals for psychological interventions a careful matching of psychopathology, preferred treatment modality and practical resources all need to be balanced. However, in this work it is rarely, if ever, the case that one can say that a certain individual is ideally suited to a certain intervention and no other.

Further reading

Bott Spillius, E. (ed.) (1988) *Melanie Klein Today. Volume 1: Mainly Theory; Volume 2: Mainly Practice*. The New Library of Psychoanalysis. London: Routledge.
Hinshelwood, R.D. (1991) *A Dictionary of Kleinian Thought*. London: Free Association Books.
Hinshelwood, R.D. (1994) *Clinical Klein*. London: Free Association Books.
Segal, H. (1986) *Introduction to the Work of Melanie Klein*. London: Hogarth Press.

Bibliography

Anderson, R. and Segal, H. (eds) (1992) *Clinical Lectures on Klein and Bion*. The New Library of Psychoanalysis. London: Routledge.
Bion, W. (1962) Learning from experience. In: *Seven Servants: Four Works by Wilfred R. Bion*. New York: Jason Aronson, pp. 1–111.
Bion, W. (1967) A theory of thinking. In: *Second Thoughts*. London: Heinemann, pp. 110–119.
Britton, R., Feldman, M. and O'Shaughnessy, E. (1989) *The Oedipus Complex Today*. London: Karnac Books.
Hinshelwood, R.D. (1991) *A Dictionary of Kleinian Thought*. London: Free Association Books.
Joseph, B. (1985) Transference: the total situation. *International Journal of Psycho-Analysis*, **66**, 447–454.
Joseph, B. (1989) *Psychic Equilibrium and Psychic Change: Selected Papers of Betty Joseph*. The New Library of Psychoanalysis. London: Routledge.
Klein, M. (1935) A contribution to the psychogenesis of manic-depressive states. In: *The Writings of Melanie Klein*, vol. 1. London: Hogarth Press (1975).
Klein, M. (1940) Mourning and its relation to manic-depressive states. In: *The Writings of Melanie Klein*, vol. 1. London: Hogarth Press (1975).

Klein, M. (1946) Notes on some schizoid mechanisms. In: *The Writings of Melanie Klein*, vol. 3. London: Hogarth Press (1975).

Klein, M. (1955) The psycho-analytic play technique: its history and significance. In: *The Writings of Melanie Klein*, vol. 3. London: Hogarth Press (1975).

Milton, J. (1997) Why assess? Psychoanalytical assessment in the NHS. *Psychoanalytic Psychotherapy*, **11**, 47–58.

Patrick, M., Hobson, R.P., Castle, D. *et al.* (1994) Personality disorder and the mental representation of early social experience. *Development and Psychopathology*, **6**, 375–388.

Rosenfeld, H. (1965) *Psychotic States*. London: Hogarth Press.

Segal, H. (1986) *The Work of Hanna Segal*. London: Free Association Books.

Steiner, J. (1993) *Psychic Retreats*. The New Library of Psychoanalysis. London: Routledge.

Stern, D. (1985) *The Interpersonal World of the Infant*. New York: Basic Books.

4
Bion

Samuel M. Stein

I don't know the answers to these questions – I wouldn't tell you if I did. I think it is important to find out for yourselves.

W. R. Bion (Sao Paulo, 1978)

Introduction

Wilfred Bion was one of Britain's most significant psychoanalytic thinkers. His highly original writings were in a direct line from Freud to Klein, but also encompassed theology and mathematics. Whilst he had no objections to classical analysis, he would not accept being told 'you must think so far and no further'. Bion (1978) said, 'We learn these theories – Freud's, Jung's, Klein's – and try to get them absolutely rigid so as to avoid having to do any more thinking.' He believed that psychoanalysts need to be able to ask questions as often and as long as they are unsatisfied, without being limited by their lecturers, teachers, analysts or parents.

As Bion's writings were largely aimed at the practising analyst, he assumed that the reader was already familiar with basic psychoanalytic approaches. Similarly, this chapter cannot stand alone but needs to be read in conjunction with the preceding chapters on Freud, Jung and Klein. In developing his ideas, Bion did not try to replace existing psychoanalytical theory but concentrated on observation, psychic transformation and the critical appraisal of psychoanalytic practice. He felt that psychoanalysis could be described by six basic theories, with subsidiary models to meet a wide range of contingencies, and sought to identify the relatively few elements required to express, by changes in combination, nearly all of the theories essential to the working of psychoanalysis. Bion felt that, by sharpening of the senses and perception, psychoanalysts could find a method of excluding what was irrelevant and concentrating on what was fundamental. One advantage of this model is that it does not commit the psychoanalyst to the formal rigidity of a theory, but presents him with a tool which he can discard when it has served its purpose.

Bion did not think that his explanations mattered, except in drawing attention to the nature of the problem, and tried to give others a chance to fill the gaps left by him. He believed that answers were not to be found in textbooks but only in the process of psychoanalysis itself, and that a book failed for the reader if it did not become, in addition to an object of study, an emotional experience in itself. The value of Bion's work therefore depends very much on the skill and patience of the reader, who will need to read and re-read the text until a pattern begins to emerge which brings all the disparate elements together in a synthesized whole. This is the experience which Bion described as O.

Historical perspective

Wilfred Bion (1897–1979) was born in Muttra, India where his father was serving as a civil engineer. He described his mother as 'a little frightening', and sought his father's admiration and approval. Bion spent his early childhood in India but left at the age of eight to attend Bishop's Stortford College preparatory school in England. He excelled at rugby, swimming and waterpolo and, on leaving school, Bion enlisted for military service. He served in France during the First World War as a tank commander and was awarded the DSO and the Legion of Honour for bravery. After demobilization, he read history at Queen's College, Oxford. Whilst at university, he first heard mention of Freud and talk about psychoanalysis, but on enquiring further was persuaded it was better not to get involved as there were 'Jews and foreigners' mixed up in it. Bion later studied medicine at University College London, where he won the Gold Medal for Surgery and qualified as a doctor in 1930.

Bion's first analysis, which he found extremely illuminating, was with John Rickman. He was subsequently analysed by Melanie Klein. To his surprise, psychoanalysis seemed to have a distinct relationship to what he thought was common sense. As he said, 'I found that what Melanie Klein said, while seeming very often to be rather extraordinary stuff, had a kind of common sense about it – not altogether what I would have regarded as obvious or clear to me, but on the other hand not divorced from what I knew about myself or other people, or even about my war experience.'

Shortly before the Second World War, Bion married the actress Betty Jardine. She gave birth to their only daughter, Parthenope, whilst Bion was on active service in Normandy, and tragically died three days later from a pulmonary embolism. Bion returned to London where he served as the Senior Psychiatrist on the War Office Selection Board. He participated in the Northfield Experiment and his attention was directed towards the study of group processes which culminated in the publication of a series of influential papers later produced as *Experience in Groups*.

Bion was Chairman of the Executive Committee of the Tavistock Clinic, London in 1945. He was also Director of the London Clinic for Psycho-Analysis between 1956 and 1962, before serving as President of the British Psycho-Analytical Society from 1962 until 1965. In 1968 an offer to work in Los Angeles provided the opportunity to escape from what Bion called the 'cosy domesticity' of England. He returned to England in 1979, just two months before his death in Oxford, less than a week after he was diagnosed as suffering from myeloid leukaemia. Several of Bion's works have been published posthumously by his second wife, Francesca, who still lives in

Oxfordshire and who played an active role in editing his work prior to his death. Their son read medicine at university and their daughter trained as a linguist. Bion's eldest daughter, Parthenope, lives and works as a psychoanalyst in Turin.

Principles of theory and practice

Dreams

Dreams, which originate from emotional experiences, are central to the conscious and unconscious processes on which ordered thought depends. Dreaming is the mechanism by which streams of unconnected impressions and events are made suitable for storage as memory. Dreams act to provide a barrier against mental phenomena which might overwhelm the patient's awareness, and help to moderate frustration by making the intolerable tolerable. Dreams may also serve to evacuate undesired thoughts, feelings and images. According to Bion, dreaming is a continuous process which belongs to both waking life and sleep as there are numerous activities carried out when awake which are reminiscent of dreams. The content of the dream is not important as it is only a transitive act, a symptom of mental indigestion.

Although the dreamer disguises the dream thoughts so that the manifest content bears little resemblance to the latent content, dreams always mean something. Dream-work renders the dream comprehensible by transforming the latent content into manifest content. Both external and internal reality are thus made readily accessible to the personality. Similarly sense impressions can only come to be associated with either conscious or unconscious processes if they are transformed by dream-work, which renders stimuli and impressions storable and communicable. Dream-work therefore makes abstraction, symbolization, memory and naming possible, and is rapidly destroyed as part of an attack on linking.

Bion extended Freud's concept of 'dream-work' and called it dream-work-α. Whilst dream-work relates to the interpretation of dreams, dream-work-α relates to the capacity to dream as it operates on stimuli arising within and without the psyche, day and night, to promote synthesis. Dream-work-α transforms sense impressions and experiences into α elements so that they can be ideogrammatized, stored and remembered as suitable material for dream thoughts. However, β elements are not amenable to being used in dreams. Sleep is often essential to make possible sufficient suspension of consciousness to allow an emotional experience that the personality would not permit itself in conscious waking life to be submitted to dream-work-α for conversion into a narrative capable of being worked on by rational thought processes. Dream-work-α was later simplified by Bion into the concept of α-function.

Ignorance and the unknown

According to Bion, unknown ideas are hated and feared as we do not like coming across something which is novel and which we do not understand. Yet every emotional experience of knowledge gained is at the same time an emotional experience of ignorance illuminated. As being ignorant is unpleasant, we therefore have an investment in knowing the answer and are pressured from within to close the discussion and fill the free space, reaching out for the nearest psychoanalytic theory, for example, rather than not having the faintest idea of what the patient is saying or doing. There seems to be a constant warfare between the attraction of something new and one's wish to remain in a familiar state of mind. However, as Bion said (New York, 1977), 'I do not know' is not the same as 'I am confused'.

The context of psychoanalysis relates to these unknown emotional experiences that are only known to be unknown, and therefore must be recognized as such. The absolute facts of the session can never really be known, and analysts may become frightened of their own ignorance when confronted with unique and therefore unknown situations. It is especially difficult for inexperienced analysts to tolerate doubt, and the temptation is to terminate prematurely the stage of uncertainty about what the patient is saying by giving an interpretation. It is similarly fatal to good analysis if premature application of theory becomes a habit which places a screen between the psychoanalyst and unknown material.

Psychoanalysts must therefore develop a capacity for tolerating their analysands' statements without rushing to the conclusion that they know the correct interpretation. The psychoanalyst should be aware of the aspects of the material that, however familiar they may seem to be, relate to what is unknown to both the analyst and the analysand. The problem is to ignore the coherence that facts may have in the patient's mind, allowing the analyst to experience the incomprehension of what is presented to him. This state of incoherence and incomprehensibility must endure until a new coherence emerges within the analysis.

No matter how thorough an analysis, the person will be only partially revealed and, at any point in the analysis, the proportion of what is known to what is unknown is small. Defences are inevitably instituted to put a stop to the disagreeable feelings of ignorance, and there is pressure to escape into what is already known. If the conflict between the need to know and the need to deny becomes acute, it may usher in attacks on linking. After many years of effort, Bion felt he had at last achieved the capacity to be awed by the depths of his own ignorance. He said, 'I know enough to know that I am ignorant' (Rio de Janeiro, 1974).

Intuition

The psychoanalytic situation is intuited as a form of analytic observation parallel to the physician's use of 'see', 'touch', 'smell' and 'hear' (Bion, 1970). By listening both to what the patient says and to what he does not say, the psychoanalyst has to intuit what is being communicated in the session. The problem for the practising psychoanalyst is how to match his hunch, intuition or suspicion with some formulation or conceptual statement. Giving an interpretation demonstrates that the analyst is capable of verbalizing his intuitions and primitive reactions to what the patient is saying. Psychoanalysts who develop their capacity to intuit the constantly changing pattern of emotional experiences soon become aware that there are certain experiences which are constantly conjoined.

The conditions in which intuition operates are opaque. The analyst is required to bring intuition and reason to bear on an emotional experience between two people in such a way that not only the analyst but also the analysand gains an understanding of the analysand's response to that emotional situation. The psychoanalyst must therefore undergo a training which develops and intensifies intuitive capacity, allowing the analyst to give patients help which they cannot get in any other way. The psychoanalyst should prevent his intuition being damaged by the intrusion of memory, desire and understanding which obstruct unknown phenomena and harm analytic intuition. It is fatal to good analysis if the premature application of theory impedes the analyst's exercise of his own intuition. Difficulties often arise if the analyst replaces his own intuition in this way with theory and other analysts' experiences. Bion developed the Grid as an exercise to develop intuition (see below, p. 101).

Linking

A link is an emotional experience which establishes the nature of the relationship between phenomena or objects. The term 'link' is specifically employed to discuss the patient's relationship with a function (endurance, fortitude, patience, danger, sympathy, love) rather than with the objects which are related. The prototype for all links is the primitive breast; however the breast and mouth are only important in defining the bridge between the two. When the 'anchors' (e.g. breast or mouth) usurp the importance which belongs to the bridge (relationship or link), growth is impaired.

Love (L), hate (H) and knowledge (K) are links which represent the dynamic relationship between psychoanalytic objects and between container: contained. The link may change in character, and there are an infinite number of links which any one object can have with other objects. β elements lack a capacity for linkage with each other, whereas elements of normal projective identification may form an important link. The link may also imply a model or abstraction, and symbols require linking in their formation as there has to be a relationship between one ideograph and another. The linking of images leads to narrative, and struggling to make a connection leads to thinking.

Attacks on the linking function of emotion originate in the part-object dominated paranoid–schizoid (Ps) phase, and that-which-links is minutely fragmented to prevent coherence. The psychotic patient extends the splitting process to the links between thought processes themselves, and makes destructive attacks on anything which functions to link one object with another. The psychotic patient attacks thought because it links sense impressions of reality with consciousness whereas he wishes to sever links with reality. Destruction of dream-work is an attack on linking, as are concretization, stimulation of memory and desire, and a hatred of common sense.

Psychoanalysis attempts to elucidate links that hinder or promote relationships. Such a link is provided by the patient's free associations and the analyst's interpretations, and is expressed in psychoanalytic theory by the term transference. The link between the analyst and patient should not be love (L) or hate (H), but knowledge (K). However, this link is constantly imperilled by deliberate attacks, and may be subjected to splitting and evacuation.

Combination of elements

There exists a tendency in the human mind for certain ideas to be associated together in the pursuit of meaning. Elements long since known, but scattered and seemingly foreign to each other, are united and introduce order where the appearance of disorder reigned. These elements are combined according to certain rules and come together to initiate a process of change. The nature of the link is determined by accompanying emotions. Thoughts too can be combined in a series of derivations from an underlying basic pattern, and the struggle to make such connections is an instance of thinking and learning.

The constellation of elements precipitates a constant conjunction between certain discrete and previously incoherent phenomena by binding specific attributions. These constant conjunctions may be marked by one word, a phrase or an entire deductive system. The configuration receives its meaning by virtue of experience, and the question of meaning only arises after the term or name has served to bind or fix the constant conjunction. Similarly hypotheses, concepts, models, narratives and myths all maintain that certain elements are constantly conjoined.

The selected fact is essential to this process of discovery. It is an α element which reveals the relatedness of unconnected elements, and gives coherence to the object as a whole by unifying these elements into a single function whose relatedness had not previously been seen. The selected fact terminates the dispersal of β elements and initiates a transition from the paranoid–schizoid to depressive position (Ps→D). The selected fact describes the emotional experience which accompanies a sense of discovery of coherence, making it possible to both think and talk about it.

Psychoanalysis helps people to recognize constantly recurring configurations. The analyst needs to stare at the unknown situation until a pattern begins to emerge whilst the patient is in the consulting room. The constant conjunction should become manifest after a period of time through the analyst's ability to select unifying facts from the constantly changing pattern of emotional experience. Interpretations should draw together a number of apparently unrelated facts in a way that demonstrates their relationship. The task is to abstract elements by releasing them from the existing combinations in which they are held and imposing a new pattern which makes order appear where none was before. However caution must be exercised as the connections may be in the analyst's own mind and not proper to the material. As the psychotic patient cannot identify unifying facts, objects may join together in a destructive and hostile manner. In response, the psychotic patient attacks thoughts and thinking until finally two objects cannot be combined, thus preventing coherence and destroying reality.

Symbol formation

Sensations are converted into α elements by α-function, which renders the elements suitable for use and allows them to be stored as ideograms or pictorial images. These pictorial symbols can subsequently be recovered by the individual, and memory is thus a pictorialized communication of an emotional or physical experience. For example, the psyche represents pain by holding a visual image of rubbing an injured elbow or a tearful face.

Symbol formation therefore represents the constant conjunction of elements, and depends on the ability to abandon the paranoid–schizoid position and grasp whole objects. Symbols are thus compatible with a capacity for thinking and, in keeping with the mechanism Ps↔D, must be capable of an interplay between abstraction and concretization. Abstraction, which converts elements into ideas via symbol formation so that experiences can be reapplied in various parallel situations, is the process of moving from the specific to the more general by releasing elements from the particular concrete image with which they are associated.

Symbol formation may be disordered and can give rise to deep disturbances of personality. The breakdown in symbol formation relates to an inability to transform the actual union of elements into an abstraction, and these individuals have to exist by introjection and projective identification of β elements. If emotional links are dominated by hatred and envy, then the individual is unable to form symbols. Similarly, the psychotic patient cannot symbolize and has to employ concrete images as units of thought. The patient has to wait until the occurrence of an apt event in external reality before he feels in possession of an ideograph suitable for use in communication.

Reverie and containment

The relationship between container (♀) and contained (♂) is established by the nature of the emotional link. The contained evacuates unpleasure in order to get rid of it or to have it transformed into something that is pleasurable, and the container takes in the evacuations for the same motive. Primitive emotions are contained by a container whose task it is to detoxicate incoherent, unrelated phenomena and transform them into a coherent and meaningful pattern. The usual product of container:contained (♀:♂) is meaning, and the relationship provides the basis for learning from experience. The configuration of an event may often be represented by this relationship between container and contained, and may show itself to a striking degree in many of the individual's activities. According to their background, an individual will describe various objects as containers including their mind, their personality, the unconscious, the nation, money, ideas, thoughts and actions.

This theoretical concept of container:contained (♀:♂) underpins Bion's description of maternal reverie. The infant's own feelings are too powerful to be contained within his personality and, by projective identification, he arouses in the mother feelings of which he wishes to be rid. Reverie describes the mother's capacity to receive the infant's projective identifications and yet retain a balanced state of mind. She accepts the projective identifications (or β elements) and modifies them so that they can be taken back by the infant in a more tolerable form. This shared activity becomes introjected by the infant as the container:contained (♀:♂) apparatus that is essential for α-function. The mother's ability to take in and hold the infant's projected thoughts and emotions thus determines his later capacity for thought and the ability to differentiate between conscious and unconscious elements.

However, conflict may occur in which either the container gets split apart or the contained object gets destroyed. For example, if the infant perceives the mother's anxiety and impatience, he is compelled to take back his own anxiety and the tasks which the breakdown in the mother's capacity for reverie have left unfinished are imposed on his rudimentary consciousness. These anxieties are made even more terrifying by the mother's rejection, as the infant's rudimentary consciousness cannot carry the burden placed on it by the mother's inability to accept projective identifications. A disturbance in understanding follows with an inability to grow mentally as the failure to establish a relationship between mother and infant in which normal projective identification is possible precludes the development of α-function.

The psychoanalytic situation will evoke the container:contained configuration ($♀:♂$). The individual's personality can be represented by container:contained, as can the relationship with the psychoanalyst. For example, a patient who cannot be contained within the analytic situation will engage in acting-out behaviour. To rid himself of powerful fears which his personality cannot contain, the patient splits them off and projects them into the analyst where the patient anticipates they will undergo modification before being safely re-introjected. Bion stressed the importance of the psychoanalyst's capacity to absorb and contain the discarded, split-off aspects of other personalities whilst retaining a balanced outlook. Like the mother, the analyst is required to intuitively accept the patient's fears and make interpretations conducive to α-function. The therapist is required to contain the unthinkable, unknowable and indescribable experiences of the patient and survive, allowing appropriate separation and individuation to take place.

Psychosis

Psychosis, according to Bion, is comprised of a mass of apparently unrelated facts and the psychotic's personality is a mosaic of improvised fragments. The psychotic patient can compress these fragments but cannot fuse them and, as a result, splitting and projective identification are used as substitutes for repression and denial. By taking a minutely fragmented view, the individual can avoid feeling the seriousness of the situation as hallucinations and delusions promise an instantaneous solution to the existence of unwanted emotions. These hallucinations are not representations; they are things-in-themselves, born of intolerance of frustration. Psychotic splitting also causes difficulty in the formation of symbols and the development of abstract thought. The psychotic patient thus deals with the functions of the personality as concrete objects and is unable to profit by experience. Unfortunately, 'the patient can no more make use of an hallucination than he could get milk from an imaginary breast' (*Cogitations*, 1992).

As the psychotic patient has no α-function, even thoughts and ideas are treated as concrete objects. If someone moves a table, it is to the psychotic as if someone had interfered with his mind. Phantasies are also felt to be indistinguishable from facts, leading to an internal universe populated by inanimate objects. The psychotic patient employs these concrete images as units of thought, and needs the thing-in-itself as he cannot manipulate words and thoughts to do work in the absence of the object. The patient needs the actual object into which to project split-off parts of himself in order to allow their existence. The psychotic patient therefore has to wait for external representations in order to 'think' about something as he cannot simply imagine a situation.

Psychoanalysts are concerned with seeing the relatedness of unconnected elements in the analytic situation. This evidence may be scattered in the material over a period of time, and the analyst must demonstrate the fragments that the patient is attempting to juxtapose. To achieve this, the analyst must participate in the state of hallucinosis and place himself in a position to intuit the elements and the laws which govern their changes. Bion believed that psychotic patients would never accept an interpretation, however correct, unless they felt that the analyst had passed through a similar emotional crisis as a part of the act of giving the interpretation. The psychotic patient will also pay little attention to a communication unless it is on exactly the right wavelength. He is very precise, and does not like interpretations which are 'off the beam' (Bion, 1978).

The psychotic patient may set out, specifically during the sessions, to attack the production of α elements in himself or in the analyst. The patient denies the analyst conditions to fulfil α-function in an attempt to destroy the links with reality and between objects. The mechanisms of splitting, projective identification, depersonalization and hallucination are often part of the analysis of psychotic patients who forcibly push parts of themselves into the analyst. Thought is also attacked as a link which provides coherence and the analyst's 'rules' will be under constant attack. However, Bion (Sao Paulo, 1974) repeatedly advised that, if the minimum conditions for analysis still exist, the analyst should continue to analyse the patient even after they have suffered a psychotic breakdown and have been hospitalized.

The non-psychotic part of the personality

Bion developed the hypothetical concept of a non-psychotic part of the personality as even the most disturbed patient can show flashes of intuition and common sense. Bion postulated that the patient, no matter how psychotic, will have an accessible, rational, responsible and mature part of the personality with which the therapist can make contact. Bion (Sao Paulo, 1978) differentiated between sane psychotics (who had vestiges of rational, conscious behaviour) and insane psychotics (who deteriorated and were admitted to mental hospitals). Attacks on linking lead to an ever-widening divergence between the psychotic and non-psychotic parts of the personality until the gulf is felt to be unbridgeable. The aim of analysis is to help the insane psychotic to progress towards psychotic sanity.

Differentiation of the psychotic from the non-psychotic personality depends on a minute splitting and fragmentation of the part of the personality that is concerned with awareness of internal and external reality. Where the non-psychotic part of the personality resorts to repression, the psychotic part of the personality employs splitting and projective identification. The non-psychotic part of the personality is also associated with assimilation of sense impressions, α-function and α elements. It must be capable of tolerating frustration, guilt and depression as well. The non-psychotic view impels towards further discovery and synthesis, and there is a shift towards a higher valuation of the external object at the expense of the hallucinated internal object. In the analysis of the psychotic patient, all interpretations should be addressed to the non-psychotic part of the personality even though there may be little evidence for its existence.

Learning from experience

Both emotional and physical experiences may give rise to meaning, especially if a significant constant conjunction is identified. This constant conjunction of disparate elements is initially devoid of specific meaning. The named conjunction only accumulates meaning as a result of personal experiences from which the individual can learn. Learning from experience is therefore based on container:contained ($\female:\male$), Ps$\leftrightarrow$D and the interplay between concretization and abstraction. β elements cannot be made unconscious and therefore no learning can take place without α-function as only undigested facts will be retained.

It is inevitably frustration which initiates the procedures necessary for learning by experience, which entail the storing of experiences and the making of internal and external reality available to thought. Stored emotional experience is essential to understanding and allows the experience to be used in conscious waking thought, in unconscious waking thought and in dream thoughts. Visual imagery and the K link are germane to learning from experience, and the necessary transformation takes place more readily if the reality principle is dominant. According to Bion (1961), there is a hatred of having to learn by experience at all and a lack of faith in the worth of such learning. Omnipotence is preferred to thoughts or thinking, and the longed for alternative to learning from experience is 'arriving fully equipped as an adult fitted by instinct to know without training or development exactly how to live and move and be in a group'. The psychotic proves unable to learn from experience in exactly this way.

Transformations

Transformations operate at several different levels of sophistication. α-function transforms sense impressions into emotional experiences which can be stored and later used in dreaming and other thoughts. By means of α-function, β elements too are transformed into α elements that are more suitable for psychological use. Converting an experience into a pictorial image serves as a transformation, and the report of a dream is the verbal transformation of a visual image. Dream-work-α (later described as α-function) transforms sense impressions to make them suitable material for dream thoughts. The latent dream thoughts are transformed into manifest content by dream-work. In this way, dream-work-α is able to transform conscious material into unconscious material suitable for unconscious waking thinking. Abstraction is also an aspect of the transformation of an emotional experience into α elements by α-function. Similarly, a state of 'knowing' (K) may be transformed into a state of 'being' or 'becoming' (O). Transformations in O are more conducive to psychological development than transformation in K.

Transformations may be scientific, aesthetic or religious, and may be prevalent in hallucinations, painting, music or mathematics. Psychoanalysis is itself a transformation and tries to help the patient to transform that part of an emotional experience of which he is unconscious into an emotional experience of which he is conscious. As the facts of an analytic experience are transformed into an interpretation, interpretations too are transformations. The analyst needs to be able to transform what the patient is saying into a usable form and, likewise, the patient must be able to transform what the analyst has said to allow it to seep from conscious rational levels to other levels of the mind. As any element involved in a transformation may effect any other element, transformations may occur in cycles and Bion's theory thus illuminates a chain of phenomena in which the understanding of one link helps in the understanding of others.

Transformation therefore represents constant conjunctions and the shift from the paranoid–schizoid to the depressive position may elucidate a pattern that brings together disparate elements, making visible both coherence and meaning. However, if the emotion is psychotic in nature, it cannot be transformed by α-function but instead remains a mental event which is characterized by pleasure or pain. The psychotic patient deliberately attacks his α-function to prevent the transformation of psychical qualities into α elements.

Interplay between the paranoid–schizoid and depressive positions

There is an underlying harmony and interplay between the paranoid–schizoid (Ps) and depressive (D) positions. The paranoid–schizoid position is characterized by internal psychic incoherence, splitting and fragmentation. In D, the disparate elements of Ps are brought together. Ps↔D thus represents the interplay of fragmentation and integration. D→Ps leads to dispersal of particles with feelings of persecution, while Ps→D leads to integration with feelings of depression. The dispersal of β elements, for example, may be controlled by Ps→D. In contrast, fragmentation is used to substitute persecutory anxiety for the dread of depression. There should be freedom of mental movement between Ps and D as this successful transition is essential to mental development and critical in the process of psychoanalysis.

When hitherto unrelated elements are discovered to be coherent by the operation of Ps→D, their relationship with one another is fixed by naming the relationship. It is this selected fact or name which unifies and precipitates the coherence of Ps elements, and which marks the transition from Ps→D. As the Ps phase, dominated by part-object relationships, may give rise to whole-object relationships, the depressive position can also be represented by the combination of container (♀) and contained (♂). The interplay between Ps and D precedes the development of container:contained (♀:♂), which in turn leads to the development of meaning. A meaningful relationship with the whole object can only be attained on achieving the depressive position and the successful completion of container:contained (♀:♂).

The interplay between Ps↔D is related to the development of thought and thinking. Ps and D are vital factors in converting the unknown to the known, and the individual's capacity for learning depends throughout life on the ability to tolerate the dynamic and continuing interaction between the two positions. The foundations of primitive thinking should be laid in the paranoid–schizoid position, leading to more sophisticated thoughts as Ps→D brings together elements to form signs and symbols. The capacity to form symbols is dependent on the ability to grasp whole objects, which requires the abandonment of Ps with its attendant splitting and a capacity to tolerate depression arising from the synthesizing function of D.

Ps→D also involves a movement from concrete to abstract thinking. Both dreaming and unconscious waking thinking are occupied with transitions between Ps and D. Attaining the depressive position may lead to the development of rational depression at discovering how little one knows about one's self. The successful interpretation may likewise, whilst bringing relief, push the patient into a state of depression. Individuals may therefore try to obstruct the Ps↔D mechanism, and attacks on linking may inhibit α-function to reduce the synthesizing (and hence depressing) function of D.

Knowledge (K)

To 'know' the truth is a matter of psychic need as we hate being ignorant and have an active investment in finding answers. Knowledge (K), the state of knowing, trying to know or knowing about, is therefore conducive to mental health. Curiosity, synthesis, memory, model-making, container: contained, Ps↔D and abstraction are associated with K. Knowledge equals the sum total of α elements and β elements, and covers everything the individual knows and does not know. However, K is a state of knowing, and not a state of becoming or being.

Knowledge (K) is an assertion of relationship, and the earliest and most primitive manifestations of K occur between mother and infant. The breast fulfils a K function by moderating the fear that has been projected into it and allowing the infant to re-introject a tolerable and growth-stimulating part of its personality in due course. The K link thus operates against a background of the senses and is capable only of yielding knowledge 'about' something. In the basic K relationship 'X knows Y', X is not in possession of knowledge about Y but rather X is in the state of getting to know Y and Y is in the state of getting to be known by X. However, the word 'know', as in 'I know X', has a constantly changing meaning which is determined by its context.

Self-knowledge is the aim of psychoanalysis. It requires courage on the part of the patient because he is terrified of learning something about himself which has never wanted to know and of which he has spent his life not being aware. By means of interpretation, the analyst uses all clinical material to illuminate a K relationship. However, in ordinary life, our interest is chiefly in the nature of what we are trying to know and not in the process by which we try to get to know it. We often use what we 'know' to avoid 'becoming' – K as opposed to O. Every emotional experience of knowledge gained is at the same time an emotional experience of ignorance illuminated. In analysis, every gain in self-knowledge appears to reveal how little is known until we find ourselves having to ask whether we are capable of knowing at all and are not merely under the illusion of thinking we know.

O

O represents emotional experiences which may be otherwise described as ultimate reality, absolute truth, the Godhead, the infinite or the thing-in-itself. O is 'darkness' and 'formlessness', and represents unknowable psychic reality. O is therefore a state of 'becoming' which can be felt but it cannot be 'known' as it does not fall within the domain of knowledge (K) or learning. Verbal, musical and artistic modes of communication are all transformations of O as they achieve contact with psychic reality and allow the characteristics of O to evolve. Objects known or knowable by man are all evolutions of O which have been transformed into thought. O may be represented by a constant conjunction, with myths and dreams emerging where O has evolved sufficiently to be represented by sensuous experience. Change is therefore a component of O which may enter the domain of K when it has evolved to a point where it can be known.

The patient's presentation will be significant in representing his view of O. As the analyst's attention is focused on the unknown and the unknowable, O represents the central feature of every psychoanalytic situation. The analyst must therefore achieve a frame of mind in which he is receptive to the O of the analytic experience. The analyst is particularly concerned with evolved elements of O which are represented in a form that can be known, such as dreams and myths. However, there may be a difference between the patient's experience of O and the analyst's experience of O. The analyst should therefore wait for evolution to take place in the session so that O becomes manifest in K through the emergence of actual events. O may also be transformed to K using the objects of memory and desire to mark a new constellation and precipitate a constant conjunction. For example, interpreting hallucinations by transforming an unknowable emotional experience into a sensuously apprehendable event is a transformation from O→K. Psychoanalytic discovery also requires transformations from K→O which represent a move from 'knowing' to 'being'.

O in any analytic situation is equally available for transformation by the analyst and the analysand, and any O not common to both is incapable of psychoanalytic investigation. Transformations in K are feared when they threaten the emergence of transformations in O, and resistance to K→O manifests itself as a preference for knowing about something instead of becoming something. As change in the direction of O is painful, and unity with O is a fearful prospect, defences are erected against 'becoming' O. However, the value of interventions will be therapeutically greater if they are conducive to transformations in O rather than transformations in K. The more the analyst is in contact with O, the more real will be their interpretation.

Love (L) and hate (H)

Love (L) and hate (H), like knowledge (K), are dynamic links between psychoanalytic objects. Terms such as 'love' and 'hate' are hypotheses expressing a constant conjunction between feelings which are not directly related to the senses. Bion considered only love and hate because he regarded them as comprising all other feelings. They do not represent facts or discrete happenings but represent interactional processes between X and Y. H is a hostile link and represents the basic relationship of X hates Y. L represents the basic relationship of X loves Y. However, L and H are only substitutes for O or the ultimate relationship. Although it is important to feel love as well as hate, strong feelings of love and hate tend to decrease our ability to discriminate and learn.

α elements, β elements and α-function

Neither α nor β elements are real or observable. Bion defined β elements as unassimilated sense impressions which yielded only pleasure or pain. They are unprocessed elements which are incapable of abstraction and which cannot provide meaning. As β elements cannot be made unconscious, there is also no scope for repression and intolerance of frustration leads to the immediate evacuation of β elements which are employed as projectiles to rid the psyche of accretions of stimuli. Although β elements represent the earliest matrix from which thoughts can be supposed to arise, they are not thoughts and are confined to the domain of action. As β elements lack a capacity for linkage, they seek cohesion through a container and are only employed where α elements do not exist. Compulsive actions are examples of β elements. In contrast α elements are the most genetically primitive elements of thought proper. They are the processed products of α-function, and form the units of dream thought and narrative. Without α elements, it is impossible to know anything.

α-function, initially called dream-work-α or just α, occurs whether awake or asleep. It allows mental digestion of sense impressions by producing α elements which are capable of association. α-function is thus a synthesizing process which modifies frustration and operates to store conscious emotional experience in the unconscious. α-function is therefore essential for the operation of unconscious waking thinking, narrative, attention, memory, dreaming, judgement, abstraction and generalization. Increased α-function also increases the dominance of the reality principle, whereas decreased α-function encourages projective identification and omnipotent phantasy.

Hostility and destructive attacks lead to fragmentation of α-function, and thought becomes impossible as the patient retains only undigested facts which are antithetical to a sense of reality. If α-function is disturbed, sense impressions and emotional experiences remain unchanged and are evacuated as β elements by projective identification as a result of frustration. In the psychotic patient, the contact barrier of α elements is destroyed and replaced with a β-screen of β elements which are unable to differentiate between conscious and unconscious states of mind. As a result, α-function is reversed with dispersal of psychic elements and the creation of bizarre objects.

Interpretation

From the incomprehensible, inaudible, ineffable part of the session comes the material for interpretations. Interpretation does not use conscious material to interpret the unconscious; it is using the unconscious to interpret a conscious state of mind. As analysts interpret situations which are beyond comprehension or experience, there are an enormous number of possible interpretations depending on whether the analyst works with the common root of the interpretations or the different varieties which subsequently emerge. An interpretation should not be given on a single association, but should be related to clinical material as it unfolds in the analysis with emphasis on feelings rather than words.

To give an interpretation, the analyst has to be capable of verbalizing a statement about his sense impressions, his intuitions and his primitive reactions to what the patient says. The task confronting the analyst is to bring intuition and reason to bear on an emotional experience between two people in such a way that not only the analyst but also the analysand gains an understanding of the analysand's response to that emotional situation. Bion would often remain silent, hoping to become aware of or observe something which could be interpreted. If possible, he would leave the initiative to the patient. However, it is necessary to have some agreement between analysand and analyst on what material requires interpretation. The problem is to know which of possible interpretations is at a given time correct, and the analyst has to find a method by which to establish an order of preference. The psychoanalyst's interpretation should always be of a state of mind, keeping to the ordinary conversational system of verbal communication. An inherent difficulty in analysis is that any interpretation also tells the patient something about the analyst, who may harbour a desire to see further than either the analysand or some of his colleagues.

The interpretation should draw together a number of apparently unrelated facts in a way that demonstrates their relationship. There is a value in listening to the associations until, in due course, a pattern emerges which can be interpreted to the patient. The analyst should do his best to assimilate the information made available to him, derived from the emotional experience with a unique individual, and transform it into an interpretation. Interpretations therefore make us aware of coherence and order where, without them, incoherence and disorder would reign. In this sense, interpretations are identical with the selected fact. It is not enough for the analyst to be convinced that there is evidence for the truth of his interpretations; he must have enough evidence available to afford the analysand the opportunity of being persuaded by the cogency of the interpretation.

No interpretation is any good unless it is reminiscent of real life. When an analyst makes an interpretation, he causes the universe of discussion to expand. Each free association and each interpretation therefore represents a change in the situation which is being analysed. In this sense, the interpretation is merely setting a formal seal on work that has already been done and is no longer of much consequence. Whilst the successful interpretation brings relief, it also takes the patient into the depressive position and confronts him with yet wider vistas of unrelated elements. Thus correct interpretations may be followed almost immediately by a sense of depression. The patient may therefore offer every inducement to bring the analyst to interpretations that leave the patient's defences intact, and may try to deprive the analyst's interpretation of meaning. The analyst needs to be aware of bizarre responses to interpretations which would appear to be quite correct.

Memory and desire

Memory involves objects that are past, internal and possessed. Desire involves objects that are future, external and coveted. Both intrude into the analyst's state of mind when observation is essential, blinding him to the point at issue and distorting his judgement. Memory is always only a partial aspect of experience, and is distorted by the influence of unconscious forces. Memory and desire derive from experiences gained through the senses; they are evocations of feelings of pleasure and pain, and generate sensuous greed. Hallucinations, for example, are born of desire and memory of satisfaction is used to deny its absence.

Memory has no place in the practice of psychoanalysis, and the impulse to 'remember' what has been said or done must be resisted. The desire for results, for understanding and even the wish to be a good analyst may prove obstructive. For example, the analyst may be forced to delve into memories and desires as a defence against uncertainty. Memory and desire also give projective identification a direction, and prevent transformation. Theories too may increase memory and desire. Attention should not be focused on elements that are already known as this occludes the presence of unknown and therefore more relevant elements. Also, whilst the analyst waits for material that he has been led to expect, he fails to observe material that is actually presenting itself. Memory and desire are therefore opacities that obstruct the intuition of unknown phenomena, eroding the analyst's power to analyse. Bion made no notes, and resisted any attempts to remember a particular session or have desires regarding a patient's well-being. To mark a new constant conjunction, the analyst needs to be able to discard the evocative characteristics of memory and desire. If memory could be dispensed with, desire would likewise disappear, and vice versa.

Receptiveness achieved by excluding memory and desire is an extremely penetrating procedure, and must be regarded as an essential discipline for psychoanalysts. The analyst must free himself by being vulnerable to the facts, by discarding what he already knows, by creating space for new ideas and by leaving room for the patient. The psychoanalyst's own analysis is important in denuding memory and desire as he will be more likely to experience painful emotions and anxieties which are usually screened by analytic theories. A changed order of analytic phenomena also occurs, with increased awareness of the unique nature of every psychoanalytic experience. As memory and desire are discernible as elements in the transference, the analyst must resist any impulse to gratify the analysand's desires or to crave gratification for his own desires. In time, the psychoanalyst will become more aware of the pressure of memories and desires and will become more skilled at avoiding them.

Bion tried hard to start the session with as blank a mind as possible, without trying to remember what the patient had said on previous occasions. He advocated that the psychoanalyst should aim to achieve a state of mind in which, at every session, he feels that he has not seen the patient before. If the analyst feels that he has seen the patient before, he is treating the wrong patient, as the patient whom he saw yesterday, or last week, month or year, will not be the same person as he is seeing today. Every session attended by the patient must have no history and no future as the analyst who comes to the session with an active memory is in no position to make observations of mental phenomena.

Experiences in groups

The individual is a political animal and the group is essential to mental life. Bion sought to extend psychoanalysis into group settings as he felt that analytic approaches to the individual and the group simply dealt with different facets of the same phenomena. This included the Kleinian theories of projective identification and the interplay between the paranoid–schizoid and depressive positions. As groups benefit from a common purpose, unconscious tendencies will find an outlet in the mass action of group behaviour. The group may therefore be perceived as one fragmented individual, with each person representing a different state of mind. Loss of individual distinctiveness is the price for group membership, and group mentality is hostile to individual thought as the group needs to preserve its coherence and identity.

Group culture will always show evidence of basic assumptions in which shared opinions held to be essential to group integrity and cohesion may pass unchallenged as fact. Participation in a basic assumption group requires no training, experience or mental development and the group does not need or use organization, cooperation, symbolization or rational verbal communication. Bion described three basic assumptions – flight–fight (BaF), pairing (BaP) and dependency (BaD). In BaD, the basic assumption of dependence, one person is always felt to be in a position to supply the needs of the group, and the rest are in a position in which their needs are supplied. In BaP, the basic assumption of pairing, there is a premonition of sex and reproduction as the basic assumption. In BaF, the basic assumption of flight–fight, the group has met to fight or to flee. All three basic assumptions contain the idea of a leader and, when the group is pervaded by one basic assumption, the emotional states related to the other two groups are in abeyance. Unorganized groups are more easily submerged by basic assumptions which are opposed to development and obstruct the work function of the group. The basic assumption must be evaluated at any given moment as group culture may change from one basic assumption to another.

The work group (W) is a sophisticated group which serves to translate thought and feelings into behaviours which are adapted to reality. Development is an important function of work groups, and the leader needs to mobilize emotion without mobilizing the accompanying basic assumptions. The characteristics of the work group are similar to those attributed to the ego by Freud, and involve mental functioning designed to further the task in hand. The effort put into maintaining a sophisticated structure indicates the strength of emotion associated with the basic assumptions. The sophisticated structure is precarious and, as contributions to the work group decrease, so contributions to the basic assumption group increase.

Bion's concept of group therapy is psychotherapy of the group and not simply public psychotherapy of individuals in a group. Group psychotherapy is focused on the tensions within and the actual experiences of the group whose therapeutic occupation is the study of the afflictions from which they individually and collectively suffer. The clinician needs to turn his attention to the structure of the group, and to the forces operating in that structure. The psychoanalyst should establish no rules and put forward no agenda or structure for the group. Behaviour is interpreted in terms of the group's attention to the analyst as a form of group transference, and interpretations have to be made on the strength of the analyst's own emotional reactions.

The Grid

The analyst must be able to measure change, and psychoanalysis thus requires a frame of reference and a system of coordinates to measure progress. Bion developed the Grid as an instrument with which practising psychoanalysts could assess and think about material from the psychoanalytic session using signs that could be manipulated like numbers in mathematics. The Grid aimed to help the transition between theoretical background and consulting room phenomena, including dreams and oedipal material. It also served to discriminate psychoanalytic elements from one another by allowing the analyst to scrutinize the patient's associations and the analyst's own subsequent interpretations. Doubtful material could be referred to the Grid for extra-analytic meditation with the analyst placing conflicting statements into separate categories and then comparing them. The dynamic link between these phases on the Grid was represented by L, H or K. Bion hoped that reviewing analytic work by means of the Grid would lead to a facility in the unconscious for immediate assessment of evidence as it unfolds in the session.

The Grid is analogous to a ruler in physical science and is not a substitute for observation. The coordinates on the Grid apply equally to process and content; what matters is both the communication and the use to which it is being put. The content of knowledge and the acquisition of knowledge belong to different axes, and thus elements have a character both by virtue of the row and the column of which they are a member. The links between rows and columns on the Grid are provided by container:contained, the interplay between the paranoid–schizoid and depressive positions, and the concept of the selected fact. The vertical column (A–H) indicates developmental status and expresses differences in sophistication rather than function. Movement towards H represents increased sophistication and is used when emphasis is on growth of the patient's thoughts. The horizontal axis (1–6) states the use to which the elements are being put, and the function that an element is being made to perform.

The Grid categories make it possible to draw attention to and find shades of difference in meaning in a way which would be difficult or impossible without them. By regarding the patient's statements as transformations, and categorizing them by means of the Grid, one can do something towards understanding what is taking place. The analyst recalls the session and speculatively places a given statement in the category which he thinks is correct. This gives direction to his speculations and, by binding a number of elements in this way, the analyst can discover the meaning of these elements' conjunction. The possibility that the episode might be better placed elsewhere on the Grid helps to stimulate the analyst's capacity for attention to the elements of psychoanalysis.

Bion did not intend for the Grid to be used during the working psychoanalytic session. He elaborated the Grid for his daily 'cogitations' as an imaginative exercise, similar to the musician who practises scales. The Grid aimed to sharpen and develop intuition until it became increasingly possible to arrive at conclusions instantaneously which were at first the fruits of laborious intellectualization. Bion later described the Grid as an inadequate attempt to produce an instrument made up of psychoanalytic theories. However, he hoped that someone would be able to turn it to good account and develop a more satisfactory and improved version that could be of some use to practising psychoanalysts.

Clinical example

Kathleen is a seventeen-year-old girl who presented with overtly psychotic symptoms. She was 'hearing voices', and had lived much of her life in an 'internal world' of her own making. She was allocated a male therapist for individual therapy and, following an introductory meeting, the first session was arranged. However, the therapist inadvertently missed the scheduled session and arranged a second session several days later. Having made a clear mental note to remember the session, he again forgot the planned arrangements and began to wonder how the two missed appointments were related to the patient. With careful monitoring of his own feelings, the therapist managed to attend the third session as planned but, within twenty minutes, he fell asleep.

This was repeated for the next three sessions, alerting the therapist to a pattern that was emerging in regard to the patient which could not be explained away by tiredness. On beginning to feel sleepy in the sessions, the therapist started to describe his feelings to the patient and, as the therapy progressed, he was better able to detect the impending sleepiness and respond to it verbally. The therapist slowly came to understand that Kathleen's life was governed by significant internal and external threats which proved psychologically unmanageable and which led her to withdraw into her 'own private world' where she felt safe. A similar pattern had engulfed the therapist who would avoid the patient's unconscious sense of fear and despair by missing sessions or falling asleep. As the therapist proved more and more able to cope with Kathleen's difficult feelings and thoughts, the therapy took a turn for the better.

Kathleen remained silent for many of the initial sessions and responded little to the therapist's comments or questions. She seemed very absent from the room, as if having escaped into her internal world. Direct attempts by the therapist to find out more about this internal world were unsuccessful. It gradually emerged that Kathleen heard voices, which had been present for many years and which belonged to images of her childhood toys. These 'voices' lived in her head and maintained a running commentary throughout the day. Although the voices were at times punitive and frightening, by and large they were welcome company and Kathleen had little desire to change the status quo.

Instead of persisting with fruitless attempts to relate to this 'psychotic' world, the therapist instead engaged the non-psychotic part of Kathleen's personality which had been able to establish friendships and gain academic success. The non-psychotic part of her personality was readily engaged, and the sessions became more animated and lively. Kathleen was able to discuss many of her concerns relating to her 'internal world' and, whilst the therapist was denied access, Kathleen was willing to act as go-between when difficulties arose. She was able to express some of the therapist's concerns about the intentions of the 'voices' directly to them, but also conveyed to the therapist those experiences in which the voices were scathing of an interpretation or laughed at an error made by the therapist.

Kathleen's voices remained active, and no attempt was made to engage directly with them. Instead, the more sane part of her personality was engaged and the therapy progressed as if working with a neurotic patient. As a result, the 'volume' of Kathleen's voices decreased and they were often silent. She was more able to express herself verbally, having learnt that the therapist could contain her anxieties, moderate them, and return them to her in a more manageable form. Her general demeanour improved, as did her capacity to think for herself and maintain social relationships. She was felt to live in the real world for greater periods of time, only withdrawing to her internal world at times of severe stress. She became increasingly animated, more in touch with her own feelings and the therapy progressed with beneficial effects.

Further reading

Bion, W.R. (1982) *The Long Week-End, 1897–1919*. Oxford: Fleetwood Press. (Reprinted London: Free Association Books, 1986.)

Bléandonu, G. (1994) *Wilfred Bion: His Life and Works, 1897–1979*. London: Free Association Books.

Bibliography

Bion, W.R. (1961) *Experiences in Groups and Other Papers*. London: Tavistock. (Reprinted London: Routledge, 1994.)

Bion, W.R. (1962) *Learning from Experience*. London: Heinemann Medical. (Reprinted London: Karnac Books, 1991.)

Bion, W.R. (1963) *Elements of Psychoanalysis*. London: Heinemann Medical. (Reprinted London: Karnac Books, 1989.)

Bion, W.R. (1965) *Transformations*. London: Heinemann Medical. (Reprinted London: Karnac Books, 1991.)

Bion, W.R. (1967) *Second Thoughts*. London: Heinemann Medical. (Reprinted London: Karnac Books, 1993.)

Bion, W.R. (1970) *Attention and Interpretation*. London: Tavistock. (Reprinted London: Karnac Books, 1993.)

Bion, W.R. (1977) *Two Papers: The Grid and Caesura*. Rio de Janeiro: Imago Editora. (Reprinted London: Karnac Books, 1989.)

Bion, W.R. (1978) *Four Discussions with W.R. Bion*. Strathclyde: Clunie Press.

Bion, W.R. (1980) *Bion in New York and Sao Paulo*. Strathclyde: Clunie Press.

Bion, W.R. (1982) *The Long Week-End, 1897–1919*. Oxford: Fleetwood Press. (Reprinted London: Free Association Books, 1986.)

Bion, W.R. (1990) *Brazilian Lectures*. London: Karnac Books.

Bion, W.R. (1991) *Cogitations*. London: Karnac Books.

Bléandonu, G. (1994) *Wilfred Bion: His Life and Works, 1897–1979*. London: Free Association Books.

5

The Independent British School

Michael van Beinum

> *This is the place that I have set out to examine, the separation that is not a separation but a form of union.*
>
> Winnicott, 1971, p. 115

Historical perspective

Within the British Psycho-Analytical Society there are three groups, each with its own characteristics. These are the Kleinian Group, the Contemporary Freudian Group and the Independent Group. This division occurred as a result of what has become known as the 'Controversial Discussions', which took place in the Society between January 1943 and May 1944. On one side were Anna Freud and her followers, outlining the different stages of psychosexual development (e.g. Abraham, 1924) and claiming the mantle of Sigmund Freud. Disagreeing with this group were Melanie Klein and her supporters who, although at pains to demonstrate their faithfulness to the theoretical lines suggested by Freud, were developing a new metapsychology.

There were a great many differences between the two sides, such as theoretical beliefs, in what they each saw as the aims of psychoanalysis and in the manner of giving transference interpretations to the patient (Kohon, 1986; Sandler and Dreher, 1996). Anna Freud, for example, emphasized the different stages of psychosexual development (oral, anal, phallic and oedipal), the role of the ego and the analysis of the mechanisms of defence. Klein, in contrast, saw psychopathology as being laid down in the first few months of life and stressed the persistence throughout life of early infantile unconscious phantasies. She was concerned with describing the different positions – the paranoid–schizoid and depressive positions – that she saw as present throughout life and reflecting different forms of object-relating. The aim of analysis was to promote a developmental movement towards, and working through of, the depressive position, with particular emphasis on the therapeutic value of mourning.

The major differences between the two groups led to a difficulty in training candidates. Following the mediating influences of John Rickman, Sylvia Payne and William Gillespie, a 'Gentleman's Agreement' was arrived at, where two parallel training courses, A and B, were set up under one training committee. Seminar leaders for Group A were drawn from the society at large, whereas Anna Freud and her followers would lead seminars for the B group. A student's first training case was to be supervised by an analyst of their own group, while their second case was to be supervised by an analyst who was neither a Kleinian nor an Anna Freudian, but a member of the Independent Group.

Thus, following the Controversial Discussions, a 'Middle Group', or Independent Group, came into being, made up of analysts who had refused to belong exclusively to either the Kleinian or Freudian alignment. The Independent Group therefore consisted of a diverse and broad range of therapists, many of whom were strongly influenced by both Freud and Klein. The main figures include Fairbairn, Winnicott and Balint, although many other notable analysts come under its umbrella.

Principles of theory and practice

General principles

It is not possible to give a brief definition of the core beliefs of the Independent tradition, and this chapter will focus primarily on one aspect of their work, namely a stress on the relation of the subject to his object. Such an object relationship may be either internal or external, where internal objects are phantoms, images occurring in phantasies which are reacted to as though they were real (Rycroft, 1972). It describes a way of relating that is considered as an interrelationship: the individual effects his objects as much as his objects effect him. Within this broad definition, different members of the Independent Group have widely divergent views. They 'do not constitute a "school" by virtue of subscribing to a shared set of beliefs but, like a school of painters, by virtue of a shared set of problems and sensibilities' (Greenberg and Mitchell, 1983, p. 220). They have in common an innovative and open approach, and are rooted in empiricism.

Many Independent analysts take classical psychoanalytic theory and technique as axiomatic. Thus much of the analytic work is taken up with analysing defences against anxieties arising out of the oedipal, or three-person, situation. From Klein, the Independents took the concept of projective identification and hence the need to contain such projections by the therapist providing a holding environment. Projective identification, where the patient splits off an unacceptable part of himself and has the illusion that it belongs instead to the therapist, can also be used in the service of unconscious communication. The therapist may become aware of unusual feelings and thoughts arising in himself which are the product of the relationship with the patient, and which *may* be a means by which a patient lets the therapist know something which cannot be communicated, at that time, in any other way. The Independents stress the importance to later adult pathology of early traumatic episodes occurring in the first two years of life, and therefore an understanding of their developmental theories is important.

Michael Balint

Michael Balint completed his analytic training with Ferenczi in Hungary in 1926. He moved to Manchester in 1939, and later to London, to avoid the political persecution in his own country. After the death of his first wife, Alice, he married again. His second wife, Enid, was also an analyst and they jointly developed 'Balint groups in general practice'. Groups of GPs would meet on a regular basis with a psychotherapist to facilitate discussion of particular patients and their responses to those patients. The overall aim was to promote deeper insight by GPs into the (often unconscious) negotiation between doctor and patient about symptoms and their meaning. Michael Balint died in 1970.

Freud proposed the concept of primary narcissism, meaning that in the beginning the infant loves himself and is pleasure-seeking, before going on, in the oedipal phase, to develop the capacity to love others. In contrast, Balint advanced the view that the psychological growth of the infant, from the beginning, was absolutely dependent upon an intense relatedness with his primary caregiver. Based on analytic work with deeply regressed patients, he described a condition he termed 'the basic fault'. By this he meant a geological fault, in the sense of there being a disturbance in the structure of the patient's mind. Patients said that they felt there was something missing inside themselves, rather than having a feeling of something dammed up and needing to be released (Sutherland, 1994). Balint assumed that this fault, or scar, was caused by a failure of fit between the needs of the infant and the response of the mother. The mother might have met the physical needs of the infant, such as for food and warmth, but she might not have related to the baby as a person in his own right, with emotional needs for love and understanding.

During analysis, patients might regress to the level of the basic fault. Balint saw this as regression to a pre-oedipal stage, a stage at which the infant was not yet able to cope with a three-person relationship. Balint was here referring to the stage theory of infant development, where the infant expresses innate drives for pleasure through different bodily parts according to his stage of development – namely oral, anal, phallic and, finally, oedipal (Abraham, 1924). At the oedipal level, analyst and analysand communicate with a common language and verbal interpretations of the material are in order. But, at the level of the basic fault, such verbal communication would be inappropriate, and a different technique is called for (Quinodoz, 1993). Balint postulated two types of regression. In 'benign regression' patients are seeking recognition, the fulfilment of primary relational needs, while in 'malignant regression' the patient is seeking gratification of instinctual cravings. If the needs of a patient with a benign regression are met, the patient can grow and develop. But if the instinctual cravings of a patient in a malignant regression, such as the need to physically hold the therapist, are succumbed to by the therapist, psychological growth does not take place and leads instead to further, and insatiable, demands for gratification.

Lastly, Balint postulated two types of personality resulting from attempts by the patient to deal with an internal basic fault. In ocnophilia the subject, still seeking emotional support and understanding, clings to others for security and is afraid of open spaces. In philobatism, however, one sees the opposite – namely an attempt to do without others and instead relate to inner objects. Both these object relations were seen by Balint as a defence against the failure of the perceived environment.

Balint, in 'The Unobtrusive Analyst' (*The Basic Fault*, 1968), described a patient who had been in analysis with him for over two years.

> *'The patient remained silent right from the start of the session for more than 30 minutes; the analyst accepted this and, realizing what possibly was happening, waited without any attempt at interference; in fact, he did not even feel uncomfortable or under pressure to do something ... The silence was eventually broken by the patient starting to sob, relieved, and soon after he was able to speak. He told his analyst that at long last he was able to reach himself; ever since childhood he had never been left alone, there had always been someone telling him what to do.'*
>
> *Balint went on to explain how verbal interpretations of the silence might have been correct, but would have broken the silence; furthermore, there was no conflict in the silence which had to be interpreted. Instead, the patient needed a silence and an analyst who, at that moment in time, understood this. The task of the analyst was to provide the right circumstances where such a silence could occur, by means of an uninterrupted analytical session and a long period of good analysis, and then to provide the empathic, silent, support which allowed the patient to find himself.*

D.W. Winnicott

Donald Winnicott (1896–1971) came from a middle-class Plymouth background. He became a prominent paediatrician in London, and his detailed and humane understanding of mothers and babies pervades his psycho-analytical work (Greenberg and Mitchell, 1983; Clancier and Kalmanovitch, 1987). He did a great deal to popularize psychoanalytic insights by a series of radio broadcasts and articles for the popular press on aspects of child-rearing. He was analysed first by Strachey, and later by Riviere, one of Klein's closest collaborators. Winnicott used a playful, and often poetical, style of writing. He could make use of established theoretical concepts in an idiosyncratic manner, often developing them into startlingly original ideas.

Winnicott stressed the primacy of the mother–child relationship from birth. For him, there was 'no such thing as an infant, meaning of course that whenever one finds an infant one finds maternal care, and without maternal care there would be no infant' (1960, p. 39). Infants come into the world with an inherited potential, but the development of this potential in the infant is intimately linked up to maternal care. When the baby is born, the mother, by virtue of her 'primary maternal preoccupation' – an intense preoccupation with her infant – is able to create for the baby the illusion that he has omnipotent control of his world. At this early stage of development, the infant has not separated out a self from the maternal care on which he is utterly dependent in a psychological sense.

Important for the subsequent healthy psychological development of the infant is what Winnicott called holding; this refers not just to the mother physically holding the infant, but also to her managing the total environmental provision, including the psychological and physiological experiences of the infant. She needs to hold the infant, not only in her arms, but in her mind as well. This requires a 'good-enough mother'; a mother who pays sufficient attention to both meeting the instinctual need for feeding and also to understanding other psychological needs, such as for security and to discover the world. A good-enough mother is reliable and empathic, taking account of the infant's sensitivity and uniqueness, and is in touch with the subtle physiological and psychological changes in her infant from day to day. As a result of such holding by a good-enough mother the infant begins to develop a sense of integration and wholeness, of becoming an individual in his own right. This includes the perception of 'me' and 'not-me', the development of a personal or inner reality for the infant, the dawning of intelligence and the beginning of the mind as something different from the psyche. In turn, this allows for the development of symbolic functioning and for living relationships.

If good-enough mothering is provided, which Winnicott felt was normally the case, then the developing baby would pass through two early maturational stages. During the first few months the baby develops a 'sense of being' through primary identification with the breast, facilitated by the illusion that the breast could be summoned omnipotently whenever the baby felt the need for it, such as feeling in need of comfort. At this stage infant and breast are, as far as the infant is concerned, one and the same thing. Winnicott names this sense of being the 'female element'. It forms the basis for self-discovery and a sense of existing. This contrasts with the 'male element' of the next stage, that of 'doing', where object relatedness proceeds to differentiate self and object. Here the object is discovered to be beyond omnipotent control, and the infant develops a capacity for virtual objectivity. It is not that the male element supersedes the female element, but rather that development allows for both to exist together.

What Winnicott called transitional phenomena lie between these two stages, allowing the infant to move from subjectivity to objectivity, from having the subjective experience of being merged with the mother to also being separate from her. The infant moves between, on the one hand, having the illusion of having omnipotent, internalized control over the environment and, on the other, exploring the vicissitudes of the real world. The infant is all the time moving between illusion and reality, between invention and discovery, holding both, as it were, in mind at the same time (Phillips, 1989). The infant can cross the potential transitional space between mother and infant, between inner psychic reality and outer objective reality, by use of a transitional object. This can be anything, but often is something like a teddy bear, a toy, or a piece of cloth, which the child imbues with meaning and with which it has a very special relationship. Through use of this transitional object, the infant begins to explore the world. It is affectionately cuddled, excitedly loved and hated, and mutilated – all of which it has to be able to survive. At the same time, it is also seen as having a vitality of its own. There is a tacit understanding that it is both created by the infant and a part of the real world. The prototype of the transitional object is the mother's breast, provided by the good-enough mother at the moment that the infant is about to create in his own mind the breast that she offers in reality. With time, the original transitional object becomes diffused across a whole variety of objects, which thereby acquire meaning for the infant. Thus the teddy bear may come to symbolize the breast, but is also important for being a teddy bear, and not a breast. It is both at the same time, and thereby allows the link between me and not-me.

The good-enough mother starts off with an almost perfect adaptation to her infant's needs, but with time adapts less completely. This 'failure' allows the developing infant, gradually more able to withstand mother's failures, to begin to use mental activity, such as remembering, thinking and fantasizing. If all goes well, the infant is thus helped to tolerate frustration and to use mental activity instead of demanding instant gratification. Important here is the gradual diffusing of transitional phenomena across the whole intermediate territory between inner reality and the external world.

Explorations by the infant of the potential space between his internal psychic reality and the outside world are characterized by play. For Winnicott, such play was a very serious and essential process in development, and was critically dependent upon the mother reliably providing the security that play would neither be interrupted unnecessarily, nor get out of hand and become frightening. A marvellous example of such play, and of good-enough mothering, is given by the children's book *Katie Morag and the Tiresome Ted* by Mairi Hedderwick (1991).

If the mother provides a good-enough facilitating environment, then the infant goes on to develop a 'true self', grounded in a sense of being, and confident in his explorations of the world. The true self remains hidden and secretive but is the source of all spontaneous living. Such infants are able to relinquish the illusion of having created external objects, and are able to play creatively and spontaneously with transitional phenomena. Winnicott notes that such individuals go on to develop the capacity to be alone in the presence of another. If, however, the mother repeatedly is not able to meet the needs of the infant, Winnicott postulates that the infant gradually develops a 'false self', based on an identification with the mother's wishes and desires, in preference to its own. The child does not develop the illusion of creating the world, as the real world, in the form of mother's own needs and desires, has intruded before the infant is able to withstand it. Such individuals develop little capacity for play, and rather than joyously exploring their own being in the world are instead anxiously trying to identify what the other wants and fitting themselves into that mould, thereby stunting any natural development.

The model of 'good-enough mothering' and the holding environment provides a theoretical framework for the analytic situation. In the same way as a good-enough mother creates the conditions that allow for the spontaneous development of her infant, the therapist aims to provide a facilitating environment which allows maturation to proceed and one where both therapist and patient can play. The therapist attempts to hold the patient psychologically, which includes accepting his projective identifications. Interpretations can be seen as transitional phenomena, providing a bridge between the inner, subjectively conceived world and outer objective reality. Just as the mother must not be perfectly adapted to her infant's needs in order to allow her infant to develop, Winnicott suggested that the patient needs the therapist to fail him, in a subtle way, by not being perfect. This allows the patient to create their own reality which is different from that of the therapist. A notable feature of Winnicott's technique was letting patients discover their own insights, rather than the therapist intruding by making the interpretation just before a patient was about to come upon it spontaneously for himself.

W.R.D. Fairbairn

Ronald Fairbairn was born in 1889, in Edinburgh, as an only child in a middle-class and Calvinistic family. He studied philosophy in Edinburgh, and subsequently divinity in London. It was only at the end of military service in the First World War that he embarked upon a medical training with a view to becoming a psychotherapist. He spent his entire professional life in Edinburgh, in relative isolation from professional colleagues with whom to share his ideas, and lacking the opportunity to obtain a conventional psychoanalytic training, such as supervision and a training analysis. Despite this, he developed strikingly original ideas, working particularly with schizoid patients, and, with allowances made for the earlier work of Freud, Abraham and Klein, can be considered the founding father of object relations theory (Grotstein and Rinsley, 1994). His earlier training in philosophy was vital here as it gave him the theoretical rigour to develop a general psychology based upon twentieth-century, post-Einsteinian principles of relativity, where energy and matter were interdependent, as opposed to nineteenth-century notions of mechanism, used by Freud, where energy and structure were separate (Sutherland, 1989).

According to Freud, the infant seeks out the mother and her breast in order to satisfy his instinctual drive for pleasure; the relationship is in the service of pleasure-seeking. Fairbairn, however, saw the infant's primary aim as seeking a relationship. What the infant seeks is to be loved for himself, as a person. The main defences were against the painful affects of not being loved by a parent figure with full acceptance.

An inevitable consequence of the primary need for a relationship is dependency upon others. In the beginning is the immature dependency of the infant upon his mother, where the infant looks towards his mother to meet all his needs. This infantile dependence is based upon a primary identification with the mother, and in particular that part of her that meets the infant's physical needs, namely the breast. This means that right at the beginning the infant and the breast, from the infant's point of view, are one. In this state the infant cannot tolerate ambivalence, and has a relation to a part-object (the breast) and not to a whole object (the mother with all her complex needs and feelings as a whole person). If all goes well, and the developing child knows that both his love for his parents is accepted and that he is loved as a person by them, he will eventually, in early adulthood, grow into a state of mature dependence. Total independence from other people is seen as pathological, for at all times an autonomous person requires to be related to others for effective functioning. In a state of mature dependence upon others, based upon a differentiation of the object from the self, he is able to tolerate ambivalence; the other person is seen as a whole person, and their feelings and way of life are respected. Such a capacity for good relationships is the product of a continuous interactive process between the developing child and his parents.

When, however, the mother–child relationship (and later the father–child relationship) is not satisfactory, and the mother does not accept the child as a person in his own right, but instead imposes her own needs and wishes upon him or in other ways rejects his love – such as not being available when needed – a process of splitting occurs. According to Fairbairn, under the pressures of deprivation and frustration, the infant splits his imperfect mother into three components – the 'rejecting object', the 'exciting object' and the 'ideal object'. The self is likewise split into three, as different parts of the self relate to different parts of the split-off object, leading to three sets of relationships. There is a 'central ego' in relation to an ideal object. The central ego is that part of the self that is concerned with reality testing, conscious thought and reflection. The central ego directly represses both an 'antilibidinal ego' (or 'internal saboteur') related to the rejecting object (sadistic primitive superego), and a 'libidinal ego' related to the exciting object. Both the latter sets of relationships are repressed by the central ego because they are seen as intolerably bad.

All three sets of relationships are internalized and constitute an active and dynamic system, and comprise the 'endopsychic structure of object relations'. Thus 'the internalization of bad objects represents an attempt on the part of the child to make the objects in his environment good by taking upon himself the burden of their apparent badness, and thus to make his environment more tolerable. This defensive attempt to establish outer security is purchased at the price of inner insecurity, since it leaves the ego at the mercy of internal persecutors; and it is as a defence against such inner insecurity that the repression of internal bad objects arises' (Fairbairn, 1952, pp. 164–165).

The result is that the infant has inside him a set of relationships that reflect his experiences with his real parents. The exciting object entices in the same way that the real parent appeared to offer contact; the rejecting object withholds in the same way as the parents failed to offer contact; and the ideal object provides contact through the pleasures and values of the real parents (Greenberg and Mitchell, 1983).

Splitting the ego is the fundamental schizoid phenomenon. The child, as a result of emotional frustration, comes to feel that he is not loved, and that his own love for his mother is not accepted. The child thus both comes to see his mother as a bad object and to regard his own love as bad, and then attempts to retain his 'bad' love inside himself. Fairbairn termed this protection of others from the bad love of the self as the 'moral defence'. Love relationships with external objects come to be seen as dangerous, and the patient focuses on internal object relations instead. There is thus a withdrawing from external relationships, becoming socially aloof, and a preoccupation with inner reality; this is accompanied by an attitude of omnipotence, where the person may feel superior. Underneath, however, he still wants and needs relationships, either external or internal, and is fearful of having no relationships, which would represent a psychic death.

A further consequence of splitting of the ego is that the work of the ego, such as integrating the personality and adapting to the external world, is compromised. This means that, according to the degree of splitting, there is poor reality testing and sudden shifts of mood. An example of this would be found in the borderline patient.

Fairbairn proposed that different forms of psychopathology were aetiologically related to difficulties arising in object relationships during development. Thus a schizoid defence was related to difficulties arising in the very early object relations of the baby sucking (loving), and depression to subsequent difficulties over biting (hating). Obsessional, paranoid, hysterical and phobic symptoms resulted from defences against the emergence of schizoid or depressive tendencies (Fairbairn, 1952).

Relationships with inner objects are acted out in the external world, so that another person is coerced into the role of the inner object in such a way that they are not permitted to have much independence or individuality. For instance, the other may be placed in the role of the harsh and punitive authority figure, or as a temptress who, by withholding and teasing, leaves the individual feeling angry and resentful. Tragically, because the systems of both the libidinal ego and the antilibidinal ego are actively repressed from consciousness, they remain largely insulated from the modifying influences of experience in the real world. They thus come to constitute a closed system, so that little or no learning normally takes place. One of the tasks of the analytic work is to bring such processes into consciousness so that they can be worked through.

Fairbairn's therapeutic aim was to promote a maximum synthesis of the structures into which the ego had been split. This is achieved by breaking into the closed system which constitutes the patient's inner world, and thus making it accessible to the influence of outer reality. This allows reduction of infantile dependence and reduced hatred of the libidinal object (Fairbairn, 1958).

Harry Guntrip

Guntrip (1901–1975) initially became an officer in the Salvation Army, and then entered the church as a Congregational minister. It was only in his mid-forties that he embarked upon a psychoanalytic career. At the age of 48, by which time he had already established himself as a psychotherapist in Leeds, he entered analysis with Fairbairn. He subsequently underwent a second analysis with Winnicott.

Guntrip is best known for promoting Fairbairn's ideas; Fairbairn's own writing was sparse and difficult, whereas Guntrip had a much more accessible style. In addition, Guntrip attempted to develop Fairbairn's concept of the split-off parts of the ego. He proposed that the libidinal ego undergoes a further split. Part of it remains attached to the exciting object and actively continues to seek the desired relationship with the originally disappointing mother. Another part of the libidinal ego, however, becomes split off from the exciting object and withdraws from any attempt at relating to others. This Guntrip called the 'regressed ego'. He argued that the real depriving experiences with others have led to a feeling that all attempts at relationships are useless. Instead the regressed ego turns inwards, trying to return to the pre-relationship security of the womb. For Guntrip the regressed ego continually threatens the personality with a state of nothingness, a psychological black hole that swallows up everything else. It creates a constant sense of inner dread and vulnerability (Guntrip, 1971). 'In the face of the constant threat of total depersonalization and disorganization ... the ego continually struggles to remain attached to life. All mental life and involvements with others, real or imaginary, operate most basically as a defence against regressive longing ... Oral, anal, genital fantasies reflect "a struggle to stay born and function in the world of differentiated object-relations as a separate ego", as defences against the central part of the ego that has "gone back inside"' (Greenberg and Mitchell, 1983, p. 212).

Guntrip places the responsibility for mental health squarely at the door of bad mothering, as such failures in mothering lead to a traumatized part of the self that takes flight from all object relations. He also argued that the role of the therapist, through his understanding, was to provide the good mothering that the patient had failed to get from his original experiences with his real mother (Guntrip, 1969). In Guntrip's view the therapist becomes a heroic figure who can rescue the victimized patient by his kindly omniscience (Greenberg and Mitchell, 1983).

Guntrip has been criticized by a number of commentators, who argue that he failed fully to understand Fairbairn's work, that he subtly distorted it to suit his own ideas, and that his notion of a regressed ego that turns away from all attempts at relating is incompatible with Fairbairn's central tenet of the primary importance of the baby being at all times in search of a relationship (Greenberg and Mitchell, 1983; Grotstein and Rinsley, 1994). It also seems as if Guntrip would like to place all responsibility for the negative feelings that an infant has for his mother as being the fault of poor mothering, and deny the baby any active role in this.

Bowlby and attachment theory

John Bowlby (1907–1990) was the son of an eminent surgeon. He trained in both psychology and psychiatry, and after the Second World War moved to the Tavistock Clinic in London to become chairman of the Department for Children and Parents. He was commissioned by the World Health Organization in 1951 to investigate the mental health of homeless children. His report concluded that a warm, intimate and continuous relationship between the infant and his mother was essential for mental health. This subsequently led to his researches on the vicissitudes of this relationship, summarized in his three-volume work *Attachment and Loss* (1969, 1973, 1980). Bowlby found the formulations of Freud and his followers unsatisfactory and, in an attempt to make sense of the rival theories, he turned to the new disciplines of ethology, control theory and information processing. He was much influenced by the work of Fairbairn and Winnicott, but also based his theories on the direct observation of young children.

Bowlby argued that behaviour is grouped into a series of discrete, and partially pre-programmed entities, such as feeding behaviour, attachment behaviour and sexual behaviour (Bowlby, 1988). He suggested that such instinctive behavioural systems determined much of the emotional life of a person, and that they evolved as a result of natural selection.

In his work, he focused almost exclusively on attachment behaviour in the child. Attachment is mediated by sucking, smiling, crying, clinging and following. The effect is to keep the child in close proximity to his mother-figure. It may be triggered by pain, fatigue, anything frightening or the mother appearing inaccessible. It is terminated by contact with the mother, either by sight or sound, or, if anxiety is high, by touching or clinging. The biological function is protection, especially from predators.

Confidence in the availability of attachment figures underlies emotional stability. Problems arise when the attachment is either insecure in some way, as a result of inadequate parenting, or if the infant loses his attachment figure. This leads to feelings of anxiety and anger in the child and, if prolonged or repeated, may lead to adult pathology. 'Whether a child or an adult is in a state of security, anxiety or distress is determined in large part by the accessibility and responsiveness of his principal attachment figure' (Bowlby, 1973, p. 23).

Bowlby describes three main stages of behaviour when a child is separated from his attachment figure: protest, despair and detachment. This closely follows the processes observed in adult grieving. Bowlby argues that much adult pathology is the result of loss and pathological mourning originating in childhood, as well as from insecure attachment.

The major contribution of Bowlby's work has been to provide a route, based upon the direct observations of young children and their mothers, whereby psychoanalytic theories about the early origins of pathology can be prospectively tested. A criticism, however, has been that his work is not about psychoanalysis but is a form of developmental psychology. Bowlby does not appear to have a notion of a dynamic unconscious, and at times gives the impression that the behavioural systems he describes act blindly, with no account taken of the influence of the meaning of the experiences of loss for the individual (Greenberg and Mitchell, 1983).

Bowlby's work has proved to be a fruitful area for research, notably in the work of Ainsworth and Main on attachment theory (see e.g. Main, 1986). Ainsworth developed an experimental situation which could reliably measure the infant's quality of attachment to his or her mother – the Strange Situation Procedure (Ainsworth et al., 1978). She identified three types of attachment: secure attachment, insecure resistant attachment and insecure avoidant attachment. More recently Mary Main and her colleagues identified a fourth group, which they called disorganized and disoriented attachment (Main and Solomon, 1986). An important recent finding has been that a mother's attachment classification, as measured by the Adult Attachment Interview (Main, 1986), can reliably predict the attachment classification of her, as yet unborn, infant in the future. The Adult Attachment Interview looks at the coherence of the story the mother tells about her own upbringing. It is thus hypothesized that the attachment patterns that both infants and adults show reflect qualitative differences in internal working models of relationships, similar to those of object relations.

Although Main and Ainsworth are developmental psychologists, and not analysts, their approach is beginning to influence theoretical developments in psychoanalysis. For instance, Peter Fonagy, a Contemporary Freudian analyst, is attempting to integrate findings from attachment theory and experimental psychology into analytic thinking (e.g. Fonagy et al., 1994; Fonagy and Target, 1996).

Another example of the integration of research findings from experimental developmental psychology and psychoanalysis is found in the work of Daniel Stern, an American psychoanalyst (and therefore not a member of the Independent Group). Stern argues that infants differentiate themselves from birth and then progress through increasingly complex modes of relatedness (Stern, 1985). Throughout the infant is seen as intensely social, with a continuous dialectical inter-relatedness between what the infant brings to a relationship and what the mother, or environment, contributes. He describes four different senses of the self, each one defining a different domain of self-experience and social relatedness: 'They are the sense of the emergent self, which forms from birth to age two months, the sense of a core self, which forms between the ages of two and six months, the sense of a subjective self, which forms between seven to fifteen months, and a sense of a verbal self, which forms after that . . . Once formed, each sense of self remains fully functioning and active throughout life. All continue to grow and coexist' (Stern, 1985).

The emergent self relates to the sense of coming into being, of becoming aware of self-organizing processes. All learning and all creative acts begin in the domain of emergent relatedness. The core self is a sense of self as being a separate, cohesive, bounded physical unit, with a sense of agency, affectivity and continuity in time. Mother is seen as having a separate physical existence, as being a core other. During the development of a subjective self the infant learns that the subjective contents of one's mind can be shared with another, and also that the other has thoughts and feelings of her own, which regulate the encounter. Lastly, during the development of a verbal self the infant learns to use language, with which to relate both to others and with oneself. The acquisition of language, however, is problematic, as it 'drives a wedge between two simultaneous forms of interpersonal experience: as it is lived and as it is verbally represented. Experiences in the domain of emergent core and intersubjective relatedness, which continue irrespective of language, can be embraced only very partially in the domain of verbal relatedness' (Stern, 1985, pp. 162–163). Stern suggests that adult pathology can be understood as arising from deficits in these different senses of self, which themselves arise out of adverse experiences.

Aims of therapy

Independent analysts take the techniques of classical psychoanalysis as almost axiomatic, including the use of the couch. The aim of therapy can be broadly summarized as helping the client become more aware of the influence of their internal world on their daily functioning. Balint tried to achieve a benign regression to the level of the basic fault to allow a new beginning. Much analysis is at the oedipal level, consistently interpreting intrapsychic conflict at the three-person level, in order to reveal the painful and earlier conflicts behind them. Winnicott, by providing a holding environment, tried to foster the development of the True Self and spontaneity. Important here was the patient's own process of self-analysis and self-discovery, as well as the analyst's self-analysis. Both patient and therapist should become healthily creative and be able to surprise themselves, working in the area of transitionality. Fairbairn echoed this by stating that the therapeutic aim was to help the patient change from being a closed system, where the intrapsychic world was unable to learn from experience, to becoming an open system. This would allow the integration of the different split-off components of the inner world.

How does the Independent School differ from other therapies?

There are a great many continuities between the object relations therapists and the work of both Freud and Klein, but also a number of notable differences, some of which have already been mentioned.

Freud and Klein saw pathology as the result of an excess of instinctual drives, and the infant as essentially demonic, attacking and demanding (see Grotstein and Rinsley, 1994). In contrast, the authors discussed here see pathology as being the result of a relationship between the infant and the environment, and stress a failure of environmental provision. Fairbairn and Klein also differed in their understanding of the nature of internal objects; Klein saw them as phantasies whereas Fairbairn conceptualized them as structures. Furthermore, Klein argued that bad internal objects originated out of internal drives, whereas Fairbairn argued that they were the result of internalizing an external, emotionally unsatisfactory relationship (Perlow, 1995).

A fundamental stumbling block was Klein's insistence upon the death instinct. Fairbairn, for instance, did not feel it was useful as an explanatory principle, understanding the hatred found in patients as being the result of frustration at not having satisfying relationships rather than the expression of a basic instinct. Furthermore, Kleinian analysts would see envy as being a primary emotion; object relations analysts would see envy as complex and requiring a 'theory of mind'. The infant needs to be able to see the other as having feelings which are different from himself, including the feeling of enjoying the thing that the infant wants but cannot have.

Kleinian analysts would argue that all material produced in a session is considered to be a manifestation of transference, and that a mutative interpretation is always a transference interpretation. Object relations therapists, however, would argue that there are other experiences which are mutative as well, and that not everything in the session is transference; there is always a real environment with which the patient has to interact. An example is given by Balint, who had a patient who, during a session, told of how he had never been allowed to do a somersault. Balint replied 'Why not now?', whereupon the patient got up and performed a somersault in the room for the first time in his life.

For both Kleinians and Independents, working with the counter-transference is an important component of the analytic encounter, particularly the part of it that could be understood as an unconscious communication from patient to therapist. In the transference, Kleinian analysts would concentrate upon the hate and destructive impulses of the patient. Many Independent analysts, however, would feel that by concentrating on this aspect of transference one could make the patient adopt a false conformity to the treatment as they tried to protect themselves against punitive interpretations. They would therefore tend to err towards empathy rather than severity.

Which patient and why?

A wide variety of patients may be considered for an 'Independent' analysis as it is a form of therapy particularly suited to helping patients with difficulties in long-term relationships.

Winnicott identified three categories of patients:

- those patients, the majority, whose difficulties are in interpersonal relationships;
- patients whose wholeness as people is at times in doubt;
- patients who have suffered severe early trauma and who have, in an attempt to deal with total disintegration, developed a false self.

With regard to patients whose difficulties are in interpersonal relationships or those whose wholeness as a person is at times in doubt, Winnicott believed that a classical analysis was the treatment of choice. In the analysis of the latter, one is dealing with an emotional weaning of patient from therapist, and analysis of mood is of primary importance. The mood states of the patient can be extreme, and the therapist has to be able to survive the emotional attacks of the patient and remain a functioning analyst.

If the patient had developed a false self as a result of severe early trauma, Winnicott believed that only a modified form of analysis was possible. With such patients much of the work consists of managing the patient and the therapeutic encounter, and the analysis of such patients is fraught with danger, including disintegration into psychosis.

The only significant contraindication to treatment is a history of severe mental illness, such as psychosis, as an intense analysis may precipitate further breakdown. However, this form of psychotherapy is expensive, both in time and money. If the patient, or therapist, is unwilling to make such a commitment, other forms of psychotherapy may be more appropriate.

Which therapist and why?

Therapists usually come from the helping professions, such as medicine, psychology or social work. All therapists undergo a rigorous training under supervision, including a lengthy personal analysis. This helps make the therapist more sensitive to their own internal world, as part of an ongoing process of self-analysis. It also develops the capacity in therapists to think about and work through, rather than act out, the countertransference (the feelings aroused in therapists by the patient). An important contribution of the Independent School has been to focus on the contribution that the therapist makes to the dialogue between patient and therapist.

Stressing that therapists must be available emotionally to their patients, the Independent School argues that the analyst needs to be able to work with their own True Self, being creative, spontaneous and intuitive in the service of the patient. The patient will make use of the analyst's internal responsiveness in order to compel the analyst to re-live elements of the patient's infantile history. The analyst must be able to be available to the patient in an authentic way, and only subsequently use an analysis of the countertransference to try to understand what happened (Bollas, 1987). This requires emotional strength, sensitivity, honesty and great courage from therapists.

Therapeutic setting

Therapy requires a safe and secure setting which is comfortable and free from all interruption. Traditionally a couch is used for the patient, with the therapist sitting at the head, out of sight of the patient. This minimizes visual cues for the patient, and allows the inner world of the patient to become more accessible. This is less rigorously insisted upon by the Independent School, and some Independent therapists, such as Rycroft, would routinely see patients sitting face to face.

Winnicott saw the therapist as being a host who stage managed the therapeutic encounter, in terms of reliably providing a safe, comfortable and secure setting, and who could be relied upon to behave himself. Particular attention is paid to maintaining strict boundaries, such as starting and finishing sessions on time. Breaks in therapy and the approaching ending of therapy are key areas, since here the relationship between patient and therapist is threatened. Such breaks are of particular importance in cases of severe regression, where there is a merging between therapist and patient.

The Independent analysts have been in the forefront of taking the analytic endeavour from the privacy of the consulting room into the wider community. Examples include the Tavistock Institute of Human Relations, which adapted ideas from psychoanalysis to consultancy work with large organizations, and the work of Michael and Enid Balint in pioneering Balint Groups in General Practice (Rayner, 1990).

Clinical example

The following clinical example is quoted from the work of Patrick Casement, including Casement's own reflections on the material, illustrating a patient's use of the therapist's availability (*On Learning from the Patient*, 1985, pp. 176–179).

A female patient came for her first session after a holiday break. She arrived ten minutes late, and explained to her therapist (a man) that there had been a lot of traffic on the way which had held her up. She poured out details of what had happened to her since her last session. She had been feeling unsupported by her husband, having had to cope with the demands of the children on her own and they had been very difficult.

The therapist sensed that the patient was alerting him to the possible impact upon her of the holiday break. Because of the pressure to talk, which was the most obvious aspect of her communication, he continued to listen.

The patient gave further examples of feeling alone, having no one to turn to, feeling cold, etc. There were still no pauses in her narrative. The therapist was beginning to feel redundant in the session, in that the patient was not leaving any room for comment, and he wondered whether he should intervene to make his presence felt. But, lacking any clearer cue from the patient, he chose to remain silent.

After further outpouring of holiday details the patient began to describe an incident with her husband. He had been depressed recently and unresponsive. She was feeling in particular need of his support one night, but he didn't reach out to her – even when she was crying. After a pause she added: 'He didn't even speak to me.' There was a slight pause in the flow of talk from the patient at this point. The therapist, therefore, took his cue from her silence and used the themes presented to provide a bridge towards eventual interpretation.

Therapist: 'You have been telling me details of what you have been dealing with since your last session. You now tell me about somebody who has been depressed, who did not respond to you, and you add that he didn't even speak to you.'

Casement noted that 'the therapist is here replying to the patient from a position of unfocused listening. He therefore does not focus the patient's anxiety immediately upon himself; that would be pre-emptive. Instead, he leaves room for the patient to make her own reference to him, if she is ready for this. This guards against a transference interpretation being thrust at her.'

Patient: 'I was beginning to wonder why you weren't saying anything. It occurred to me that perhaps you were sorry to be back at work, or you might be feeling depressed.'

Therapist: 'I realized you were anxious, but I was waiting to see if you could let me know more about this. [Pause] I think you may have been trying to let me know about your own depression, which you have been needing somebody to be in touch with; and the holiday break has added to your sense of being left to deal with this alone.'

The patient began to cry: the flood of her talking had stopped. After a while she began telling the therapist about her mother's moods, when she was small. There had been times when the patient could not find any way to get through to her mother, who had been too preoccupied with her own depression.

Therapist: 'I think you may have experienced my absence during the holiday, and my silence in this session, as reminders of being with your mother – her distance from you and your difficulty in being able to get through to her.'

The patient recalled more about her relationship to her mother, and began to get angry with the therapist for being like her. By the end of the session, however, the patient was able to notice that her therapist was not being defensive or retaliatory in response to this anger. Her closing comment was: 'I expected you to object to my being so angry with you.'

Casement sees this as an example 'of a therapist who is prepared to wait, to be found by the patient in whatever way that happens. The patient is therefore not prevented from making use of the therapist to represent a bad experience in childhood. Having attacked him for being like her mother she finds that he has remained unchanged by this. So, through this non-retaliatory survival of her treating him as a "bad object" she re-discovers the therapist as a "good object".'

Casement notes that 'it is all too easy to cut across a patient's spontaneous finding of the therapist's presence by intervening too quickly. A similar error is to bring the patient's communications to a premature focus onto the therapist, which is often done in the name of transference. This deadens the experience by lessening the sense of immediacy in the transference. By not allowing more time for this to develop in the session, a patient can be blocked from arriving at the more specific details that are often contained in a patient's further associations (if they are not interrupted).'

He further reflects: 'It also deflects from the patient's experience of feelings towards thinking about feelings, before the actual experience has been more fully entered into. This invites the patient to intellectualize and can also be evidence of a countertransference defensiveness on the part of the therapist. When this happens, patients will often respond to this as a cue from the therapist to avoid what may have been difficult for the therapist to stay in touch with for longer.'

Problems in therapy

The therapist becomes extremely important to the patient, a fact that may be overlooked by the inexperienced therapist, and calls for careful thought and attention to details of technique. Problems are likely to occur when the patient is deeply regressed. Such patients can place great demands upon an analyst's ability to survive and retain his analytic stance. Powerful feelings may be aroused in the therapist by the patient and this requires regular supervision; even senior therapists will obtain this throughout their working lives. Without such supervision the analyst may find himself acting out the countertransference, with possible disastrous consequences for the patient.

For example, a detailed attention to interpreting the minutiae of the transference by an analyst can be felt by some patients as an intrusion, which does not meet their need to be known. Similarly, the appearance of all-knowingness on the part of the analyst can be anti-therapeutic. Winnicott remarked that in his opinion inexperienced trainee analysts could sometimes do better work than their elders. Trainees were often acutely aware of their not-knowing, and were therefore led by their patients, rather than seeming to know what their patients were trying to say before they had said it, based on an extensive academic knowledge.

Evaluation of therapy

Outcome studies are extremely difficult and beset by methodological difficulties since treatment is not standardized. There are numerous individual case studies attesting to the effectiveness of this form of psychotherapy, but rigorous large scale outcome studies are still required. Malan has conducted extensive research demonstrating the effectiveness of brief dynamic psychotherapy. He found that good outcome was correlated with an intense emotional involvement between patient and therapist, high motivation for change, enthusiasm on the part of the therapist and repeated use of transference interpretations (Malan, 1976). Peter Fonagy and his colleagues demonstrated the effectiveness of psychoanalytic treatment in brittle diabetes (Moran et al., 1991). Bowlby's work gave rise to a large body of research, some of which has already been mentioned (Stern, 1985; Main and Solomon, 1986; Main, 1986; Fonagy and Target, 1996). Although these studies are grounded in developmental psychology rather than psychoanalysis, they are having a marked impact on psychoanalytic research and may play an increasingly important part in the future evaluation of psychoanalytic treatments.

Alternatives to therapy

This largely depends upon the problem for which the patient is seeking help. Longstanding personality difficulties are unlikely to yield to less intensive therapies, but focal problems such as a phobia or depression would, in the absence of underlying difficulties, be better treated by, for instance, cognitive behaviour therapy. It also depends upon what the patient is looking for, as a number of patients want a focused solution to a particular problem, and are not prepared to undergo lengthy analysis.

Also, a number of patients are referred for therapy who experienced severely damaging childhoods and have little capacity for reflective work, in the hope that therapy can somehow undo many years of abuse and deprivation. Such patients are best managed by means of firm limit-setting and strengthening of existing defences, rather than exploring what lies behind the defences by means of analysis.

The Independent tradition in psychoanalysis is entirely compatible with biological interventions, such as medication. There are difficulties, however, combining it with other psychotherapies administered by other therapists. This may lead to a split transference, where the patient may idealize one therapist at the expense of the other as a manifestation of their difficulty in interpersonal relationships. This may lead to a breakdown of therapy if no psychological space is provided where the patient can be helped to explore the meaning of such splits.

Further reading

Greenberg, J.R. and Mitchell, S.A. (1983) *Object Relations in Psychoanalytic Theory.* Cambridge, MA: Harvard University Press.
    A good introduction, placing the work of the British independent tradition in an American context.
Phillips, A. (1989) *Winnicott.* Fontana Modern Masters. London: Collins.
    The best introduction to the work of Winnicott.
Rayner, E. (1990) *The Independent Mind in British Psychoanalysis.* London: Free Association Books.
    The best text on the subject, easily accessible to the beginner.
Winnicott, D.W. (1980) *The Piggle.* Harmondsworth: Penguin.
    A very readable and moving account of the analysis of a five-year-old girl.

Bibliography

Abraham, K. (1924) A short study of the development of the libido viewed in the light of mental disorders. In: *Selected Papers on Psychoanalysis.* London: Maresfield Reprints (1979), pp. 418–501.
Ainsworth, M.D.S., Blehar, M., Waters, E. and Walls, S. (1978) *Patterns of Attachment: A Psychological Study of the Strange Situation.* New York: Lawrence Erlbaum.
Balint, M. (1968) *The Basic Fault: Therapeutic Aspects of Regression.* London: Tavistock.
Bollas, C. (1987) *The Shadow of the Object.* London: Free Association Books.
Bowlby, J. (1969) *Attachment and Loss. Volume I: Attachment.* London: Hogarth Press.
Bowlby, J. (1973) *Attachment and Loss. Volume II: Separation, Anxiety, and Anger.* London: Hogarth Press.
Bowlby, J. (1980) *Attachment and Loss. Volume III: Loss, Sadness, and Depression.* London: Hogarth Press.

Bowlby, J. (1988) *A Secure Base: Clinical Application of Attachment Theory*. London: Tavistock/ Routledge.

Casement, P. (1985) *On Learning from the Patient*. London: Tavistock/Routledge.

Clancier, A. and Kalmanovitch, J. (1987) *Winnicott and Paradox*. London: Tavistock.

Fairbairn, W.R.D. (1952) *Psychoanalytic Studies of the Personality*. London: Routledge and Kegan Paul.

Fairbairn, W.R.D. (1958) On the nature and aims of psycho-analytic treatment. *International Journal of Psycho-Analysis*, **39**, 374–385.

Fonagy, P. and Target, M. (1996) Playing and reality: 1. Theory of mind and the normal development of psychic reality. *International Journal of Psycho-Analysis*, **77**, 217–233.

Fonagy, P., Steele, M., Steele, H., Higgit, A. and Target, M. (1994) The theory and practice of resilience. *Journal of Child Psychology and Psychiatry*, **35**, 231–257.

Greenberg, J.R. and Mitchell, S.A. (1983) *Object Relations in Psychoanalytic Theory*. Cambridge, MA: Harvard University Press.

Grotstein, J.S. and Rinsley, D.B. (eds) (1994) *Fairbairn and the Origins of Object Relations*. London: Free Association Books.

Guntrip, H. (1969) *Schizoid Phenomena, Object Relations and the Self*. New York: International Universities Press.

Guntrip, H. (1971) *Psychoanalytic Theory, Therapy and the Self*. New York: Basic Books.

Hedderwick, M. (1991) *Katie Morag and the Tiresome Ted*. London: Collins.

Kohon, G. (ed.) (1986) *The British School of Psychoanalysis*. London: Free Association Books.

Main, M. (1986) Introduction to the Special Section on Attachment and Psychopathology: 2. Overview of the field of attachment. *Journal of Consulting and Clinical Psychology*, **64**, 237–243.

Main, M. and Solomon, J. (1986) Discovery of an insecure, disorganised/disoriented attachment pattern: procedures, findings and implications for the classification of behaviour. In: M. Yogman and T.B. Brazelton (eds), *Affective Disorders in Infancy*. Norwood, NY: Ablex, pp. 95–124.

Malan, D.H. (1976) *Towards the Validation of Brief Psychotherapy*. New York: Plenum Press.

Moran, G., Fonagy, P., Kurtz, A. and Bolton, A. (1991) A controlled study of the psychoanalytic treatment of brittle diabetes. *Journal of the American Academy of Child and Adolescent Psychiatry*, **30**, 926–935.

Perlow, M. (1995) *Understanding Mental Objects*. London: Routledge.

Phillips, A. (1989) *Winnicott*. Fontana Modern Masters. London: Collins.

Quinodoz, J-M. (1993) *The Taming of Solitude*. London: Routledge.

Rayner, E. (1990) *The Independent Mind in British Psychoanalysis*. London: Free Association Books.

Rycroft, C. (1972) *A Critical Dictionary of Psychoanalysis*. Harmondsworth: Penguin Books.

Sandler, J. and Dreher, A.U. (1996) *What do Psychoanalysts Want?* London: Routledge.

Stern, D.N. (1985) *The Interpersonal World of the Infant*. New York: Basic Books.

Sutherland, J.D. (1989) *Fairbairn's Journey into the Interior*. London: Free Association Books.

Sutherland, J.D. (1994) Balint, Winnicott, Fairbairn, Guntrip. In: J.S. Scharff (ed.), *The Autonomous Self: The Work of John D. Sutherland*. NJ: Jason Aronson, pp. 25–44.

Winnicott, D.W. (1960) *The Maturational Process and the Facilitating Environment*. London: Hogarth Press.

Winnicott, D.W. (1971) *Playing and Reality*. London: Tavistock.

6

Other Psychoanalytic Developments

Chris Evans

This chapter addresses some specific developments in psychodynamic thinking, considering the work of Kohut, Lacan, Kernberg and Matte Blanco. It is not intended to provide a complete overview of the individuals and schools involved, but it should flag up nodes in the network of psychodynamic ideas that are under development.

Kohut

Heinz Kohut (1913–1981) was born into a Jewish family in Vienna. His father was an excellent musician, whose career as a concert pianist was curtailed by the onset of the First World War. Kohut qualified as a doctor before specializing in neurology. After fleeing Austria in 1939, he planned to continue with his neurology studies in the United States but he later switched to psychiatry and trained as a Freudian analyst.

Heinz Kohut had two analyses; the first in Austria by August Aichorn, the second, after his emigration, in America, by Ruth Eissler.

Kohut's two main works were *The Analysis of the Self* (1971) and *The Restoration of the Self* (1978). Based on his early experiences, Kohut used musical metaphors to describe the psyche in many aspects of his work. He could be a meticulous theorist, and had read broadly and critically within and around psychoanalysis before he started formulating his own views.

Kohut taught a 'classical' approach to Freud's work at the Chicago Institute of Psychoanalysis from 1958 for about a decade. This was primarily the ego-psychological approach developed in America by Hartmann, Jacobson and others out of the work of Anna Freud. It is often characterized as a 'drive–defence' model in which the ego attempts, through the 'defences', to inhibit expression of, or even experience of, energy from the unconscious. Kohut was brilliant at teasing out the various aspects of Freud's work.

Through the late 1960s, until his death in 1981, Kohut struggled on three levels with the prevailing analytic views around him. The first was his attempt to understand narcissism, which was a vexatious concept in classical theory with two stages: primary narcissism, in which others are not experienced as separate; and secondary narcissism, which is the cathexis of the self with libido (i.e. investing one's own libido in oneself). Both are seen as pathological alternatives to true object love, which involves the libidinal cathexis of another person as a whole object with whom one is in a full, genital relationship.

Kohut's second struggle was to separate analytic theory from social moralizing. He came to see the prevailing understanding of narcissism and emotional development as the imposition of a moralistic model on to what should have been an objective and scientific study of continuing psychological growth.

His final theme was to keep arguing that what makes the analytic (and, he would say, any psychological) project different from other sciences is that the empirical data are those of empathy and introspection.

Kohut's 'The two analyses of Mr. Z' is a summary of his conversion. His new theory of self-psychology proposed that the internal world contained 'selfobjects'. Selfobjects are internal structures, fusions of a sense of self and the image of an object. They are internalized qualities of a relationship which perform a function, and are experienced as part of the self as we experience a limb or our eyes and ears as part of the self.

Kohut suggested that our sense of self is built out of these selfobjects, particularly out of the gradual recognition of our separateness when the functions of the selfobjects (or, more specifically, the function of the object in the selfobject relationship) fails to perform as we would wish. This idea of development of the self out of these inevitable but manageable frustrations is similar to that of Winnicott. However, Kohut postulated two separate and coexisting developmental lines of healthy narcissistic development. One involves idealization of the object and, if not traumatized, leads to ideals; the other involves the development of self-respect, through admiration from the object ('the gleam in the mother's eye') and, again if not traumatized but only manageably disappointed, leads to ambitions.

His model of 'trauma' is psychoeconomic, in which intense experiences are too strong to be metabolized successfully into the development of an unconflicted self. This is reminiscent of Fairbairn. Trauma is thus a function of both the object/environment and the interaction between the object/environment and the subject. All deficits in the self arise therefore through traumata and failures of objects – parents or others – to provide manageable disappointments and frustrations.

Kohut's self is a tripartite structure with self-assertive ambitions from the 'grandiose' line of healthy narcissistic development at one pole; values and ideals from the 'idealizing' line are at the other pole. Skills and talents, developed out of the functions of the selfobjects, are organized in the 'field' between the two. These, or more precisely their damage and distortions, are linked with three forms of transference: mirroring, idealizing and twinning.

Mirroring transferences are those where the therapist is sought as an admiring mirror in which the patient/child can see his or her self-assertive ambitions admiringly reflected by a supportive and attentive parental object. Idealizing transferences leave the ideal achievements located in the other. Twinships represent attempts to link or fuse with the other to take over or share their perceived skills or talents. A crude parallel with the structural model of id (self-assertive ambitions), superego (values and ideals) and ego (talents and skills) can be seen, but it is also clear that the model is radically different from Freud's.

Kohut was clear that treatment consisted of 'transmuting internalization'. This 'working through' process was brought about by the manageable frustrations arising from the neutrality of the analyst and the boundaries of the relationship, coupled with interpretation. For Kohut, interpretation should have both a dynamic (conflict) and a genetic (historical) component. Where he differs from others, notably Kernberg and most Kleinian analysts, is in his belief that the working through of narcissistic damage *can only come after* the establishment of sufficient selfobject transference. Few who do not have narcissistic damage will come for therapy or analysis in Kohut's model. For the selfobject transference to become established, it is necessary for the analyst to be experienced as a rosy mirror of the patient's grandiosity, or to become idealized by the patient, or to be successfully twinned with the patient and merged. Kohut argued that early interpretation of these transferences would be traumatic, and prove resistant to psychological transformation rather than lending themselves to internalization and mutative change. This remains contentious but few would now deny that Kohut helped to focus on many problems by developing the ego-psychological model and theorizing about narcissism.

What is often lost in discussion of Kohut's contributions are his themes about the epistemology of analysis: that it should be separated from any social morality or politics, and that it rests on empathy and introspection. The former lays a strong claim to traditional scientific status for the field. The latter puts the empirical basis of that same science on a very unconventional footing. The conceptualization of empathy and introspection as the empirical data of analysis led to personal attacks, specifically that Kohut's entire theoretical structure and technical methods rested on his own (insufficiently analysed) narcissism. This is captured well in an obituary by an admirer: 'Later in life he became so convinced of the diminishing of his resources that he refused almost every honour or request to speak or even to appear in order for him to work as long as possible. Unfortunately so many of these rejections were read as refusals to confront the issues or as personal insults. Hardly a week passed in the long period of glowing praise from others that was not matched by the meanness of spirit that was hard to comprehend and painful to bear.

'And so he came to study narcissism. Heinz would be the first to admit his personal preoccupation with that peculiar state, but he often said that his work in administration best high-lighted the overwhelming primacy of hurt feelings and rageful response. When finally he began to publish his ideas, they were clearly a product of his lifelong intense concern with the task of understanding another human being' (A. I. Goldberg [1982] Heinz Kohut (1913–1981) *International Journal of Psycho-Analysis,* **63**, 257–258).

The claim that Freudian theory is permeated by a complex mixture of Judaism and Christian morality seems undeniable. However, it seems just as clear that Kohut, with many other American analysts, replaced or combined this with a more expansive, individualistic morality of the 'American dream'. For someone who had to flee Nazi Vienna for his life (although his family were secular rather than religious), and who found the security in Chicago to explore the music and culture that his father had been prevented from enjoying, to not have shown some support of what he clearly liked in American culture would have been unrealistic. To ridicule classical theory for moralizing and yet to not detect an admixture of the societal and moral in one's own work, can seem strange in our postmodern world. There exists a tension regarding the dyadic individual situation and its narcissistic avoidance of the social world that many analytic theorists find hard to acknowledge or explore, and Kohut's struggles served to raise awareness of it.

Lacan

Jacques Lacan (1901–1981) was initially unsympathetic to analysis and held an eminent and responsible position in Parisian psychiatry. However, he later wrote a doctoral dissertation examining psychoses and delusions from a phenomenological and, rather covertly or intuitively, from a psychodynamic point of view. He qualified as an analyst in 1934, and was closely associated with the Surrealist movement. He survived the Second World War in Paris by keeping a low profile, whilst continuing to develop his ideas about surrealism and psychoanalysis, both of which were considered seditious and un-Aryan by the occupying Nazi regime.

Lacan's early work developed the notion of the 'mirror phase' in which the infant becomes aware of 'seeing' himself or herself. He argued that the literal image in a mirror is experienced as whole and competent at a time when the child is acutely aware of its own uncoordinated 'specific prematurity of birth', as Lacan called our long period of extra-uterine dependency. In this model he was referring not just to concrete experiences of our image in a mirror but to the general process in which we create a sense of self, and hence a capacity for control of our functions, through identifications with others around us and their capacities.

This is convincingly demonstrated by observing a five-month-old child's frustration when he cannot manipulate things, as compared with his explosion of pleasure when he is in a good mood and 'mirrors' himself with his image in a mirror, in his parents' eyes, or in play with a sister in all her competence *and* her mirroring of him.

The similarity with Kohut's notions of selfobjects as the only route to healthy narcissism is obvious. However, in radical distinction from Kohut, Lacan goes on to frame all self-awareness as denial of incompetence and fragmentation, and as alienation and illusion. This is quite unlike Kohut's positive framework of ambitions, ideals, talents and skills.

Lacan summarizes the functions of the ego as the maintenance of 'negative hallucinations'. This term is given to the experience when hypnotized to believe that things around you are not there. For example, someone hypnotized in this way will avoid the articles of furniture they have been persuaded are not there, and will give confabulatory explanations for the route which they took around the room to avoid bumping into the furniture they cannot see. Lacan argues that any analysis conducted through the ego is doomed to do no more than polish our false images of ourselves, our self-alienation. A similarity with Klein's, at first sight rather negative, metapsychology is present.

In his later work, Lacan drew upon structuralist linguistics and anthropology. He argued that language, or the capacity for language, like the unconscious, is present from birth. He replaced his earlier, bipartite separation of the ideal (which is identified with and which creates the illusory self) and the real (which is fragmented, unintegrated and uncontrollable) with a threefold model of the real, the symbolic and the ideal registers.

In this new formulation, the ideal is illusory and identificatory otherness which is experienced as the self and as the ego. The symbolic is the creation of meaning by its representation in imagery and language. These leave the real as, in typically Lacanian paradoxical fashion, exactly that of which we are unaware because we have not replaced it with what we can experience: the illusory and identificatory, or the symbolized. For Lacan, the real is only attributed to the fact of death and to the indescribable, transcendent experience of *jouissance*, a word with no strict equivalent in English but equating with any experience which is too stimulating to be experienced and symbolized. Jouissance is equated at times with orgasm, but is certainly not confined to this experience and may be reminiscent of Fairbairn's 'exciting object'. Lacan seems to have discarded the hydraulic model of the Freudian dual-instinct or dual-drive theory, and recreated eros and thanatos as transcendent – the only real, unsymbolized, unsymbolizable experiences.

Lacan extended these ideas, addressing both gender and the Oedipus complex. In his model, the triad of mother, father and baby is less defined by loving and hating relationships, jealousy and castration anxiety. Instead it is defined by the sense that the father, by his otherness and prohibitions, is always the framework of language, symbolization and separation. His 'no' acts as a symbolic castration. Emptiness and alienation, rather than concrete affects and relationships, are recurrent themes throughout. Lacan also developed his ideas by drawing on mathematics and network theory, forms which seem to have had less influence on his work than linguistic formulations.

Lacan is renowned not only for his complex and abstruse theory, but also for the technical development of the short or variable analytic 'hour'. Whereas the traditional analytic 'hour' lasts precisely fifty minutes, Lacan saw this prior specification as a defence against a true encounter with the unconscious – a defence for both the therapist and the patient. He reserved the right to terminate the session at the point of maximum affective impact or the point of maximum self-analytic impetus for the patient. The variable analytic hour is often reviled as an extreme of abuse of the analysand by the analyst. However, it also expresses the powerlessness of the analyst, and the need for the analysand to be free to leave the session at the point of maximum impact. The patient's decision to depart or to remain in the session can then be explored within the analysis.

Lacan radically challenged the dominant ideas about the nature of analytic training, and the criteria for qualification. His method of 'the pass' was that trainees would qualify through a complex process. First the trainee would select a number of peers and present to them a summary of how he saw himself and what he had learned, both personal and theoretical, during the training. His peers would present this to a committee of qualified analysts, who then would decide whether the trainee should 'pass' or not. Although radical and convoluted, it represents an extraordinary test of individual narcissism, of the ability to communicate in the symbolic and of faith in the foundation of peer relationships. Certainly it represents an extreme focus on a problem, something Lacan never seemed to evade.

Lacan's early work offers a radically reframed model of object relations, and of the self as an illusion. His later work was equally radical, one hallmark being his phrase 'the unconscious is structured like a language'. In these explorations, Lacan proposed a return to Freud with rejection of the mechanical and reductive models that had failed to capture just how profoundly complex Freud's notion of the dynamic unconscious was.

Like Kohut, Lacan too was rethinking and challenging the complacent view of analysis as science, and forcing it to explore links with philosophy, linguistics, anthropology and the whole network of ideas in the social and human sciences.

Kernberg

Otto Kernberg (born 1928) is Professor of Psychiatry at the Cornell University Medical College. He was Director of the Psychotherapy Research Project for the Menninger Foundation, and is President of the International Psychoanalytic Association (1997–1999).

Kernberg, like Kohut, considers narcissism seriously in his work and, like Kohut, he uses object relations as his framework. Unlike Kohut, he has always worked within general psychiatry as well as psychoanalysis, and has written on group, milieu and therapeutic community treatments as well as individual work.

Along with Kohut, Hartmann, Jacobson and the object relations theorists of the British Independent School, Kernberg is concerned with object relationships and the relationship between the self and the agencies of the structural model. Both Kohut and Kernberg see internal objects as representations of a subject and an object linked together. In Kohut's selfobjects, the representations of subject and object are linked by a function; in Kernberg's theory of internal objects the link is an affect.

Kernberg views object relations as drive-related; they are organized by aggressive or libidinal drives. Unlike Kohut, Kernberg seeks to retain a dual drive theory and the structural model of ego, id, and superego. Like Klein, and to a lesser extent like Fairbairn, Kernberg attributes a fundamental importance to aggressive drives. By contrast, Kohut sees aggressive drives as the attempts, which may be constructive or ill-organized and destructive, to repair trauma and as the condensates of intolerable affects. What is distinct about Kernberg's theory is that he preserves the entire structural model but radically reorganizes Freud's model of narcissism, and addresses the constant tension between the words *Selbst* and *Ich* in Freud's German, and their translations as 'I', 'me', 'self' and 'ego' by Strachey.

Kernberg argues that part of the ego is made up of internal objects (the fusional representation of subject and object with an 'affective trace'). Based on this, he suggests that the self is comprised of those internal objects in the ego in which a representation of the person takes the place of the object. For Kernberg, like Freud, these self and object condensates are parts of the ego, complemented by a primary narcissistic component in which there is no distinction of subject and object. Another, not very well-defined, component is made up of perceptual capacities such as early sensations of skin and touch, vision, hearing and kinaesthetic experience.

Like Kohut, but deviating somewhat from Freud and classical ego psychology, Kernberg acknowledges *healthy narcissism*. Unlike Kohut, he sees pathological narcissism as something quite different, not simply an arrested form of the healthy variant. For Kernberg, pathological narcissism is a developmental diversion; a completely pathological organization that requires confrontative interpretation if the therapy is not to flounder in a dead end.

Following Klein, and taking something from Bion, Kernberg sees projective identification as a crucial and problematic process which uses actions in the external world to locate unwanted internal objects, suffused with excessive destructive drives and/or painful affects, and carrying their self and subject representations, into another person. Like most others who write about projective identification, he sees this as a dangerous process which depletes the self, which damages the clarity of personal identity and which weakens the capacity to handle aggressive drives. Excessive projective identification is, in Kernberg's model, a threat to the formation of a healthy ego and self, and something which leads to borderline personality organization. The contrast with Kohut's idea of the fundamental and positive role of selfobjects, is stark.

Kernberg sees the function of therapy as the immediate and clear interpretation of projective identifications in the transference. This depends on the therapist separating their experiences into:

- those which result from these projections;
- those which arise from disturbances that are the therapist's; and
- those which are not specific to either person, but are inevitable concomitants of a relationship with someone in pain, anger and confusion.

Matte Blanco

Ignacio Matte Blanco (1908–1995) graduated as a medical doctor in Chile at the age of twenty, and became a professor of physiology by twenty-five. He came to London in the mid-1930s to undertake a psychoanalytic training and entered analysis with Walter Schmideberg, son-in-law of Melanie Klein. Though Schmideberg had a classical 'Viennese' Freudian training, Matte Blanco's main influences were the leading figures of the Independent Group. Matte Blanco went on to practise psychiatry and psychoanalysis at the Johns Hopkins Hospital in the United States, and worked in New York from 1940 to 1944. He regularly attended Courant's weekly seminar in the Mathematics Department at Columbia University. He then returned to Santiago to take up the chair in psychiatry, and remained there until he emigrated to Italy with his second wife, a Kleinian training analyst, in 1966. Matte Blanco stayed in Italy until his death in 1995.

Against that multi-lingual and well-travelled background, Matte Blanco is mainly famous for one book, *The Unconscious as Infinite Sets*, and is perhaps most important for his own 'return to Freud' and to the 'structure of the unconscious'. He noted that Freud characterized the logic of the 'system unconscious' by five features:

- Absence of contradiction
- Displacement
- Condensation
- Absence of time
- Replacement of external by psychic reality.

Matte Blanco argues that these features are seen most vividly in acute psychosis and that all can be subsumed under the first heading; they all represent a failure to find the contradictions we normally expect to find by '(external) reality testing'. Displacement is a failure to link something more directly with one thing rather than another. Condensation is a failure to see as different two (or more) things normally seen as different. Absence of time is simply failure to note the contradiction in experiencing as simultaneous things that are separated in time (for example, the scrambling of memories from different points in one's history is a common feature in dreams). Finally, replacement of external by psychic reality is precisely this failure to apply the distinctions normally attended to by the conscious, perceptual, cognitive and organizing capacities of the ego.

Matte Blanco, or his admirers, created a verb: to symmetrize. This is to replace one thing by something else, typically to replace something by its opposite. This is easily seen in the classical defences of reaction formation or identification with the aggressor. However, almost all initially bizarre experiences, slips of the tongue, dream reports and so on become easier to understand if one explores them with an eye for where reversals or substitution of opposites might alter the text.

Matte Blanco linked this basic idea with mathematical set theory, particularly the ideas of infinite sets, but also with other mathematical ideas such as the collapsing of multidimensional to fewer dimensional representations. He is perhaps most persuasive when decoding and presenting subject–object reversals and part–whole reversals in the speech of psychotic patients. His work conveys very clearly how the analyst needs to have, as part of Freud's 'evenly suspended attention', the capacity to hear things and their opposites at the same time. This can apply to reversal of the meaning of whole sentences: for 'I can win' hear also 'I can't win'. Sometimes the reversals can be more complex and subtle. Perhaps a more apt reversal of 'I can win' is 'I *can* lose', with the implication that losing is an active process that might be consummated. Perhaps this flags up the question 'to whom?', shifting to a dyadic view from the previously non-specific or monadic 'I'. Perhaps too the idea of losing something is flagged up, or even of losing something to someone. Unfortunately the prosaic richness, and the humanity, of the analytic process may be easily lost in the mathematical and logical abstraction.

Matte Blanco postulates that a full understanding of people, a full psychology, must use a bi-logic model. This is a system of dual logic with one side structured by conventional logical principles, and the other by symmetrization (replacement by opposites) of some points of difference in the conventionally logical argument. This latter side of bi-logic is Freud's logic of the unconscious.

Matte Blanco has much in common with Lacan. There is the belief that analysis is not sufficient unto itself and must link with other sciences. Both draw heavily on mathematics, Matte Blanco much less formally than Lacan. Matte Blanco also draws on theology and many other disciplines. Both, perhaps partly because they draw on other languages and disciplines, can seem unreadable and seem to lose a sense of the humanity and struggle of the analytic process. Both, with Kernberg, do not see psychotic processes as necessarily unanalysable.

With Lacan and Kernberg, Matte Blanco puts *thanatos* as a central issue. For Matte Blanco, this is the ultimate of all symmetrization. It represents the triumph of the symmetrizing side of bi-logic when there are *no* differences; there is only death, annihilation or nothing. This is a very different thanatos from that of an 'aggressive drive'. Instead it is a logical process similar to Freud's rather metaphysical idea of thanatos as an urge in all living things to return to a static 'inorganic' form.

It is easy to perceive Matte Blanco as separating the two halves of his bi-logic rather clearly, like Freud's conscious and unconscious, or primary and secondary processes, or Lacan's symbolic and real. However, there is another reading in which one sees that all symbolization involves non-contradiction, the allowing of one thing (a symbol) to stand for another. As Segal, in a Kleinian tradition suggests, it is precisely the ability to equate something and its symbol, *and to know*, somehow, that the two are not the same, that distinguishes normal from psychotic symbolization. In this reading bi-logic is something prosaic and necessary to all logics, the holding of a dual position on identification of one thing with another. It remains something, like normal thinking and psychosis, of which we have very little understanding, despite all Freud, Klein, Segal, Lacan and Matte Blanco have done to remind us of its bizarreness and to help to schematize it.

Summary

All four theorists and practitioners discussed in this chapter have reshaped the network of ideas that make up modern psychodynamic thinking. They alert readers to the difficulty of theorizing, and to the difficulty of the human process of therapy. They struggle to help with the core paradox of psychodynamic work: how to use your own unconscious, by definition beyond your conscious apprehension, to become empathically and introspectively aware of the unconscious of the patient. There is a core theorem in mathematics (Gödel's Theorem) which shows that any number theory, as we currently understand such a thing, cannot be both coherent and complete. Most mathematicians now accept that any mathematical system draws on extra-mathematical cues or schemes of representation within which it is embedded. Some psychodynamic theorists accept a similar position that their theories can never be sufficient *and* complete accounts. Some have started to explore the complex mixture of levels with which language is used to capture things, such as the poetics of the technical language.

Kohut used a 'Standard Edition' technical English for much of his writing, though it is suffused with a Germanic facility with compound nouns (selfobject) and with very complex sentences. His approach demonstrated his familiarity with Freud's own German, and his personal experience of two analyses in two different cultures. Kohut was as private as an analyst can be, and hardly refers to either of these analyses in his work.

This complexity often makes Kohut difficult to read, but there is a thread of rhythm, form and tone in his writing which is important. It is probably no accident that Kohut was interested in music, a gifted pianist and musicologist, and that his early publications were reviews of analytic books about music and composers. His model of the analytic process has something of the idea of a benevolent conductor melding the selfobjects, the analyst and the patient, with all their deficits, into a functioning orchestra. At an interpersonal and intrapsychic level, this was one of the metaphors used by Foulkes in his evolution of the group analytic method.

Lacan is very different. He published relatively little himself but sanctioned an authorized transcription of his 'seminars' by his son-in-law, who in turn has sanctioned a translation into English. Both the transcription and the translation are incomplete. (There is an interesting parallel here with the fact that although most of Freud's work was written by him in German, the only complete and approved edition of his work is that of Strachey's translation. The *Gesammelte Werke* (Collected Works) did not have Freud's explicit stamp of approval and completeness in the same way as the 'Standard Edition', though neither is a truly complete collection of Freud's writings.) Lacan drew on philosophy in a way Freud eschewed, but by contrast he made little overt use of his profound knowledge of surrealist and other literature. The contrast with the way that Freud gains layers of metaphor and power from literature is stark; Sophocles, Shakespeare, Goethe, and more covertly the Old Testament, New Testament and Talmud, vie for position in Freud's writings.

Kernberg writes in clear American English. Theory is spelled out, occasional uncertainties and contradictions are noted politely or not at all. Clinical material is presented very readably, and Kernberg often reveals a reassuring uncertainty about what to do for the best in the more difficult work he describes. The location of his work is also generally made clear and interdependence with other, including medical, interventions is acknowledged.

For all his fluency in Spanish, German, English and Italian, or perhaps because of it, Matte Blanco's work is not easy to read. The text leans heavily on mathematical thinking, though most mathematicians would be disparaging of both Matte Blanco's and Lacan's depth and grasp of mathematics. The first book is a confusing collection of earlier writing, with no real treatment of the developments in his thinking over the period of the work. On the other hand, the clinical material is clear and the sense of some very simple tools to grasp the logic of the unconscious and the form and content of psychotic thinking rewards even a skim over the surface of the book.

These four theorists represent, link up and show some very different approaches to the loose ends and tangles in the weave of analytic thinking. Only Kernberg is alive to continue to shape the form of his own developments.

However, there is a body of secondary and developing literature arising from the work of all four analysts which continues to tackle the problems they highlighted – problems which are still to be solved.

Further reading

The following are shorter works or secondary source books which provide an overview of the work published by Kohut, Lacan, Kernberg and Matte Blanco.

Benvenuto, B. and Kennedy, R. (1986) *The Works of Jacques Lacan. An Introduction*. London: Free Association Books.

Kernberg, O.F. (1982) Self, ego, affects, and drives. *Journal of the American Psychoanalytic Association*, **30**, 893–917.

Kernberg, O.F. (1986) Identification and its vicissitudes as observed in psychosis. *International Journal of Psychoanalysis*, **67**, 147–159.

Kohut, H. (1979) The two analyses of Mr Z. *International Journal of Psycho-Analysis*, **60**, 3–27.

Kohut, H. and Wolf, E.S. (1978) The disorders of the self and their treatment: an outline. *International Journal of Psycho-Analysis*, **59**, 413–425.

Lacan, J. (1994) *The Four Fundamental Concepts of Psycho-Analysis*. Harmondsworth: Penguin.

Rayner, E. (1981) Infinite experiences, affects and the characteristics of the unconscious. *International Journal of Psycho-Analysis*, **62**, 403–412.

Rayner, E. (1995) *Unconscious Logic. An Introduction to Matte Blanco's Bi-logic and Its Uses*. London: Routledge.

Schneiderman, S. (1983) *Jacques Lacan. The Death of an Intellectual Hero*. Cambridge, MA: Harvard University Press.

Siegel, A.M. (1996) *Heinz Kohut and the Psychology of the Self*. London/New York: Routledge.

Wooster, G., Hutchinson, D. and Evans, C. (1990) Two examples of supervised weekly psychotherapy, illustrating bi-logic in relation to birth. *International Review of Psycho-Analysis*, **17**, 445–453.

7

Psychodynamic Psychotherapy

Kate Lockwood

Introduction

'Psychodynamic' psychotherapy is a specific individual treatment for adults that is underpinned by psychoanalytic theory. It is not associated with one particular school of psychotherapy but refers to a treatment of at least a year, at a frequency of one to three sessions per week. Psychodynamic psychotherapy is also referred to as 'psychoanalytic' psychotherapy which differentiates it from psychoanalysis (four to five times a week) and brief dynamic psychotherapy (once-weekly treatment of up to a year). It is a distinct modification of psychoanalysis that was developed within a particular clinical and social context, which aims to be accessible and jargon-free.

Historical perspective

The history of psychodynamic psychotherapy overlaps with other developments within psychoanalysis, such as therapeutic communities, group psychotherapy, brief dynamic psychotherapy and humanistic psychotherapies, both within and without the National Health Service (NHS).

MacDiarmid (1990) reviewed Ellenberger's *The Discovery of the Unconscious* and highlighted the charismatic personalities who constructed a theoretical and clinical history riddled with divisions. Janet's 'psychological analysis', Freud's 'psychoanalysis', Adler's 'individual psychology' and Jung's 'analytical psychology' describe the four main schools of thought, each based on the prevailing European philosophies, their family backgrounds and the type of patient they saw. However, despite the established notion of the 'unconscious', at the turn of this century British psychiatry was dominated by organic models of the mind, exemplified by Aubrey Lewis and Henry Maudsley.

The First World War recognized that 'shell-shock' could be treated psychotherapeutically, and the experience of army psychiatrists facilitated the use of psychodynamic methods in in-patient settings. These approaches are exemplified by the Cassel Hospital, founded by Ross in the 1920s, and Good's work with psychotic patients at Littlemore Hospital in the 1930s. The Ministry of Pensions funded out-patient departments to treat ex-serviceman, heralding accessible psychotherapy clinics, including the Tavistock Clinic which was founded by Crichton-Miller in 1920.

The Second World War stimulated further therapeutic developments, including the Northfield experiments in which the psychoanalysts Bion, Rickman, Foulkes and Main were asked to identify and treat recoverable cases of war neuroses. Their work laid the foundations for group and institutional dynamics, and informed models of group psychotherapy and therapeutic communities. Winnicott's work in paediatrics, Bowlby's work with delinquents and the Balints' work with general practitioners also helped to establish psychoanalytic ideas within health, social and probation services. Important out-patient psychotherapy departments were set up at the Maudsley Hospital, the York Clinic at Guy's Hospital and the Davidson Clinic in Edinburgh. The Tavistock Clinic, which joined the NHS in 1948, played an important role in the development of psychodynamic psychotherapy and retains an important role as a training and treatment resource.

Until 1950, the Institute of Psycho-Analysis and the Society of Analytical Psychology (SAP) were the only formal training organizations in the United Kingdom. However, the highly specialized nature of these trainings did not meet the needs of many who wished to work as psychodynamic psychotherapists in various other settings. As a consequence, a group of individuals formed the Association of Psychotherapists in 1951. Although they received personal analyses and supervision from members of the Institute of Psycho-Analysis and the SAP, their aims were different and included seminars for practitioners previously working in isolation, more access-ible and affordable training, and advocacy for greater psychodynamic psychotherapy resources.

The subsequent development of the British Association for Psycho-therapy (BAP), the London Clinic for Psychotherapy (LCP) and the Association for Group and Individual Psychotherapy (AGIP) is well documented by Scarlett (1991). In 1967, the Lincoln Centre was founded and others followed, establishing a network of independent centres offering training and treatment in a variety of geographical locations to people from all walks of life. Training also developed through regional post-graduate courses affiliated to universities and teaching hospitals. NHS psychodynamic psychotherapy was further shaped by Department of Health initiatives. In 1965, conditions were laid down regarding the work of lay psychotherapists and, in 1975, psychotherapy was recognized as an independent medical specialty.

These historical links between NHS and private trainings developed amidst a number of 'newer' psychotherapies such as cognitive, humanistic and systemic therapies. The Association for Psychoanalytic Psychotherapy in the NHS (APP) represents psychodynamically oriented psychotherapists working in the NHS, providing a forum for communication and professional development.

Principles of theory and practice

Principles of theory

'No single psychodynamic conceptual scheme can possibly have a monopoly on clinical truth' (Cox, 1974), and different schools are united in their emphasis on the interpersonal nature of human experience that is reflected in practice despite a sometimes confusing divergence of descriptive language. Psychodynamic psychotherapy draws on principles common to all the analytic schools and encompasses a model of the mind and human development that acknowledges an unconscious mental life which influences conscious perception, feeling and behaviour. It also uses the concept of an internal world populated by internalized representations of past relationships, elaborated by imagination or phantasy. It thus comprises constellations of ideas, conflicts and wishes which are symbolized, and which demand, a language of metaphor and meaning that may be universal or personal. Unconscious contents become external through projection and colour the perception of reality. This is described by the general concept of transference, a temporal dynamic whereby the past influences the present.

Psychological containment defines a state in which internal anxieties do not threaten to overwhelm the individual. It is facilitated in the infant by appropriate care that provides a balance of nurturing and frustrating experiences. This relationship provides the infant with a sense of security, from which it can explore without feeling threatened by separation anxiety. However the infant's growing awareness of two-person relationships brings fear of abandonment and loss of control, which can evoke rage and persecutory anxiety. Inadequate containment and a fear of disintegration facilitates a reliance on defence mechanisms such as denial, splitting, projection and retreat into a narcissistic world of phantasy. When the child recognizes itself as part of a three-person world with the parents, fears of rivalry, inadequacy and loss evoke anger and guilt, which are defended against by 'neurotic' defences such as depression.

Defence mechanisms are associated with developmental stages as unconscious, adaptive strategies to contain anxiety and protect self-esteem. They keep disturbing experiences from conscious awareness as the infant attempts to get rid of anxiety-laden emotions and take in identity-enhancing experiences. These primitive defences imbue subsequent relationships with patterns of behaviour which range from the immature (e.g. acting out) to the mature (e.g. sublimation, humour). Defensive styles are considered maladaptive if they restrict an individual's life or reveal primitive patterns of coping in the face of overwhelming anxiety. In both cases, they serve to distort reality and impair insight.

Psychodynamic psychotherapy is interpersonal, non-directive, interpretative, integrative and insight-oriented. It is one of a range of psychotherapies available in the NHS and other mental health settings. Psychodynamic principles may also be applied to general psychiatry practice in an attempt to understand and describe the meaning of mental illness, of whatever aetiology. It can be used to inform the management of difficult patients who may not be able to engage in regular psychodynamic treatment.

For example, psychodynamic principles have been used to understand the primitive mental mechanisms evident in psychosis. The experience of countertransference may illuminate the difficulties of mental health work and enhance clinical management. An understanding of severely disturbed patients' reaction to the experience of hospitalization and care can be helpful in alleviating staff burnout and preventing iatrogenic deterioration. The theory of psychological containment is also relevant to community care and the management of anxiety in institutions. Such work can help patients with very intractable behavioural difficulties to move out of hospital and receive more appropriate clinical management.

Aims of therapy

The aims of psychodynamic psychotherapy are:
- Internalization of the therapist as a containing figure
- Generalization of internal experience to external reality
- Increased capacity for self-reflection
- Better tolerance of frustration
- Improved self-understanding
- Increased awareness of maladaptive defences and capacity to modify them
- Raised self-esteem
- Improved interpersonal relationships
- Symptom relief

Principles of practice

Containment is provided by the boundaries of the setting, and by the therapist–patient relationship. The external setting includes the institution, room, day, time and frequency of sessions, breaks and ending date. The therapist maintains the continuity of these features and is sensitive to their impact on the patient. The relationship is guided by the 'rule of abstinence' – the therapist does not comply with requests for reassurance (e.g. physical contact) and the patient does not seek anxiety relief outside of the therapy (e.g. alcohol abuse). The therapeutic alliance, based on a mutual commitment to the work of therapy, provides an internal boundary.

Psychodynamic psychotherapy makes use of both transference and countertransference experiences. Infantile anxieties and defences come alive in the 'here and now' of the transference and illuminate previous relationships. 'Countertransference' describes the therapist's response to the patient and is a complex phenomenon that is comprised of conscious affects complicated by unconscious feelings. It is distinct from empathy which is the therapist's capacity to tune in to the patient's affective state. Adequate containment by the therapist enables the patient's problems to be revealed in the transference, and renders them available for working through without resort to defensive manoeuvres such as acting out.

Working through draws on a repertoire of non-specific and specific techniques. The therapist maintains a countenance of 'free-floating attentiveness and responsiveness', observing the patient's non-verbal behaviour and listening to what the patient is saying, trying to understand it's meaning in the transference and simultaneously monitoring counter-transference reactions. 'Passivity' is thus more apparent than real, as acknowledged by Bion in his military metaphor of 'thinking under fire'. The patient is encouraged to talk about whatever is on their mind as the dynamic view understands nothing as 'random' (e.g. slips of the tongue), but rather as conveying unconscious meaning about some aspect of the patient and their relationships.

Specific techniques comprise a group of interventions collectively described as 'taking up', classified by Greenson (1967) as confrontation, clarification and interpretation. Confrontation involves pointing out what the patient is doing, for example repeatedly arriving late at sessions. Through clarification the therapist explores what the patient means, using questioning and re-phrasing. Interpretation offers new understanding by making links between past events and experiences in the patient's current life or in the 'here and now' of therapy. A mutual exploratory style is favoured, using clear, brief and jargon-free language. An accurate, well-timed interpretation is met with relief and an opportunity to reflect on new meaning with potential for growth. It is preferable to wait for adequate 'evidence' to support an interpretation, especially when it is just below the surface, and ideally the patient should be encouraged to make the interpretation themselves. An untimely interpretation may galvanize the patient's defences, and may leave the patient feeling misunderstood.

Psychodynamic psychotherapy is initially open-ended. The date of termination is usually set by mutual agreement, but with not less than a three- or four-month period of notice. This enables the powerful transference responses related to separation and loss to be adequately acknowledged and worked through.

Psychodynamic psychotherapy achieves its aims by bringing previously hidden feelings, behaviours, experiences, connections, conflicts and intentions into awareness. This is achieved by understanding the unconscious barrier of defence mechanisms. Improved self-understanding may then be employed in the service of change.

How does psychodynamic psychotherapy differ from other therapies?

Psychodynamic psychotherapy is differentiated from other forms of psychotherapy by the techniques employed and by the aims of treatment. Supportive psychotherapy, crisis intervention and counselling employ ventilation and exploration in the service of restoration and reinforcement of defences. Non-specialist dynamic psychotherapy in mental health work uses clarification and confrontation of defences in the service of re-education and insight. Specialist psychotherapy employs interpretation of the trans-ference in the service of integration and change (Brown and Pedder, 1991; Holmes, 1991).

One of the key differences between psychodynamic psychotherapy and psychoanalysis is the reduced frequency of sessions and the use of face-to-face interaction rather than the use of a couch. This has been well described by Coltart (1993) who, in her practice of psychodynamic psychotherapy, uses non-specific techniques, facilitates greater spontaneity of emotional expression and uses a different balance between extra-transference and transference interpretation.

Brief focal psychotherapies use similar techniques but differ in that the aim is more circumscribed, the therapy is shorter and separation issues are more prominent.

Cognitive behavioural psychotherapy (CBT) does not acknowledge the unconscious or transference phenomena, and does not use interpretation. Cognitive therapy employs clarification and confrontation, and behaviour therapy uses modelling. They are more directive and concerned primarily with cognitive restructuring, behaviour modification, re-education and symptom removal. Cognitive analytic therapy (CAT) combines aspects of psychodynamic therapy (interpretation of transference issues) in a cognitive framework. These therapies are once-weekly and usually brief. However, it is important to acknowledge that there are cognitive and behavioural elements at work in psychodynamic psychotherapy in terms of cognitive learning and modelling.

Humanistic therapies form a broad group whose theoretical base combines psychoanalytic principles with humanistic psychology, especially the emphasis on equality. They acknowledge the unconscious and transference, but rarely employ interpretation. The rule of abstinence is eschewed so there are major differences in technique, including massage, body work, role play of past trauma and directive elements such as guided fantasy in the service of integration and self-acceptance. Therapy is usually once-weekly, open to changes of times, and frequently shorter.

Which patient and why?

Modern developments in the practice of psychoanalytic psychotherapy, particularly in the modification of setting and technique, render treatment available to a considerably wider group of patients than the strict assessment criteria might suggest. Psychodynamic assessment is instead concerned with understanding psychiatric disorder in the context of the patient's personality, attending to both internal and external factors. It is based on the view that interpersonal themes are central to understanding a patient's presentation. The assessment is distinct from therapy, demanding modification of technique in pursuit of its differentiated aims.

The assessment interview is a collaboratively produced 'snapshot'. Through a balance of structured and unstructured aspects it constructs a picture of the patient's internal and external worlds. By providing the patient with a glimpse of what therapy would be like it also tests motivation, and capacity to work interpretatively. However, the assessment begins before the interview itself. Particularly in health service settings, it is often relevant to consider the unconscious meaning of the referral as this may suggest lack

The aims of psychodynamic assessment
- To make a psychodynamic formulation
- To assess the patient's ability to work interpretatively ('psychological mindedness')
- To gauge motivation (particularly a patient's autonomous decision to engage in therapy)
- To make an appraisal of ego strength (the ability to withstand the rigours of therapy)
- To evaluate and include external factors (such as sources of support and reasons for referral)
- To include patient preference
- To recommend appropriate treatment(s)
- To recommend the appropriate external setting for treatment
- To give other treatment options
- To consider prognostic issues relating to treatment and outcome
- To write or communicate with the referrer about the evaluation made.

of adequate containment in the referral setting (often primary or mental health care). Referrer expectations may also include unrealistic expectations of care or cure.

Letters to patients inviting them to assessment interviews, in addition to appointment details, should at least indicate the purpose and length of the interview. Patients are frequently very anxious prior to the interview, and a considerable proportion will fail to attend. This part of the engagement process needs to be thoughtfully considered as part of the complex interaction between patient, referrer and therapist – including the transferential issues of seeking care and the expectations and reactions that this arouses.

A written questionnaire is often used which asks potential patients to describe their presenting problems, current situation, personal biography and family history. The written factual information can help to prevent the interview becoming dominated by external themes at the expense of internal and emotional ones. In addition to the facts, it also conveys information by the manner in which it is completed – for example, at some length or very briefly. The postal return of questionnaires may also help to assess motivation. However, these written questionnaires have been criticized for discrimination on cultural and educational grounds.

Different therapists will construct their assessment interviews differently. The assessor's opening moves vary from silence to a brief introductory preamble, an indication of the length and purpose of interview, and an invitation for the patient to start wherever they would like. Some therapists conduct an open interview in which the areas covered are only determined by the patient. Others will include focused direct questioning similar to a psychiatric history and mental state examination. The more unstructured aspects of the interview allow space for the development of both transference and countertransference feelings. Those who advocate a silent start argue that it provokes anxiety in the service of stimulating transference and access to the inner world. However, most therapists strike a balance between respectful social behaviour and a therapeutic stance. In this way, the patient is not overwhelmed by anxiety which could reinforce defences and render little contact possible. In skilful hands, this process can be monitored and adjusted throughout the interview, with anxiety being modulated by introducing or withholding interview structure accordingly. This can facilitate appropriate and clinically useful contact being made.

The 'psychodynamic formulation' draws together three related elements: (a) early significant relationships are described by the patient and hypothesized from observations in the assessment interview; (b) the patient's relationship with the therapist, which may be a manifestation of the transference, can be explored by 'trial interpretations' of the transference; and (c) the patient's current problems, which may be best described in terms of underlying anxieties and defensive styles, and links between them and early relationship patterns, can also be discussed.

The assessor 'listens past the conscious' and is always aiming to consider unconscious meaning in what is being said. The active processes by which this is done in the interview are clarification, confrontation and interpretation. Clarification is used to explore around an issue where the therapist has an impression that perhaps the situation is more complex than the description suggests or something is missing. The narrative may not be logical, and repressed material is often 'simplified out' of stories. Confrontation is used to directly challenge a patient's account: often when the therapist sees defence mechanisms being used to distort a subjective experience being described. It should be done judiciously to avoid uncovering anxiety that the assessment situation cannot hold.

'Trial interpretations' at assessment should be clear, brief and tentative. They have several functions:
- Testing a psychodynamic hypothesis which is part of a formulation
- Emphasizing the nature of therapy as a mutual exploration of meaning
- Gauging the possibility of a positive therapeutic alliance
- Helping patients to think of themselves in different ways
- Considering whether they find an interpretative approach therapeutic

Most initial assessment interviews last for sixty to ninety minutes. Some therapists offer a number of follow-up sessions, usually between one and five sessions of about an hour. This 'extended assessment' model affords the assessor more material on which to base a formulation and is particularly helpful if patients demonstrate a shift in how they see themselves or relationships between sessions. It indicates a capacity to use an interpretative approach, and to 'internalize' the process. In contrast, a patient who attends follow-up as if for the first time indicates that this approach is so anxiety-provoking that it has led to defensive forgetting. If there is likely to be a long delay before regular therapy starts, extended assessment may support the more vulnerable patients by having provided an opportunity to see the way in which the assessment process can make a difference to their anxiety, and thus provide hope that future treatment will be of benefit. Extended assessment is often in itself a therapeutic experience.

In most out-patient psychoanalytic psychotherapy settings, treatment is contraindicated if the predicted risks of treatment outweigh the benefits. This would include individuals whose defensive styles are primitive and employed in the face of persecutory anxiety and feared breakdown (frank psychosis or paranoid, schizoid and narcissistic personalities) and patients who exhibit marked rage associated with feared separation (substance misuse, suicidal behaviour, borderline, psychopathic, perverse or violent personalities). Relatively contraindicated are individuals who externalize anxiety into action and body parts to defend against guilt (obsessive–compulsive rituals and somatization).

These contraindications are not absolute, and the suitability for psychodynamic psychotherapy should be based on assessment of the following factors:

- Rigid and complex defences
- A restricted capacity to tolerate anxiety
- Limited affective availability
- Difficulty in symbolizing or verbalizing affects
- A tendency to experience transference interpretations as concrete and persecutory
- Low motivation
- Chronic dependency
- Addiction to treatment as a way of avoiding change and supporting defences
- Suitability for, and availability of, alternative treatments and settings
- A tendency towards dangerous behaviour and violent acting out

Which therapist and why?

Training attracts suitable individuals often by serendipity more than by design: there will be both conscious and unconscious factors at play. Potential trainees may have been inspired by reading Freud or Jung, fascinated by psychodynamic work as a trainee psychiatrist, or stimulated by a talented therapist. It is often the eye-opening discovery of the power and complexity of the unconscious that engages future psychodynamic therapists.

Therapists in psychoanalytic psychotherapy are both medical and non-medical. The medical training qualifying an individual for appointment as a Consultant Psychotherapist, or Consultant Psychiatrist in Psychotherapy, is overseen by the Psychotherapy Specialist Advisory Committee (PTSAC) to the Joint Committee for Higher Professional Training (JCHPT) at the Royal College of Psychiatrists. Accreditation requires familiarity with a wide range of therapeutic approaches, including cognitive behavioural and systemic treatments. Psychoanalytic psychotherapy is commonly the predominant modality in training. In common with all NHS medical specialities, it includes training in research and management. Doctors only wishing to practise psychoanalytic psychotherapy outside the National Health Service normally qualify through private training institutions. Many doctors training under the PTSAC-approved higher training schemes, particularly in London, do both; they undertake training in the private sector in addition to their NHS training.

Training for non-medical therapists is most commonly undertaken in the private sector at institutions recognized by the United Kingdom Council for Psychotherapy (UKCP) or British Confederation of Psychotherapists

(BCP). The UKCP provides a charter, a register and procedures to regulate and protect standards and ethics in psychotherapy trainings, covering a wide range of therapeutic modalities. The BCP has a more specific remit to maintain standards in selection, training and practice of psychoanalysis, analytical psychology and psychoanalytic psychotherapy. The private sector training organizations for psychodynamic psychotherapy include the British Association of Psychotherapists (BAP), the Scottish Institute of Human Relations (SIHR), the Lincoln Centre, the London Centre for Psychotherapy (LCP), the West Midlands Institute for Psychotherapy (WMIP) and several others. There are an increasing number of university-based courses which provide clinical training in psychodynamic psychotherapy.

Trainees who do not have a background in mental health (such as psychiatry, nursing, psychology, social work or occupational therapy) need a minimum of six months' experience in a general psychiatry setting. In some specialized NHS training centres, non-medical therapists work and train to receive accreditable psychodynamic psychotherapy qualifications within NHS posts and without participating in a private institution programme. Some such therapists in the NHS are designated as 'adult psychotherapists' and may remain employed in a post allocated to their core profession (e.g. nursing, social work or psychology).

Trainings have three components: personal therapy, supervised clinical work and theoretical teaching. Personal therapy aims to facilitate the trainee's self understanding, to be better able to withstand the emotional demands of working at this depth and intensity, and to gain a thorough personal understanding of transference and countertransference. It is usually required for a period before the training and then throughout it, at a frequency of one, two or three sessions weekly.

Supervision is an important tool in training. Various analogies have been described: a jug (pours knowledge); a potter (moulds); or a gardener (facilitates growth, with careful pruning). It has also been said that it should be more like a sand-pit in which to play with ideas than a court room in which to be judged. Supervision helps the trainee to understand the connections between clinical practice and theory. A trainee might specifically be helped to see what aspects of countertransference refer to the institution, to the patient or to their own experience. It also has an important containment function, in that the trainee (or experienced therapist) experiences support in the work and does not become overwhelmed, bored, stuck or dangerous. In a training, trainees should experience a variety of supervisors and formats of supervision.

Clinical case work for trainees should include the treatment of a range of patients in different settings. Therapies with frequencies between one and three times weekly should be undertaken, for different durations – normally between one and three years.

Theoretical teaching is organized differently on the different courses. All courses in psychodynamic psychotherapy will cover the many developments of psychoanalytic thought and their applications. Emphasis will vary depending upon stronger allegiances to one school of thought than another, although contemporary courses do show convergence between analytic frameworks and teach about contributions of alternative approaches that would have been unlikely some years ago. This pluralism does not always extend to the inclusion of Jungian theory, which may be a legacy of the early split between Freud and Jung. The importance of understanding early development is reflected in the infant-observation component of many courses.

The work demands a capacity for empathy, tenacity and tolerating uncertainty in what can be slow and painful work. Flexibility is important, though some therapists discover a 'talent' for working with particular groups: for example being able to work with the turbulent emotions evoked by patients who have borderline personality organization, or to make contact with psychotic patients who otherwise remain isolated. The whole experience and personality of the therapist is called upon as a therapeutic tool.

Therapeutic setting

Therapy is conducted in fifty-minute sessions, with patient and therapist usually seated to face each other. They sit at a slight angle, in a clean, comfortable, warm and quiet room. The therapy should not happen in different rooms, and the room regularly used should not contain explicitly personal items which would reveal private information about the therapist. Some psychodynamic psychotherapists use rooms which contain no extraneous items whatsoever, and so give no clue about themselves at all. In rooms that need to be booked or rented, which are used by several therapists or others, there may be little choice about the physical arrangements.

Sessions are planned for the same time each week, and this is commonly once-weekly. In more intensive forms of psychodynamic psychotherapy, sessions can be two or three times a week, and as they become more frequent the therapy comes to resemble psychoanalysis more closely – and a couch might be used with the therapist in or out of view.

Breaks in therapy are arranged in advance, commonly to fit with termly patterns of holidays. The duration of therapy is negotiated between therapist and patient. It is usually open-ended as therapy starts, and most therapies which are not terminated prematurely continue for between one and three years.

In private therapy, accounts for payment are given or sent to the patient regularly. In health service settings, agreement for providing long-term treatment may need to be secured in advance.

The organizational context

NHS psychodynamic psychotherapy services may be led by medical consultant psychotherapists, psychologists or consultant psychiatrists with an interest in psychotherapy. Psychodynamic psychotherapy is also provided by therapists in private practice, the voluntary sector, external training organizations and in other settings such as university health services. Geographically, services differ widely. In the public sector, where demand is great, the administration of resources operates to different underlying philosophies of care and an equitable and accessible service is not widely available (Holmes and Lindley, 1989; Obholzer, 1989; Maloney, 1996).

The work of a psychodynamic psychotherapy service can be seen as direct and indirect. Direct work is the assessment and treatment of patients. Indirect work refers to training and supervision, consultation and staff support through links with general psychiatry, primary care and liaison settings. Training and supervision includes that of psychiatric trainees, honorary therapists, other mental health workers and GP counsellors who employ psychodynamic principles. Consultation involves attending ward rounds and clinical meetings in psychiatry, primary care and liaison settings to psychodynamically inform patient management. Staff support aims to facilitate and support the work of ward and community mental health teams by understanding defensive procedures adopted by the staff group to contain anxiety. A well-integrated model supports links between general psychiatrists and other psychotherapists, mitigating against the defensive splitting and mutual devaluation to contain anxiety fostered by ignorance of each other's work.

The institutional setting must hold the therapeutic alliance, and NHS departments are well placed to utilize other aspects of the mental health service to provide adequate containment for more disturbed patients. Examples include day-hospital programmes, in-patient admissions and medication. Unfortunately NHS psychotherapy services are rarely well enough resourced to provide a comprehensive service and therapists in private practice are not equipped to contain such difficult patients.

Psychodynamic case-work is frequently in conflict with other service and training requirements. It can be an important experience for an interested nurse or junior psychiatrist to manage personal and interpersonal boundaries through the reliability and punctuality demanded for patients and supervision, and ensuring that others demanding their time are made to wait (McGinley and O'Reilly, 1994).

Clinical example

Brian, a 21-year-old nursing student, was referred with an eighteen-month history of moderate to severe depression, unresponsive to antidepressants, which caused him to withdraw from his studies. Brian wished to explore the possibility of leaving nursing.

Brian described feeling empty, confused and inexplicably angry. He talked blandly of his family: his father (59), a hospital porter, his mother (58), who suffered depression after his birth, and a 39-year-old married sister. As Brian relaxed he expressed some frustration that his parents only cared about his career. He recalled feeling frightened and desperate when his parents argued as he did a jigsaw behind the settee. He felt sensitive and excluded in friendships, and his depression began during his obstetrics placement. The psychotherapist assessing him was struck by a veiled hostility and a reluctance to leave the room at the end of the interview.

The psychodynamic formulation was based on an insecure childhood attachment with the possibility of his conception being a mistake, his mother's depression, his father's long work hours and their marital disharmony. This was evidenced by ambivalence in the transference (experienced as frustrated neediness and rage) and pointed to underlying anxieties that threatened to destroy others or himself. He had contained these by becoming his own 'nurse-mother' and externalizing his neediness into patients. This defensive structure was put under stress when he was faced with the reality of nursing mothers that excluded him during his obstetrics placement. This caused withdrawal into his primitive and empty narcissistic world which was devoid of good-enough relationships. This world was filled with destructive rage, inexplicable anger and confusion which he projected onto others, then seeing them as hostile. Brian's dilemma could be understood as a conflict as to whether he should 'destroy' his parents (or at least his mental image of them) by leaving nursing, or find something in his career that met his reality-based need for satisfaction in work and relationships.

Despite his fragile self-esteem, Brian demonstrated an adequately healthy capacity (he had studied and made some relationships) and he was offered once-weekly therapy with a female therapist in tandem with out-patient appointments with a psychiatrist. He attended sessions regularly and punctually but was reluctant to leave them at the end. He requested a more comfortable chair, and became irritated at the occasional noise of crying from the hospital crèche.

In the countertransference, the therapist felt pressured to extend sessions (which she resisted) but did provide the chair (perhaps her response to Brian's need for a nurse-mother). She sometimes dreaded sessions and had fantasies of cancelling them (a rejecting response to his overwhelming neediness). Brian saw her as both idealized and critical/rejecting.

Supervision and personal therapy helped the therapist to understand the contribution made by feelings about deprivation in her own childhood and her personal need to look after others as a therapist.

The therapist took up Brian's childhood themes of feeling ignored (by preoccupied parents) and having to hide his need for care (behind the settee) whilst trying to piece things together (jigsaw) in the face of destructive rage. She also made links to transference experiences and events which he described as taking place outside of the therapy. The therapist tentatively explored his need for a comfortable 'crèche' with an exclusive nurse-mother, his fear of rejection if his needs were expressed, evoking despair and rage, and his attempt to denigrate and get rid of his neediness – revealed in his contempt for the crying babies.

In the first six months, patient and therapist mainly worked through these themes extra-transferentially: Brian became anxious and denied transference interpretations, but found some relief in being heard. He expressed anger about his current situation, including his feeling that a female flat-mate hated and ignored him, and that his parents were always on his back.

After eight months the therapist had a two-week break, liaising with Brian's psychiatrist. On her return, he unusually missed a session. This worried his therapist and she rang his flat but got no reply. She informed the psychiatrist who contacted Brian's general practitioner, and they learned that Brian had taken an overdose the previous day. Supervision helped the therapist to understand her feelings of guilt (at abandoning him) and anger (at his attack on her as the rejecting parent). It was decided, in discussion with the psychiatrist, that improved containment might facilitate the work and the sessions were increased to twice-weekly.

The overdose (precipitated by perceived indifference from a flat-mate when he told her he was fed up) was taken up, as was his anger to the therapist for treating him with contempt and abandoning him. Brian became curious about transference interpretations and began to work through his angry feelings *towards the therapist and how they represented unresolved childhood fears. He frequently brought dreams full of homicidal action towards establishment figures. These were associated with his demanding yet emotionally indifferent parents. In fact, his parents were pressurising him to 'pull himself together' and get back to nursing, blaming 'too much therapy' for his overdose. He felt more contained by the therapy, but often indulged in alcohol-binges during breaks.*

After eighteen months, Brian was on a reduced dose of antidepressants, had returned to nursing part-time and was thinking of taking a research post in a distant city. Further working through enabled him to internalize the therapist as neither idealized nor rejecting, but rather as 'good-enough' though flawed. He decided to accept the post, which was taken up in his therapy as adaptive, as meeting his wish to stand up to his parents and as allowing him to research his own view of the world. The last six months explored themes of abandonment in detail, and therapy ended after two years. At the last session, Brian brought the therapist a tape of his favourite music. She accepted with a smile, interpreting it as representing his need to be heard and kept in mind.

Brian continued to have a tendency to adopt his narcissistic withdrawn state when disappointed by friends. However, maturation would now be likely to facilitate further growth, with his new capacity for self-reflection and insight.

Problems in therapy

Problems and pitfalls are inherent in psychodynamic practice, and they are complicated by prevalent misconceptions that can lead to 'mistakes'. They can be understood as related to factors concerning containment, technique or both. Most 'mistakes' have transference and countertransference contributions and are best understood in the context of the therapeutic relationship. Regular, honest supervision is essential as mistakes are more likely where therapy is practised in isolation.

Session boundaries

The therapist is responsible for protecting the continuity of the external setting. However, some problems are unavoidable and, like holiday breaks, represent separations that evoke anxiety that should be taken up with the patient. A related problem is the emergence of distressing material towards the end of a session when the therapist feels pressured to extend time. In practice, the distress should be sensitively acknowledged, the patient reminded the end is near, and the pattern taken up subsequently as possibly defending against facing painful feelings in the session. Lateness and absence on the part of the patient may represent defences or ambivalence in the face of transference anxieties, and should be taken up.

The rule of abstinence

The rule of abstinence serves to establish containment. It facilitates the patient's capacity to tolerate and verbalize anxieties rather than act on them within the session (acting in) or outside therapy (acting out). These represent a belief in the magical power of action to get a reassuring response from the external world as a substitute for working through. Such actions communicate unconscious meaning and can be a stimulus to therapy if sensitively taken up and explored.

Acting in

Acting in (for example, requests for personal contact or touching, or direct questions about the therapist's life) may be benign and the therapist may choose to answer questions or accept presents after their meaning has been understood and worked through. Not to do so in some instances (for example, being given a gift at the end of a long therapy, or a request for a glass of water) would be insensitive. Abstinence does not demand aloofness, for it can confirm transference anxieties and be counterproductive. Physical contact is very controversial and best taken up in terms of acknowledging the patient's anxieties and working through the meaning in the transference.

Acting out

Acting out includes substance misuse, deliberate self-harm and suicidal behaviour, which often occurs around separations (e.g. breaks). Self-harm is the most worrying in practice and, where the therapist is concerned about risk, it is important to act on this by contacting the family or colleagues, possibly to arrange admission. It is a misconception that confidentiality forbids any exchange with others, and real risk must be dealt with both appropriately and ethically. This will outweigh the impact on the therapeutic alliance, which can be taken up later. Serious acting out is characteristic of borderline and narcissistic personalities. It is better contained if predicted, and a contract should be drawn up with the patient at the outset as part of a coordinated treatment package including contingency plans with colleagues and family who should all be aware of the risks involved.

'Stuck' therapies and negative therapeutic reactions

When the therapist feels no contact or progress is being made ('stuck' therapies) or a patient suddenly leaves treatment ('negative therapeutic reaction'), technical problems arise. The former describes a gradual phenomenon which must be understood in terms of transference and countertransference themes and may represent faulty technique or a more subtle collusion in avoiding anxiety. Steiner (1993) describes how some patients withdraw from severe anxiety into a defensive 'psychic retreat' which may be shifted by adopting a different interpretative style. The sudden negative therapeutic reaction is characterized by hostility or a manic flight into health, and may be a defensive response to negative transference.

Medication

Another misconception is that medication interferes with treatment. In practice, many patients are on psychotropic medications that may be essential to restore and maintain the patient in a state which allows engagement in the therapeutic alliance. Requests for medication in treatment should be explored as possible acting out, but may be realistic and healthy. Prescribing should be undertaken by a colleague as the impact on the transference can be complex and troublesome.

Demographic issues

Problems can arise around issues of race, gender or sexuality, such as requests to see a therapist of particular demographic characteristics. In these cases, the meaning of the request should be explored to assess the balance of defensive and realistic components. There are real issues regarding equality and accessibility of service: most patients and therapists are white, more women than men are referred and so are more heterosexuals (Kareem and Littlewood, 1992). There are complex socio-cultural reasons for this which partly reflect social defence systems. Issues of race or sexuality may be used by both patient and therapist as a landscape on which to externalize all that is disturbing, defending against these themes being worked through and used in a way that could lead to therapeutic change.

Dependency and inappropriate involvement

Misconceptions have been expressed that dynamic psychotherapy aims to transform the patient into somebody just like the therapist and to promote dependency. Professional misconduct committees have been set up to consider serious mistakes, which may have both conscious and unconscious components, such as the financial or sexual exploitation of patients. However, these complications can be reduced by stringent selection procedures and regular peer review.

Inflexibility

Subtler mistakes include dogmatism, being too abstinent, using jargon, being too persecutory, giving untimely interpretations, being vague and baffling, and not being open to exploring possibilities – including the one that the therapist is wrong! All of these will be accompanied by decreased rapport and less useful therapeutic contact.

Evaluation of therapy

Criticism of psychodynamic psychotherapy as untested and unscientific has been rife but has met with thoughtful rebuttal (Holmes and Lindley, 1989; McNeilly and Howard, 1991). Psychodynamic psychotherapy has been challenged by evidence-based medicine, in response to which there is growing call for randomized controlled outcome trials. However, this presents complex methodological and ethical issues (Fonagy and Higgitt, 1989).

Waiting list controls are flawed by the instillation of hope, and 'placebo' sessions do not exclude non-specific factors and have questionable face validity (Malan, 1973; Prioleau *et al.*, 1983). Adequate power and sample size is difficult to achieve, not least because of the heterogeneous diagnostic group that psychodynamic psychotherapy treats, who may also be unwilling to participate. This was demonstrated in the Maudsley/Tavistock study (Candy *et al.*, 1972), where insufficient numbers were recruited due to the screening procedures to control for multiple variables. Dolan and Coid (1993) also argue that the medical model of randomized controlled trials is not applicable to the treatment of patients with severe personality disorders. Such problems have generated a vogue for meta-analysis but this also poses difficulties as psychodynamic studies rarely meet the inclusion criteria (Lambert *et al.*, 1986).

Defining treatment confronts the problem of what it is and how it is delivered, in terms of consistency between sessions and therapists that accounts for specific and non-specific factors. Psychodynamic psychotherapy is difficult to 'manualize' and session-recording introduces a variable with transference implications. Hobson (1988) describes how research has to involve measurement of therapist and patient characteristics, the therapeutic alliance and specific therapeutic techniques. Variables are complex, as opposed to the discrete components that are easier to enumerate within a cognitive behaviour framework. Process research needs to combine qualitative and quantitative methodologies which involve written, taped or video-recorded transcripts of sessions rated by a neutral observer.

Change must be evaluated over appropriate time frames to capture longer-term outcome (Siassi, 1979; Sjostrom, 1985). Study of longer-term psychodynamic psychotherapy lends itself to case studies and naturalistic field studies to inform hypotheses that can be tested using more rigorous methods. This has produced important results which assist in making the case that psychodynamic psychotherapy is an essential treatment for some of our most challenging patients (Milton, 1996). A good example of process research includes the case studies of Clementel-Jones and Malan (1988), who described eight patients in detail, both successes and failures, and illustrated how assessment material reveals cogent psychodynamic hypotheses that can be tracked in semi-structured follow-up interviews to study how anxieties have evolved or resolved over the years.

Outcome studies have demonstrated the need for long-term dynamic psychotherapy in a range of disorders, especially more severe pathology, and challenge the prevalent assumption that 'shorter is better'. A meta-analyses by Howard (1986) found that 50% of patients were improved after eight sessions compared to 75% after twenty-six sessions. Frank *et al.* (1989) found dynamic psychotherapy superior to medication in the prophylaxis of depression. Siassi (1979) compared open-ended psychodynamic therapy with other psychotherapies in fifty-four anxious patients on concurrent drug treatment. Patients and assessors focused on the medication aspect of the trial to control for bias. The drug treatment was stopped at six months whilst therapy continued. Outcome at both six months and two years favoured psychotherapy. A retrospective survey by Clementel-Jones *et al.* (1990) concluded that short-term therapy can undercut potential effectiveness in severe personality disorder where forty to sixty sessions are needed; this was reiterated by Dolan and Coid (1993). Stevenson and Meares (1992) investigated well-defined twice-weekly out-patient dynamic therapy for one year in patients with a diagnosis of borderline personality disorder. Outcome (measured in terms of prescribed medication, visits to the doctor, episodes of self-harm, hospital admission and a self-report symptom index) revealed improvement at the outset which was maintained at one year, with 30% of the sample no longer fulfilling diagnostic criteria for a personality disorder. Sjostrom (1985) completed a retrospective study of long-term psychodynamic therapy with fourteen patients suffering from schizophrenia. Outcome (measured in terms of time spent in hospital, ability to work, social contacts and symptoms) was studied at both six and eight years post-therapy by means of video-recordings which were blindly rated. Compared with a matched control group, the treatment group fared significantly better.

Alternatives to therapy

Alternative approaches need to be considered in deciding which patient is offered which type of therapy. This needs to take into account the nature and severity of the patient's problems, the defensive styles used, patient preferences and what is available. Research gives limited guidelines as to what treatment is indicated due to difficulties in generalizing to clinical settings. In practice the choice is informed by what the patient will best be helped by at this time.

Orlinsky and Howard (1986) concluded that, given a range of treatments with proven efficacy in less severe disorders (e.g. cognitive therapy in mild depression and eating disorders, behaviour therapy in obsessive–compulsive disorder and phobias), psychodynamic psychotherapy tends to be the choice for individuals with complex personality difficulties and longstanding interpersonal problems. A broad group of patients may therefore benefit from psychological treatments which are less specialized than psychodynamic psychotherapy. Supportive psychotherapy maintains stability in the chronic and seriously mentally ill: it does not cause any hazard through challenging ego defences, and it can improve social skills and general fulfilment in patients' lives. Crisis intervention and counselling help to restore individuals to effective function after situational crises.

The choice of specialist psychotherapeutic treatments for adult patients in NHS services is usually between cognitive behavioural therapies and psychoanalytically informed approaches. Systemic approaches are mostly used for families in which the referred patient is a child. The humanistic, experiential and creative therapies are not often used as treatment modalities in their own right in the health service, and they more commonly form part of a structured therapeutic programme. In private settings, the whole range of therapies are available as alternatives for those for whom psychodynamic psychotherapy may be the treatment of choice.

Patients who may be better helped by a directive approach, like cognitive behavioural therapy include those who are strongly defended against deep self-scrutiny, who blame others, or want to be told what to do: they may be better helped by an approach that focuses on symptom removal, particularly if they are motivated to engage in the active components of therapy. Cognitive analytic therapy is an alternative which provides an opportunity to combine an interpretative approach with a cognitive framework; its structure means patients work hard and fast – it can help those who have sufficient ego strength to tolerate and use a brief therapy.

Focal therapy may be preferred for circumscribed difficulties with limited goals or motivation for change. It requires capacity to tolerate early separation anxieties; an external supportive network may be important.

An analysis may be indicated for patients with longstanding difficulties concerning lifelong patterns, possibly with persistent psychiatric disorder, who demonstrate adequate motivation, ego-strength and psychological-mindedness. This may widen options for patients who can make the financial and time commitments, and can achieve rewarding results.

Group therapy may be indicated for difficulties in interpersonal relationships, or individuals who would find the dyadic intimacy of individual therapy too threatening, and individuals likely to get stuck in dependent regression. Some patients feel less exposed and threatened in a group and may develop to a stage where they could use an individual therapy. The converse is also true: a course of individual psychodynamic psychotherapy may help somebody to a position where considerable further gains could be achieved by group therapy.

There are other instances where it is appropriate for a long-term trajectory of care to include several components. For example, a patient might use one therapy to facilitate engagement in another, or may not be ready for a dynamic approach when preoccupied with current life events such as impending divorce, childbirth or college exams. A patient in the midst of such events may best be supported by an extended psychodynamic assessment, a focal piece of work or a directive symptom-relieving strategy – with an intention of reviewing treatment in the future. Examples of components of a treatment 'package' may include removal of a phobia with behaviour therapy, counselling for alcohol dependency and medication for severe depression. A period of cognitive therapy may reveal themes that the patient wishes to explore further with an interpretative approach, seeking self-understanding in addition to symptom removal.

Complementary therapeutic strategies may also be needed during a course of psychodynamic psychotherapy to hold the necessary distress and disturbance which might be released by the acquisition of painful insight. Management could include hospitalization, psychotropic medication, attendance at psychiatric out-patient clinics or day hospital care. This is particularly the case for borderline personalities with a known history of psychotic episodes where acting out or breakdown is a predicted risk.

Further reading

Bateman, A. and Holmes, J. (1995) *Introduction to Psychoanalysis: Contemporary Theory and Practice*. London and New York: Routledge.

Casement, P. (1985) *On Learning from the Patient*. London: Tavistock.

Coltart, N. (1993) *How to Survive as a Psychotherapist*. London: Sheldon Press.

Freeman, C. and Tyrer, P. (1992) *Research Methods in Psychiatry: A Beginner's Guide*, 2nd edn. London: Gaskell/Royal College of Psychiatrists.

Garfield, S.L. and Bergin, A.E. (eds) (1986) *Handbook of Psychotherapy and Behavior Change*, 3rd edn. New York: John Wiley.
Holmes, J. (ed.) (1991) *Textbook of Psychotherapy in Psychiatric Practice*. London: Churchill Livingstone.
Jackson, M. and Williams, P. (1994) *Unimaginable Storms: A Search for Meaning in Psychosis*. London: Karnac Books.
Main, T.F. (1957) The ailment. *British Journal of Medical Psychology*, **30**, 129–145.
Storr, A. (1990) *The Art of Psychotherapy*, 2nd edn. London: Butterworth–Heinemann.

Bibliography

Bion, W. (1962) *Learning from Experience*. London: Heinemann.
Brown, D. and Pedder, J. (1991) *Introduction to Psychotherapy: An Outline of Psychodynamic Principles and Practice*, 2nd edn. London: Tavistock/Routledge.
Candy, J., Balfour, F.H.G., Cawley, R.H. *et al.* (1972) A feasibility study for a controlled trial of formal psychotherapy. *Psychological Medicine*, **2**, 345–362.
Clementel-Jones, C. and Malan, D. (1988) Outcome in dynamic psychotherapy. Clinical examples of long-term follow-up following individual psychoanalytic psychotherapy. *British Journal of Psychotherapy*, **6**, 29–45.
Clementel-Jones, C., Malan, D. and Trauer, T. (1990) A retrospective follow-up of 84 patients treated with individual psychoanalytic psychotherapy. Outcome and predictive factors. *British Journal of Psychotherapy*, **6**, 363–374.
Coltart, N. (1993) *How to Survive as a Psychotherapist*. London: Sheldon Press.
Cox, M. (1974) Dynamic psychotherapy with sex offenders. Lecture to the Finnish Psychiatric Association.
Dolan, B. and Coid, J. (1993) *Psychopathic and Antisocial Personality Disorders. Treatment and Research Issues*. London: Gaskell.
Fonagy, P. and Higgitt, A. (1989) Evaluating the performance of departments of psychotherapy. *Psychoanalytic Psychotherapy*, **4**, 121–153.
Frank, E., Kupfer, D.J. and Perel, M. (1989) Early recurrence in unipolar depression. *Archives of General Psychiatry*, **46**, 397–400.
Greenson, R.R. (1967) *The Technique and Practice of Psychoanalysis*. London: Hogarth Press.
Hobson, R.P. (1988) *Psychotherapy and Research – Are They Compatible?* London: Tavistock Clinic Paper, No. 126.
Holmes, J. (ed.) (1991) *Textbook of Psychotherapy in Psychiatric Practice*. London: Churchill Livingstone.
Holmes, J. and Lindley, R. (1989) *The Values of Psychotherapy*. Oxford: Oxford University Press.
Howard, K.I., Kopta, S.M., Krause, M.S. and Orlinsky, D.E. (1986) The dose–effect relationship in psychotherapy. *American Psychologist*, **41**, 159–164.
Kareem, J. and Littlewood, R. (1992) *Intercultural Therapy, Themes, Interpretations and Practice*. Oxford: Blackwell Scientific.
Lambert, M.J., Shapiro, D.A. and Bergin, A.E. (1986) The effectiveness of psychotherapy. In: S.L. Garfield and A.E. Bergin (eds), *Handbook of Psychotherapy and Behavior Change*, 3rd edn. New York: John Wiley, pp. 157–211.
MacDiarmid, D. (1990) Books reconsidered: the discovery of the unconscious; the history and evolution of dynamic psychiatry: Henri F. Ellenberger. *British Journal of Psychiatry*, **156**, 135–139.
Malan, D. (1973) The outcome problem in psychotherapy research. *Archives of General Psychiatry*, **29**, 719–729.
Maloney, C. (1996) Setting up stall in the market place: psychotherapy in a state health service. *Psychiatric Bulletin*, **20**, 277–281.

McGinley, E. and O'Reilly, J. (1994) Psychodynamic supervision for junior hospital doctors. *Psychiatric Bulletin*, **18**, 85–87.

McNeilly, C. and Howard, K. (1991) The effects of psychotherapy: a re-evaluation based on dosage. *Psychotherapy Research*, **1**, 74–78.

Milton, J. (1996) *Presenting the Case for Psychoanalytic Psychotherapy Services: An Annotated Bibliography*, 3rd edn. London: Association for Psychoanalytic Psychotherapy in the NHS and the Tavistock Clinic/Psychotherapy Section of the Royal College of Psychiatrists.

Obholzer, A. (1989) The future of psychotherapy in the NHS. *Psychiatric Bulletin*, **13**, 432–434.

Orlinsky, D.E. and Howard, K.I. (1986) Process and outcome in psychotherapy. In: S.L. Garfield and A.E. Bergin (eds), *Handbook of Psychotherapy and Behavior Change*, 3rd edn. New York: John Wiley, pp. 311–381.

Prioleau, I., Murdock, M. and Brody, N. (1983) An analysis of psychotherapy *v.* placebo studies. *Behavioural and Brain Sciences*, **6**, 275–310.

Scarlett, J. (1991) Getting established: initiatives in psychotherapy training since World War Two. *British Journal of Psychotherapy*, **7**, 260–267.

Siassi, I. (1979) A comparison of open-ended psychoanalytically-oriented psychotherapy with other therapies. *Journal of Clinical Psychiatry*, **40**, 25–32.

Sjostrom, R. (1985) Effects of psychotherapy in schizophrenia. *Acta Psychiatrica Scandinavica*, **71**, 513–522.

Steiner, J. (1993) *Psychic Retreats: Pathological Organisations in Psychotic, Neurotic and Borderline Patients*. London and New York: Routledge.

Stevenson, J. and Meares, R. (1992) An outcome study of psychotherapy for patients with borderline personality disorder. *American Journal of Psychiatry*, **149**, 358–362.

8
Brief Focal Psychotherapy

Terri Eynon and Samuel M. Stein

Introduction

Brief focal psychotherapy is a broad-based concept which consists of a number of overlapping but different theoretical models. It has also been described as time-limited, brief or focal psychotherapy and may include all of these aspects of therapy, or may emphasize only one particular component. The method utilizes many of the principles and techniques of longer-term dynamic and analytical psychotherapies. However, it should not be seen as an abbreviated version of long-term therapy since it uses a distinctive adaptation of therapeutic principles and is a treatment modality in its own right.

Brief focal psychotherapy demands certain characteristics of both the therapist and the patient. It is based on a sophisticated theoretical model, which aims to bring about significant and permanent changes by means of the therapist and patient identifying and concentrating on a specific dynamic focus which is worked with within a limited time framework (Hobbs, 1996). Brief focal psychotherapy may also be seen to combine aspects of dynamic, cognitive, systemic and behavioural theory, and has been described 'as a meeting point between psychodynamic and behavioural approaches' (Rosen, 1986). As a consequence, the therapeutic model is relatively structured, which may be particularly helpful to patients who present with a sense of helplessness or chaos.

This type of therapy is suitable for a small proportion of patients who are carefully selected. They need the capacity to withstand an intensive, demanding and time-limited interaction with another person. It has been most effectively used with patients suffering from neurotic disturbance, but it is increasingly being employed in the treatment of more severely disturbed individuals with longstanding personality problems. For these reasons, brief focal psychotherapy has become an attractive treatment from a cost-efficiency viewpoint. Using this form of therapy it has been possible to offer a greater number of patients an exposure to dynamic psychotherapy. However, as Ashurst (1991) points out, 'Quicker is not necessarily better', and the effectiveness of this treatment is ultimately determined by careful selection of patients and a high degree of skill and activity in the therapist.

Historical perspective

Brief focal psychotherapy has its origins in the psychoanalytic movement and originated with Freud as most of the early analyses he conducted were in fact short-term therapies, and his reputation developed partly through his success in quickly relieving symptoms in his patients (Rosen, 1986). Later Freud was both concerned about, and accepting of, the inevitability of change in the established practice of psychoanalysis in order that it might be offered to a wider range of patients. He did not himself see longer treatments as necessarily being more effective. For example, in 1912 he experimented by setting a termination date for the therapy which he later described in the case of the 'Rat Man'.

In 1937, Freud wrote a paper entitled 'Analysis Terminable and Interminable', yet the problem of treatment length was not taken up by the psychoanalytic community. Instead there developed a rift between Freud and, in particular, Ferenczi and Rank. These pupils of Freud began to experiment with briefer therapies, which were more active and placed greater emphasis on time limits. Freud took exception to Ferenczi's attempts to provide a corrective emotional experience, something which was to be later explored by Alexander and French in 1946. In this work there was particular emphasis placed on the 'here and now', which was to become important for the later development of brief focal psychotherapy. This emphasis distinguished brief focal psychotherapy from the traditional Freudian emphasis on historical experience.

The birth of brief focal psychotherapy in the United Kingdom emerged during the 1950s with the work of Michael and Enid Balint at the Tavistock Clinic in London. David Malan, who was also part of the Tavistock Clinic workshop, had a significant impact on the further development of brief therapy. At the same time, though independently, there were similar developments in North America. Sifneos described a 'short-term anxiety-provoking psychotherapy' in 1972, and Mann developed 'time-limited' psychotherapy in 1973. This was followed in 1980 by Davanloo's 'short-term dynamic psychotherapy'. Both Sifneos and Davanloo emphasized an overtly active and confrontational therapy technique, while Mann emphasized the importance of the time-limited nature of the therapy.

Brief focal therapy has enjoyed a surge in popularity since the 1980s, partly in response to economic pressures and partly in an attempt to offer treatment to more patients. There has been heated debate on the necessary 'dose' of psychotherapy which might be required. Butcher and Koss (1978) showed that most therapeutic contacts, even if they were planned otherwise, usually turned out to be brief ones. Whilst Ashurst (1991) defined brief psychotherapy as 'therapy of limited duration, lasting between one and fifty sessions in total', Malan (1963) suggested forty weeks as an upper limit, although this now would be seen as a relatively long therapy within the National Health Service. As a consequence, the practice of brief focal psychotherapy tends to last between sixteen and twenty sessions. But, as Rosen (1986) points out, there is little evidence pointing to an optimum number of sessions despite careful consideration of selection and therapeutic aims.

Therapists and researchers participating in the Sheffield Psychotherapy Project have even experimented with ultra-brief therapies based on Robert Hobson's 'Conversational Model'. They have developed and evaluated a two-plus-one model, in which the therapy comprises of two initial sessions, with a third follow-up session after a period of time (Shapiro and Firth, 1987; Barkham, 1989).

Principles of theory and practice

Principles of theory

The guiding principles of brief focal psychotherapy are the presence of a core dynamic focus and the adherence to active therapeutic techniques within a specified time frame. Both patient and therapist arrive at an agreed focus, with associated goals which are relevant and acceptable to the patient's difficulties. The aim of the focus is to explore an underlying core conflict which will link formative past experiences and current therapeutic interactions (Hobbs, 1996). This core conflict is a theoretical construction which describes the way in which early experience has determined the patient's subsequent approach to the world. Brief focal psychotherapy is therefore often a good choice of treatment for patients who have a well-circumscribed set of problems with a focus which can be dynamically understood and described. This was clarified by Ashurst (1991), who said 'Unless most of the patient's difficulties revolve around a central conflict that can be defined in psychodynamic terms, it is unlikely that short term therapy will be helpful.' As a consequence of its analytic origins, brief focal psychotherapy also pays serious attention to unconscious and internal psychological processes. The therapy concerns itself both with the relationship in reality between therapist and patient, and the transference relationship, which illuminates the impact of early internalized interactions (Hobbs, 1996).

Although a patient may come for therapy with a particular problem or symptom, this does not necessarily provide a focus. The focus should be a core conflict which is connected with intense feelings originating in past relationships which are subsequently re-evoked in current relationships. This is elicited early on in the transference relationship between patient and therapist, and often manifests itself during the assessment period (Hobbs, 1996). It is this interaction, rather than the presenting symptom, which forms the focus of therapy.

Malan (1976) described the high level of motivation, in both the patient and the therapist, that is required to maintain the focality, and Balint used the term 'selective attention' and 'selective neglect' to describe the way in which a therapist concentrates on the relevant therapeutic focus. The therapist needs to be alert to attempts on the part of the patient to avoid significant issues, and should refuse to be drawn down interesting by-ways which are unrelated to the core conflict. Patients whose problems are highly complex are often unable to work with the therapist to define a clear focus, and therefore would be unlikely to benefit from this approach (Hobbs, 1996).

In brief focal psychotherapy both the patient and the therapist are constantly reminded of the time limit on the therapy. As a consequence, patterns of early experience are recruited into the therapeutic relationship through the transference with great speed and intensity. Luborsky (1984) has described such transference-related interactions in his Core Conflictual Relationship Theme (CCRT) and using this theoretical perspective with a focused core conflict, the therapy may be deeper and may have much in common with more analytic psychotherapies.

Brief focal therapy may therefore involve an intense transference, which requires a strong therapeutic alliance with a patient who is able to demonstrate sufficient ego strength to bear feelings which might be aroused without acting out unduly. Active therapeutic measures also help to break down maladaptive and established core conflicts, allowing new-found and adaptive methods to come to the fore which will enhance growth and development. According to Llewelyn et al. (1988), the relationship with the therapist as a person, and the opportunity to identify and rehearse new ways of problem-solving, are particularly important in a short exploratory therapy. Ashurst (1991) also emphasizes the importance of the cathartic effect of sharing powerful and distressing feelings with another person who is attentive, respectful and non-judgemental. The strength of the therapeutic alliance at sessions three or four has been shown by Morgan et al. (1982) to correlate positively with outcome. Such methods, however, provoke much anxiety, and it is often necessary to make sure that the patient has adequate support from family and friends while the therapy is in progress.

Termination in brief therapy is a key issue and, in time-limited therapy, a fixed end-point is negotiated at the beginning of treatment. This highlights the 'ending' and provides a focus for looking at issues of separation, loss, abandonment and deprivation (Hobbs, 1996). These limitations, which emphasize the finiteness of time, have the potential to promote acting out in both the patient and the therapist. However, the breaches of boundaries and time-keeping are all grist for the therapeutic mill.

Whilst the immediate aims of brief focal psychotherapy are of necessity more limited than those of longer-term therapies, follow-up studies have found a 'snowball' effect with improvement continuing after treatment has finished (Rosen, 1986). Much of the 'working through' initiated in a brief focal therapy will need to go on after the therapy has ended (Ashurst, 1991). As with all therapies, it is hoped that the patient will continue to maintain an introspective self-awareness, and this may be enhanced if the patient gets into the habit of linking the influences of his therapy with everyday life. By 'practising' what he has learnt in therapy, the patient may be able to develop more adaptive and coping strategies which may prevent reoccurrence of the identified conflicts which were initially responsible for the individual's presenting difficulties (Hobbs, 1996).

Alexander and French (1946) emphasized the importance of a 'corrective emotional experience' in psychotherapy. Like Rank, they suggested a need to concentrate on current issues, understanding personal functioning in the 'here and now', rather than emphasizing the importance of infantile memories. The therapist nurtures a therapeutic alliance through genuineness, empathy and concern. The inescapable failures of therapy can be acknowledged within this environment, and the patient is encouraged to feel, but not to act on, his feelings. However, a corrective emotional experience is not the same as parenting the patient. The aim of a corrective emotional experience is to provide a setting in which a patient can re-evoke early feelings to do with difficulties in relationships, and to explore better ways of responding to this, thereby gaining greater mastery and self-confidence.

Further courses of time-limited therapy may later be indicated when conflicts that were not addressed originally are activated by a new crisis. However, the structure of brief focal psychotherapy, with its acknowledgement of the limitations of time, means that the therapy will inevitably fail to provide the perfect care the patient seeks. Yet, as Winnicott (1965) said, 'In the end we succeed by failing – failing the patient's way.'

Specific developments in brief focal psychotherapy

David Malan

David Malan developed his basic theoretical concepts of brief psychotherapy through his work at the Tavistock Clinic in London, and took a leading role in systematic research work in the field of brief focal psychotherapy. In 1979, he developed a diagrammatic representation of unconscious processes in the individual, expressed as two triangles – the triangle of conflict and the triangle of person. Malan's triangles can be understood as a psychodynamic shorthand to enable a therapist to rapidly understand and grasp a patient's difficulties. The triangles also illustrate the context in which conflicts are experienced, and make visible links which can be used in transference interpretations.

The triangle of conflict (Figure 8.1): Hidden feelings or impulses (F/I) which are based on a dynamic conflict, cause anxiety (A). This anxiety, often related to the fantasized consequences of behaviour, then results in defences (D) being developed to protect the individual's psychic equilibrium by rendering forbidden feelings unconscious. When defences are challenged, anxiety is generated as hidden or repressed feelings/impulses threaten to come to the fore and into consciousness. The symptoms of neurotic illness therefore represent a defence against the anxiety generated by the emergence of hidden feelings. During therapy, the triangle of conflict is used to explore the defence (D), the anxiety (A) and the hidden feelings (F/I) in relation to the therapeutic focus. The aim of therapy is to weaken the defence, bringing unconscious conflict to the surface. Hidden feelings may then be expressed and acknowledged in the relative safety of the therapeutic setting.

The triangle of person (Figure 8.2): Once an unconscious conflict has been identified, the triangle of person is used to make links between significant figures from the past (P), current or recent life experiences with others (O/C), and a transference relationship with the therapist in the 'here and now' (T). These links are explored through transference interpretation and therapeutic progress with a deepening rapport often follows interpretation of a T–P or transference link. Malan's (1976) work suggests strongly that this is associated with a successful therapeutic outcome.

The combined triangles (Figure 8.3): In 1984, Angela Molnos combined Malan's triangles of conflict and person, allowing the core conflict (D–A–F) to be addressed simultaneously with links between relationships in the

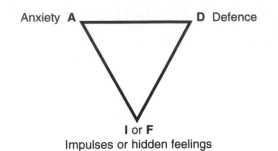

Figure 8.1   Malan's triangle of conflict

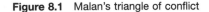

Figure 8.2   Malan's triangle of person

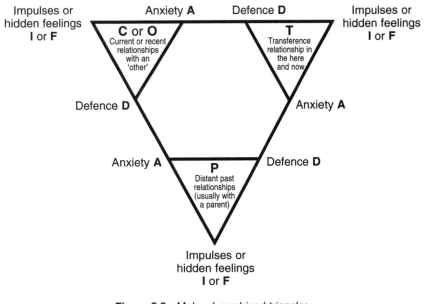

Figure 8.3   Molnos' combined triangles

present, the past and the 'here and now' or transference. This synthesis of theory represents, in diagrammatic form, a degree of the complexity of the therapeutic process which is common to all psychotherapy. The use of the diagrams, and the focus, helps to keep the therapy within manageable limits appropriate to the time constraints of the therapy. As Malan described in 1979, the aim is to reach beneath the defence and anxiety to the hidden feeling, and then to trace this feeling back from the present to its origins in the past, usually in relation to the parents.

Peter Sifneos
Sifneos, together with the Beth Israel group in Boston, developed a short-term anxiety-provoking psychotherapy (STAPP). This is a very active technique which makes use of anxiety-provoking confrontations and interpretations. Sifneos (1972) acknowledged the contribution of learning theory and behaviour modification to his model. The active repetition of anxiety-provoking situations within the therapy eventually leads to some insight and understanding of the core conflicts that prompted the original difficulties. There is less emphasis on the understanding of underlying unconscious factors and, in order for the model to be used successfully, the core conflict needs to be relatively straightforward. In addition, patients must be able to tolerate the anxiety evoked by such an active method. Sifneos encourages the patient to take responsibility for initiating an end to the therapy, using between eight and twenty sessions. According to Sifneos (1972, 1987), the therapy is most effective if the core conflict focuses on unresolved oedipal difficulties.

James Mann
Mann, also based in Boston, developed a model of time-limited therapy (1973), in which the limited time and termination are deliberately used to bring up issues of separation and loss. Mann's focus was largely on separation, and the process of establishing oneself as an independent self. Mann also saw mature emotional development as being closely related to a realistic view of time limits. In this model, therapy is offered on the basis of twelve fifty minute sessions at weekly intervals, although this may be redistributed according to patient needs – for example, twenty-four thirty-minute sessions. The focus for therapy is usually a recurring problem which is hindering growth and development. This is viewed as preconscious, and the intervention and interpretations are kept close to the patient's conscious preoccupations. The therapist's formulation includes an image of the self, a statement about feelings, the therapeutic contract and the therapeutic goal. This is intended to provide a clearly recognizable package which is readily accessible to the patient. Unlike Davanloo and Sifneos, Mann's time-limited therapy is non-confrontational.

Habib Davanloo
Davanloo developed a short-term dynamic psychotherapy model in Montreal which has similarities to that of Malan. Davanloo (1980) worked mainly with neurotic patients, and proposed an intense and confrontative therapeutic style which exposed the patient's anxieties and defences. The therapist works in the transference to reach the patient's underlying feelings with the aim of

bringing to the surface previously repressed material. The assessment tests out the patient's robustness in relation to confrontation, and willingness to both establish a good working relationship and to expose their true feelings. Once engaged, the therapist challenges the patient's defences and intensifies the therapeutic work in a way that may appear persecutory. It is necessary for the therapist to have a strong alliance with the patient in order that the confrontation may be seen to be facilitating the work of undoing the patient's defences. Davanloo encouraged the patient to experience his true feelings early on, including negative feelings towards the therapist. He believed that the experiencing of anger is beneficial in itself, and also allows the transference to be interpreted later in the therapy. Within a growing therapeutic alliance, new material emerges and maladaptive defensive manoeuvres are worked through. Davanloo's therapy is more confrontational than Malan's and less emphasis is placed on interpretation. Davanloo does not predetermine the ending, although the patient is aware that the therapy is by its nature short-term. He recommends between five and forty sessions, depending on the severity of the patient's difficulties.

Aims of therapy

Although brief focal psychotherapy aims to address the unconscious dynamic focus of a problem rather than treating the presenting symptoms, the therapy also aims to change the way in which the patient deals with conflicting feelings and expectations, thereby enabling the patient to cope more effectively with the rigours of life. It is hoped that by altering one aspect of a patient's way of coping, other components of his personality may benefit and ultimately change too. Brief therapy aims to enhance the patient's independence and autonomy, harnessing the patient's own strengths and resources in the service of continuing change and development. In this way, the patient comes to take over the therapist's task for himself. Brief therapy may thus act as a long-term prophylaxis against psychological breakdown.

Principles of practice

In practice, the application of brief focal psychotherapy is flexible and can be modified according to the needs and capabilities of the individual patient. The therapist is required to keep his interventions directly related to a realistic and short-term remit. Rosen (1986) described three phases of the therapy: (a) *beginning*, including assessment, preparation and negotiation of a contract; (b) *active phase*; and (c) *termination*.

The time limit and the focus need to be agreed between the patient and the therapist, and thereafter adhered to. Sessions are usually held weekly at a regular time. There is also an understanding established as to whether missed sessions will be made up or not – with most therapists opting for the latter. This enhances the therapeutic work as it promotes anxiety and brings previous deprivation and separation issues to the fore. The patient may suggest a termination earlier than planned but, as this often conceals considerable anxiety about loss and separation, it should be resisted.

It is the therapist's responsibility to formulate the patient's core difficulties, and to ensure that all attention is directed towards the focus. This tends to maintain the intensity of the therapy, particularly since the core conflict is likely to be directly related to the patient's current difficulties. The patient is encouraged to express thoughts and feelings openly, but classical free-floating attention is discouraged. Dreams, free associations and other material potentially tangential to the core conflict are carefully appraised by the therapist to ensure that they are not part of a defensive attempt to reduce the focus or intensity of the therapy. As Freud described in 1918, it is sometimes necessary to institute more 'active measures', but these should always have a clear function and aim (Ashurst, 1991). While the more classical therapeutic stance in psychoanalytically orientated treatment is often one of relative passivity and reflectiveness, thereby providing a 'holding' environment, the brief focal psychotherapist is not concerned with a developing transference over an extended period of time and therefore stresses the need for a more active approach (Rosen, 1986).

As with other therapies, the development of a therapeutic alliance is based on the real qualities which both individuals bring into the therapy. Although the therapist's own personality plays a greater role than in other psychoanalytic therapies, social interaction should be kept to a minimum as it tends to reduce anxiety and intensity. However, a careful balance must be drawn between facilitating a trusting relationship through interpretation of transference aspects and the undesirable development of a collusion with the patient in which the realities of the time limit and the focus set are neglected.

Although it is important not to foster dependency on the therapist, as the development of a regressive transference neurosis is antithetical to the chief principles of therapy, transference and countertransference issues play a significant role in brief focal therapy. As Ashurst (1991) writes, there is a 'relentless focus on transference interpretations, linking past with present' which 'is a powerful discouragement to regression and to the development of a symbiotic dependency resulting from transference issues which is an essential factor in long term therapy, and particularly in psychoanalysis'. Malan (1963, 1976) emphasized the importance of making interpretations early in the therapy, and suggested that interpretations related to the transference are of greater value than those which are concerned with links between current and past events. Interpretations are usually made with the idea of consolidating what has already been perceptually ordered, learned and uncovered in the therapy and not, as in other psychoanalytic therapies, to broaden the area of enquiry or to foster further uncovering. Sloane et al. (1975) found greater improvement in patients when their therapists used fewer clarifying and interpreting statements, and Rosen (1986) suggests that interpretations are better initiated at a 'here and now' level in everyday language that is understandable to the patient.

The provision of a personal and empathic relationship within the containing boundaries of a time limit and therapeutic focus may allow the patient to express previously hidden, repressed or unconscious feelings. Such emotional catharsis brings relief from internal tension and conflict, and encourages a capacity for growth and development by allowing the patient to 'work through' these difficult feelings and issues. However, brief focal psychotherapy also provides an opportunity for both cognitive learning and modelling in addition to its more dynamic focus. A 'corrective emotional experience' is promoted in which the therapist serves as a model for the patient who may adopt some of the therapist's standards or behaviour. In this way the therapy provides a forum in which the patient can experiment with new insights in a safe and secure environment.

Brief focal psychotherapy enhances communication between patient and therapist by means of face-to-face contact. A two-way interaction is encouraged, which also allows the therapist to make use of positive aspects of his own personality within the relationship. Face-to-face contact serves to maintain the intensity of the therapeutic situation, which can be enhanced by slightly less comfortable chairs which discourage relaxation and fantasy (Ashurst, 1991). This seating arrangement also allows the therapist to actively monitor the patient's state of arousal, discomfort or defensiveness in terms of appearance, facial expression, gaze avoidance, tone of voice and other overt behaviours.

Effective treatment may be marked by renewal of hope, more adaptive behaviour and an improvement in self-esteem. However, after a period of improvement, the patient may suddenly relapse, leaving both the patient and the therapist feeling hopeless and disheartened. Paradoxically, according to Rosen (1986), such a relapse during therapy is frequently associated with a better long-term outcome as it allows the patient to rehearse new approaches, insights and techniques of problem-solving within the therapeutic context.

The main features associated with a good therapeutic outcome in brief focal psychotherapy are the establishment of a therapist/parent link within the transference, the early development of a working alliance between patient and therapist, the capacity to deal with termination issues during the therapy and the absence of exclusion criteria. To this end, it is better if the wait between referral and treatment is not too long as the focus may become more diffuse and the patient's motivation to engage in brief focal psychotherapy may be impaired.

How does brief focal psychotherapy differ from other therapies?

Brief focal psychotherapy differs from crisis intervention as it does not attempt to re-establish a sense of equilibrium following an acute disturbance by bolstering existing defences or reducing arousal. In contrast, the patient is encouraged to explore a temporary loss of control in order to feel a sense of mastery, and arousal is often mobilized to facilitate the dismantling of defences (Ashurst, 1991).

Patients who suffer from early developmental disturbances of self–other differentiation are the least suitable group for brief focal psychotherapy. However, later developmental issues, particularly oedipal conflicts, appear to respond well to this type of therapy. During the course of therapy, dependence and the development of neurotic transference are not encouraged, and the exploration of fantasy through free association and interpretation is kept to a minimum. The expectation that the therapy will be brief appears to be an important difference from other therapies (Rosen, 1986).

Which patient and why?

Brief focal psychotherapy tends to benefit more psychologically-able patients and, in this regard, the requirements to undertake a successful therapy are similar to those advocated in other forms of dynamic psychotherapy. However, although brief focal therapies were initially thought of as more appropriate for the treatment of neurotic disorders, the scope of these therapies has been increased to include moderately severe personality disordered patients and even very early traumatic and developmental disorders. However, caution must be exercised as some individuals may deteriorate when treated with a more confrontative or insight-oriented therapy.

Brief focal psychotherapy may be useful in the treatment of:
- People with transitional crises (e.g. leaving home, parenthood)
- Abnormal grief reactions
- Post-traumatic stress disorder
- Adolescents with emotional or conduct problems
- Elderly people (e.g. issues of decline, retirement)

The assessment process plays an essential part in brief focal psychotherapy and may involve several interviews over a period of time. It is essential to prepare the patient for what will follow, including careful explanation of some of the feelings that may emerge within the therapy (Rosen, 1986). During the assessment it is important to establish a clear therapeutic focus, to determine the patient's capacity to withstand the intense and confrontational nature of brief focal psychotherapy and to monitor the patient's response to trial interpretations (Hobbs, 1996). It is also important to consider the patient's past life events, coping strategies, previous patterns of response to stress and reactions to current problems. The initial exploration should include an enquiry into the patient's self-esteem, and self-appraisal of both strengths and weaknesses. Assessment should also address the patient's understanding of psychotherapy, what they are hoping to achieve, and expectations regarding the role of both the therapist and the patient. It is best if a rapid assessment moves quickly into the therapy itself with limited delay.

Indications for therapy

Indications
- Evidence of ego strengths
- A capacity for meaningful personal relationships
- A capacity to establish a therapeutic alliance
- 'Psychological mindedness'
- The ability to experience affect-laden feelings
- The existence of a core conflict
- Motivation for change

In 1991, Ashurst delineated several important qualities which, in regard to brief focal psychotherapy, are 'likely to ensure that the patient has the capacity to work with unconscious intrapsychic factors, and to tolerate the anxiety and stress involved in bringing these into consciousness'. The patient needs to demonstrate evidence of appropriate ego strengths, which can be indicated by sexual, social and occupational adjustment, adaptability and the capacity to assume responsibility. Experience of at least one important and meaningful relationship with another person in the past will be essential for the success of the relationship with the therapist. The patient must also prove able to interact with the therapist, especially in regard to mobilization of transference feelings. The patient should be capable of experiencing feelings in an affectively-coloured way without resistance to the emergence of powerful underlying emotions. The existence of a core conflict is important to serve as a focus for therapy, as is the motivation to change existing patterns of thinking and behaviour. 'Psychological mindedness' refers to a patient's ability to be reflective, to think in psychological terms about current difficulties, to use interpretations, to work with unconscious intrapsychic factors and to tolerate the anxiety and distress which these processes will evoke.

Contraindications to therapy

Contraindications

- Psychosis
- Major characterological disorder or personality disorder
- Deeply depressed patient with suicidal ideation
- Lack of motivation
- Low tolerance of frustration or anxiety
- Substance misuse
- Propensity for regression
- Schizoid patients and those who fail to make positive emotional contact with the therapist
- Dependent patients

- Poor impulse control
- Psychologically fragile individuals with limited ego strengths
- Gross destructive or self-destructive behaviour
- Absence of feasible focus
- Negative response to trial interventions
- Chronic psychosomatic illness
- Rigid or primitive defences
- Problems over which the patient has little control, e.g. poverty or homelessness
- Uncritical adulation or dismissal of previous help-seeking relationships

Which therapist and why?

Although many of the individuals who helped to develop the brief focal psychotherapies were experienced psychoanalysts, analytically oriented therapists may find working in the more active and intense manner which characterizes brief focal psychotherapy uncomfortable. According to Rosen

(1986), there remains a belief that therapists should have some experience in long-term analytic therapies before progressing on to briefer models of working. However, it may simply be that for some therapists the brief focal approach is at odds with their dynamic background, or with their individual temperament and personality (Hobbs, 1996).

Whilst short-term therapies may require complex psychotherapeutic skills, brief focal psychotherapies can be safely and effectively practised by relative beginners with carefully selected cases under skilled supervision (Malan and Osimo, 1992). The emphasis on problem-identification and goal-determination provides a useful learning structure for novice therapists. However, supervision is especially important, even for experienced therapists, because of the brevity and intensity of the therapy, and the need to work efficiently and quickly. Training in brief therapy also lends itself to recently developed supervisory techniques which stimulate rapid learning and self-discovery, such as audio-recordings and video-feedback.

A variety of factors related to the nature of the therapist are thought to contribute to the success of brief focal psychotherapy. Malan (1976) attributed importance to the level of therapist enthusiasm and to the ability to adhere to a therapeutic focus, whilst Brockman et al. (1987) considered that experience was not a prerequisite for a successful outcome.

Therapeutic setting

A principal aim in brief focal therapy is to create a trusting, safe and therapeutic environment. In this sense, the therapy setting for undertaking brief focal psychotherapy differs little from that of other dynamic psychotherapies. The setting should be pleasant, quiet and comfortable, allowing the patient to feel safe in a neutral environment. It should also be private and consistent, without change or interruption, and conducive to the anxiety-provoking and intimate work to be undertaken. Of particular note is the lack of a couch as all sessions will be undertaken face-to-face. The patient and therapist sit facing one another at an angle which readily allows the patient the choice of being able to visually engage the therapist or, equally comfortably, to look away.

Clinical example

Amy, aged 50, was referred for psychotherapy by her GP. He had supported her through several prolonged periods of low mood, but now felt he could do no more. Perceiving the referral itself as a rejection, Amy was dismayed to find that she was only offered time-limited therapy of six months' duration and said so at the first meeting. At the assessment, her obesity had suggested a likely focus on issues around greed and need. She herself said that she thought her problems were due to her inability to break free from her mother. She had one child, a nineteen-year-old son, with whom she had a stormy relationship. Her husband had recently begun to work for long periods away from home, and she felt less and less able to cope. For the first few weeks of therapy she prefaced every meeting with a statement that it was all to do with her mother, but then spent most of the session talking about anything and everything else. When this behaviour was pointed out, she said 'I don't get to the point until the 49th minute but, even if I had four hours, I still wouldn't get there until the end.' After that, the nature of the sessions changed. From seeming empty, arid and pointless, they became full of life to bursting point. One session even ran over by ten minutes as the therapist felt unable to stop the rush. Before the next session, Amy rang in to say she could not come as she had a cold.

On her return to therapy, it was suggested to her that the 49th minute was the problem. At the end of the therapy she could be either deprived or indulged. She could reach the end of the session having deprived herself of the opportunity to discuss her most pressing problem, or she could induce the therapist into indulging her, even when that was not in her best interests. Over subsequent weeks, this dilemma was applied to other areas of her life. Her mother had been a hard woman who had always tried to do the right thing by her children, but who applied strict rules with an icy inflexibility. Amy was allowed no sweets or other such indulgences. However, Amy's aunt owned a sweet shop and would shower her with sweets, under the nose of Amy's mother, who would fume silently. This aunt's husband had been prescribed a low fat diet. Once when he was ill in bed, his wife and Amy's mother in attendance, he craved a cream cake. Amy's mother said no, but the aunt went and fetched him one much to her mother's disgust.

Amy, having felt deprived in her own childhood, had not wished her son to suffer in the same way. Unfortunately this had produced a 'spoilt and greedy brat' who saw no reason to get a job, or to help his mother in any way. He lazed around the house, resentful of his parent's material possessions. He expected his mother to drive him to see his friends, and to pick him up at all hours, unaware that this deprived her of any free time for herself. She resented his idleness but felt unable to deprive him, and so harboured a great deal of anger which only came out in furious rows about trivial matters. Her eating habits also showed this pattern. Very overweight, she had tried dieting but only succeeded in getting fatter. It transpired that, in order to lose weight, she would skip both breakfast and lunch, arriving home to cook a small meal for herself and her son. Whilst cooking she would be so hungry that she would eat biscuits, crisps and cake, starting off an evening binge.

In the terminology of Malan's triangles, she hid her feelings of resentment at being deprived for fear of rejection, and indulged others at her own expense. This completed the triangle as it fuelled her own sense of deprivation. The pattern of deprivation and indulgence was brought into focus by therapy, which she perceived as deprivingly short. It was also seen as a result of rejection by her GP, and would ultimately lead to rejection at termination.

When, rather than depriving her, the therapist indulged her, this was equally anxiety-provoking. From being a 'mother' who applied the boundaries with a depriving level of strictness, the therapist became like her aunt, unable to hold to the boundaries at all, and like herself in relation to her food and to her son. Amy became aware of the significance of this pattern, but still seemed unable to come to terms with the impending termination, despite her intellectual comprehension of its significance. At the end of each session, she would always be in full flow and it would sometimes take three statements of 'It's time' to get her to leave. Six weeks before the end, she presented the therapist with what seemed an insoluble problem. Her boss at work had told her she could no longer attend in work time as the office was under pressure. Next week would have to be her last session unless she could be offered a slot after 4 o'clock. This left the therapist with a dilemma: if she said no, she felt that *she was depriving Amy; if she said yes to Amy, she was depriving herself of some personal time which she had specifically set aside. Amy had succeeded in placing the therapist neatly into her own difficult dilemma.*

At the next appointment, the therapist still had no solution. She had hoped that Amy would have found one, but was disappointed. The therapist explained to Amy how she found herself in the same predicament. She could say no to Amy's request and feel she was being depriving, or she could change the time and possibly feel resentful at being indulging whilst depriving herself of her carefully set-aside time. Consideration of this seemed, almost miraculously, to resolve the problem. With minimal disruption to either timetable, a slot was found in the lunch hour. Amy left that session happily, with no need of reminders. After that session, her mood changed. She began to look after her own needs and stand up to her son, who also became easier to manage and less resentful. She began to eat sensibly and stopped gaining weight. The end of each session was no longer a battleground. Amy left therapy having experienced that boundaries in relationships can be firm but not inflexible, and that a middle way between deprivation and indulgence can be found.

Problems in therapy

Problems arise in the practice of brief focal psychotherapy if unsuitable patients are recommended for this form of therapy, or if the therapy is not carried out within the recognized remit of time-limited and focused treatments.

Inappropriate assessment and sub-optimal selection of patients may allow fragile patients who have a tenuous sense of self or serious character pathology to find their way into brief focal psychotherapy. In such patients, the intensity of the work may prove destabilizing and precipitate a breakdown. The confrontational nature of brief focal therapy may, especially if practised in an over-enthusiastic or precipitate manner, bring unconscious material prematurely to the fore with resultant anxiety, disintegration, acting out and a tendency to re-enact past relationship difficulties rather than to modify or improve them (Hobbs, 1996). Similarly, patients with a vulnerability to become psychotic, destructive, suicidal or deeply regressed may benefit more from supportive psychotherapy.

Problems may also arise if the therapist does not maintain the focal and time-limited boundaries of the therapeutic contract. Although this is made difficult by the therapist having continually to assess a rapidly changing therapeutic environment, the therapist needs to avoid collusive familiarity with the patient and prevent excessive regression or dependency from taking hold (Rosen, 1986). This can be achieved by addressing transference and countertransference issues, with experienced supervision if necessary, to monitor intrusions into the focus or time-frame of the therapy. If insufficient containment is possible within these boundaries, then the therapist needs to consider transferring the patient to another therapist within an alternative treatment modality rather than trying to adapt a very circumscribed treatment process to fit unsuitable patients or problems (Hobbs, 1996). It is therefore important that the therapist does not, intentionally or unintentionally, encourage the patient to have greater expectations of the therapeutic process than fall within the remit of brief focal psychotherapy.

Experienced long-term therapists may have difficulty in limiting themselves to a focus and responding to the rapid changes that are so much a feature of brief focal psychotherapy. The patient's progress may also be so satisfactory that the therapist is seduced into expanding the original goal of therapy. Questions therefore arise as to whether follow-up sessions are appropriate or contraindicated. Mann (1973) does not see his patients again after termination because of potential separation issues, whereas Rosen (1986) found that planned follow-up sessions at between two and six months after termination of therapy do not undermine the effect of therapy. According to Rosen, a 'wait and see' policy in regard to follow-up and further treatment is probably the best alternative rather than extending an existing therapy indefinitely or pursuing an incorrect mode of therapy without effect.

The therapist's view of brief focal psychotherapy as an effective technique for dealing with psychological difficulties is extremely important as the patient, based on past experiences of deprivation and abandonment, is likely to see time-limited therapy as a sub-optimal option. If the therapist shares this view it may be evident in transference and countertransference issues, and could have an adverse effect on the therapy. Brief focal psychotherapy therefore cannot be used successfully if considered to be 'second best' by both patient and therapist, and in this sense has little role to play as a second choice of treatment.

Evaluation of therapy

According to Malan (1976), work on a limited focus tackled within the context of the patient's everyday life creates an effect similar to the ripples caused by a pebble thrown into a pond and there is growing evidence that brief focal psychotherapy is capable of bringing about adaptive psychological processes which may result in long-term personality change.

Brief focal psychotherapy is easier to research, and is more amenable to standardization as measuring symptomatic improvement is simpler than demonstrating dynamic change. The way in which clinical outcome has been measured to date has therefore favoured behavioural interventions at the expense of psychodynamic therapies, although increasingly sophisticated scientific research is being developed to measure the outcome and process of brief focal psychotherapies. For example, the use of both audio-taping and video-taping of psychotherapy sessions for peer evaluation is commonly used.

Within the current climate of cost-effectiveness, brief focal psychotherapy is being increasingly called upon to demonstrate its efficacy and benefit. However, cost-consciousness should not drive the assessment of, and research into, clinical effectiveness, as examining only short-term outcomes may produce spurious evidence (Ashurst, 1991). Any research into brief focal psychotherapy must take into account the impact of longer-term therapies and other alternatives (such as behaviour therapy, counselling, etc.) when developing an empirical approach and clinical overview (Hobbs, 1996).

Perhaps these evaluative findings can best be summarized by Hans Strupp's (1978) comment that 'Short-term therapy should be the treatment of choice for practically all patients. On the basis of many reports, about two-thirds of patients will respond positively to such interventions; the remaining one-third can be continued if this seems indicated, referred elsewhere, or judged to be beyond currently available therapeutic efforts.'

Some important research findings

- Shlien, Mosak and Driekurs (1962) – brief therapy was not only as effective as long-term treatment but more efficient with improvement taking place at an earlier point.

- Malan (1963) – a positive outcome was reported in many cases and substantial improvement endured after the end of therapy.

- Sloane *et al.* (1975) – remarkably few differences between behaviour therapy and brief focal psychotherapy and, although behaviour therapy seemed to result in lower scores on target symptoms at one-year follow-up, by two years there was little difference between the groups.

- Luborsky *et al.* (1975) – suggest similar success rates for brief and long-term psychotherapies, as it has not proved possible to demonstrate any superiority of long-term psychotherapy over short-term dynamic therapy.

- Howard *et al.* (1986) – in centres providing long-term individual psychotherapy approximately 50% of patients showed improvement by session 8 and 75% showed improvement by session 26.

- Howard *et al.* (1986) – dose-response studies suggest that up to a point, the more therapy the better the outcome but there is also a law of diminishing returns operating so that relatively more therapeutic benefit derives from the early sessions.

- Shapiro and Firth (1987) – brief focal psychotherapy is marginally less effective than cognitive behavioural therapy.

- Crits-Christoph (1992) – short-term dynamic psychotherapy is an effective treatment.

- Whale (1992) – brief focal psychotherapy is effective in the treatment of chronic pain.

- Svartberg and Stiles (1991) – the effects of brief focal psychotherapy are comparable to other forms of treatment.

- US DHHS (1993) – brief focal psychotherapy can prevent relapse of depressive illness.

Alternatives to therapy

Patients for whom brief focal psychotherapy is inappropriate could be considered for a longer-term dynamic alternative or even for a less dynamic model, such as supportive psychotherapy. A problem-solving approach may prove preferable, as may pharmacotherapy. However, dynamic psychotherapy is a stand-alone treatment and concurrent work in one of these alternative modalities may simply increase the potential for acting out outside of the therapeutic framework.

Patients who have responded to brief focal psychotherapy may well require some follow-up treatment, and additional brief focal interventions may be called for in regard to new or as yet unaddressed foci. However, these problems may benefit from a series of intermittent brief focal interventions in preference to a more sustained therapy (Hobbs, 1996). Episodes of focal therapy offered at times of need within the framework of an enduring but latent therapeutic relationship may at times be more appropriate than either short-term or long-term traditional approaches (Ashurst, 1991).

The idea of a focus in brief focal psychotherapy is conceptually not that far removed from the definition of the problem in behavioural therapies. Patients who are suitable for brief focal psychotherapy may well respond to schema-focused cognitive behavioural therapy or cognitive analytic therapy, and may progress to alternatives such as family therapy or group therapy at a later stage in their development.

Further reading

Davanloo, H. (ed.) (1980) *Short-Term Dynamic Psychotherapy*. New York: Jason Aronson.
Malan, D.H. (1976) *The Frontier of Brief Psychotherapy*. New York: Plenum Press.
Malan, D.H. (1979) *Individual Psychotherapy and the Science of Psychodynamics*. London: Butterworths.
Mann, J. (1973) *Time-Limited Psychotherapy*. Cambridge, MA: Harvard University Press.
Sifneos, P.E. (1972) *Short-Term Psychotherapy and Emotional Crisis*. Cambridge, MA: Harvard University Press.

Bibliography

Alexander, F. and French, T.M. (1946) *Psychoanalytic Therapy: Principles and Application*. New York: Ronald Press.
Ashurst, P. (1991) Brief psychotherapy. In: J. Holmes (ed.), *Textbook of Psychotherapy in Psychiatric Practice*. London: Churchill Livingstone, pp. 187–212.
Balint, M. and Balint, E. (1961) *Psychotherapeutic Techniques in Medicine*. London: Tavistock.
Barkham, M. (1989) Exploratory therapy in two-plus-one sessions. I: Rationale for a brief psychotherapy model. *British Journal of Psychotherapy*, **6**, 81–88.
Brockman, B., Poynton, A., Ryle, A. and Watson, J.P. (1987) Effectiveness of time limited therapy carried out by trainees. *British Journal of Psychiatry*, **151**, 602–610.
Butcher, J.N. and Koss, M.P. (1978) Research on brief and crisis oriented therapies. In: S.L. Garfield and A.E. Bergin (eds), *Handbook of Psychotherapy and Behavior Change: an Empirical Analysis*, 2nd edn. New York: John Wiley.
Crits-Christoph, P. (1992) The efficacy of brief dynamic psychotherapy: a meta-analysis. *American Journal of Psychiatry*, **149**, 151–158.
Davanloo, H. (ed.) (1980) *Short-Term Dynamic Psychotherapy*. New York: Jason Aronson.
Hobbs, M. (1996) Short-term dynamic psychotherapy. In: S. Bloch (ed.), *An Introduction to the Psychotherapies*, 3rd edn. Oxford: Oxford University Press, pp. 52–83.
Howard, K.I., Kopta, S.M., Krause, M.S. and Orlinsky, D.E. (1986) The dose effect relationship in psychotherapy. *American Psychologist*, **41**, 159–164.

Llewelyn, S.P., Elliot, R., Shapiro, D.A. *et al.* (1988) Client perceptions of significant events in prescriptive and exploratory periods of individual therapy. *British Journal of Clinical Psychology*, **27**, 105–114.

Luborsky, L., Singer, B. and Luborsky, L. (1975) Comparative studies of psychotherapy. Is it true that 'Everyone has won and all must have prizes'? *Archives of General Psychiatry*, **32**, 995–1008.

Luborsky, L. (1984) *Principles of Psychoanalytic Psychotherapy: a Manual for Supportive-Expressive Treatment*. New York: Basic Books.

Malan, D.H. (1963) *A Study of Brief Psychotherapy*. London: Tavistock.

Malan, D.H. (1976) *The Frontier of Brief Psychotherapy*. New York: Plenum Press.

Malan, D.H. and Osimo, F. (1992) *Psychodynamics, Training, and Outcome in Brief Psychotherapy*. Oxford: Butterworth–Heinemann.

Mann, J. (1973) *Time-Limited Psychotherapy*. Cambridge, MA: Harvard University Press.

Molnos, A. (1984) The two triangles are four: a diagram to teach the process of dynamic psychotherapy. *British Journal of Psychotherapy*, **1**, 112–125.

Morgan, R., Luborsky, L., Crits-Cristoph, P. *et al.* (1982) Predicting the outcomes of psychotherapy by the Penn Helping Alliance Rating Method. *Archives of General Psychiatry*, **39**, 397–402.

Rosen, B. (1986) Brief focal psychotherapy. In: S. Bloch (ed.), *An Introduction to the Psychotherapies*, 2nd edn. Oxford: Oxford University Press, pp. 55–79.

Shapiro, D.A. and Firth, J. (1987) Prescriptive versus exploratory psychotherapy: outcomes of the Sheffield psychotherapy project. *British Journal of Psychiatry*, **151**, 790–799.

Shlien, J.M., Mosak, H.H. and Driekurs, R. (1962) Effects of time limits: a comparison of two therapies. *Journal of Counselling Psychology*, **9**, 31–34.

Sifneos, P.E. (1972) *Short-Term Psychotherapy and Emotional Crisis*. Cambridge, MA: Harvard University Press.

Sifneos, P.E. (1987) *Short-Term Dynamic Psychotherapy: Evaluation and Technique*, 2nd edn. New York: Plenum Press.

Sloane, R.B., Staples, E.R., Cristol, A.H. *et al.* (1975) *Psychotherapy versus Behaviour Therapy*. Cambridge, MA: Harvard University Press.

Strupp, H.H. (1978) Psychotherapy research and practice: an overview. In: S.L. Garfield and A.E. Bergin (eds). *Handbook of Psychotherapy and Behaviour Change: an Empirical Analysis*. New York: Wiley.

Svartberg, M. and Stiles, T.C. (1991) Comparative effects of short-term psychodynamic psychotherapy: a meta-analysis. *Journal of Consulting and Clinical Psychology*, **69**, 704–714.

US DHHS (1993) *Depression in Primary Care: Treatment of Major Depression*. Rockville, MD: AHCPR Publications.

Whale, J. (1992) The use of brief focal psychotherapy in the treatment of chronic pain. *Psychoanalytic Psychotherapy*, **6**, 61–72.

Winnicott, D.W. (1965) *The Maturational Process and the Facilitating Environment*. London: Hogarth Press.

9

The Conversational Model

Philip M. Brown

Historical perspective

The Conversational Model, developed by Dr Robert F. Hobson, has arisen from a number of roots. The model integrates features and approaches from different traditions of psychotherapy including psychoanalysis, psychoanalytic psychotherapies, interpersonal therapy, cognitive and behavioural therapy, systemic approaches and the therapeutic community movement. It also draws on more disparate sources of thought including philosophy, the Romantic movement, biological science and systems theory. Hobson's ideas grew partly out of his dissatisfaction with the state of psychoanalytic theory, thought and practice prevalent during the late 1940s when he began to train as a Jungian analyst. During the 1950s, 1960s and 1970s, as he practised, he found the certainty of some schools of psychoanalytic thought in their theoretical canon extremely rigid. He was particularly critical of contemporary psychoanalytic attempts to base their theories of human emotional development on retrospective material from the analysis of adult patients.

Some discrete influences on the development of the Conversational Model can be identified. Firstly, Hobson trained as an analytical psychologist and a number of ideas fundamental to the model are developments of Jung's conceptualization about the nature of psychotherapy as a dialogue, a discussion between two people in which the therapist is a fellow participant. This interaction should produce an amplification of possible meaning, rather than a reduction of clinical material to a pre-existing theoretical concept – which may only be one meaning of an event amongst many possibilities.

Secondly, the Conversational Model draws on many ideas from mainstream psychoanalysis, and is consistent with much that is current in theory and practice (though there are also some major differences and divergences). This might seem paradoxical given the origins of the model in dissatisfaction with psychoanalysis, but psychoanalytic theory and practice have also changed and developed over the past fifty years as the Conversational Model has come into being. One convergence between mainstream psychoanalysis and the Conversational Model, for instance, is that there is now less emphasis in contemporary psychodynamic practice on attempting to reconstruct the pathogenic past of the patient and instead the focus is on understanding, in some detail, the experience of the current moment in the relationship with the therapist. The Conversational Model rests firmly on psychodynamic foundations but it is clearly also an interpersonal model of psychotherapy. Another important source is the work of Harry Stack-Sullivan, the American Neo-Freudian writer, whose own interpersonal theories arose from dissatisfaction with Freud's theory of instinctual drives. There are echoes too, in Hobson's work, of John Bowlby's work on attachment, Heinz Kohut's theories of the self, and modern infant developmental theory.

Amongst Hobson's other influences are medicine, psychiatry and scientific research methodology. However, he combines this with an understanding of human beings garnered from his love and knowledge of Romantic poetry. Hobson's papers on psychotherapy draw on the work of, amongst others, Coleridge, Wordsworth and Joseph Conrad. In this way he encompasses directive, logical thought together with fantasy and imaginative thought and feeling.

Hobson's early papers outlining the Conversational Model were published in the early 1970s, and subsequently expanded on and extended in later works. According to the model, therapy is an interactive, mutual and equal but asymmetrical process, in which both therapist and patient contribute to a unique conversation. The conversation is seen as potentially encouraging the development of a new, never-before-experienced sort of relationship between patient and therapist. The model has become established within National Health Service psychotherapy departments, particularly in Manchester. It has also been taken up by academic psychiatrists as a particularly suitable model for psychotherapy research purposes, and a number of empirical studies have been published since 1984.

Principles of theory and practice

General principles of theory

According to Hobson (in an unpublished lecture), 'The model is a method of social learning and problem-solving in relationships between two people. A situation is created in which a patient's significant interpersonal problems are revealed, explored, understood and modified by testing out the possible solutions generated in the dialogue. The therapist's aim is to produce a therapeutic dialogue, a "conversation", during which the significant problems are directly expressed here and now in the relationship – not simply talked about.'

Hobson's approach is based on the belief that many of the difficulties experienced by people arise out of faulty relationships, especially those relationships in early life which involve profound intimacy and dependence between people. The Conversational Model suggests these difficulties may be remediable within and *by means of* an intimate therapeutic relationship, which is itself more therapeutic than accurate interpretative work. The relationship between patient and therapist is not only developed as a vehicle for exploring the internal world of the patient, but is also a crucial therapeutic factor in itself. Hobson regards this therapeutic relationship as the vehicle for knowing another person and becoming known in turn, rather than knowing 'about' something. Following Buber, he terms this an 'I–Thou' relationship, in distinction to an 'I–it' relationship (Hobson, 1985).

The therapeutic relationship becomes the setting for interpersonal learning about ways in which a person applies maladaptive solutions to the problems and anxieties generated by having to relate to other people, for instance, avoiding intimate contact. It can be seen as a setting in which a person can learn, within an intimate interpersonal relationship, about one's self and others in a flexible way that can accommodate change and encompass difference and conflict as well as intimacy and harmony. Difficulties and deficits within intimate relationships can be seen more clearly as they actually happen, 'live', in a meeting between two people. This relationship, involving a 'union of deep feeling with profound thought' can, through the active use of imagination, result in new ways of relating to oneself and others, and in new experience (Hobson, 1974).

These ideas include hints of cognitive learning theories and yet are not incompatible with the psychoanalytic concepts of transference and countertransference. However, the emphasis on shared experience is subtly different, and it is not assumed that everything that happens in the therapeutic relationship is a manifestation of transference – a re-enactment in the present of aspects of past relationships.

An important aspect of the model is the tentativeness with which the therapist presents his ideas about the patient and the relationship. This does not mean being vague but rather being open to correction. The process of tentative formulation, followed by mutual negotiation and adjustment, with the aim of improved communication and understanding, is seen as central to new interpersonal learning. Difficulties in this process suggest maladaptions to and distortions of interpersonal, and internalized, relationships which can then be further explored. This process of mutual interpersonal adjustment is similar to Daniel Stern's (1985) concept of attunement between mother and infant.

The Conversational Model gives more emphasis to interpersonal processes than to intrapsychic processes such as instincts, drives and defences. However, the internal world of the patient is not neglected: although the communication between therapist and patient relates primarily to what is happening in the relationship between them, this is then used to focus also on the patient's internal world, impulses and defensive structures. This facet of the model is concordant with some strands of psychoanalytic thought, such as the British Object Relations School, and the Self-Psychology of Heinz Kohut with its emphasis on the security of the self.

All therapists shape the unfolding conversation by their words and other vocal utterances, by their non-verbal behaviour and by their silences. However, the Conversational Model therapist is more active and directive than the classical psychoanalyst, aiming to focus attention actively on feelings, thoughts, words and experiences rather than allowing free association. In the Conversational Model, interventions are ideally based on what can be observed, felt or experienced.

The Conversational Model examines and defines the microscopic processes of interaction between patient and therapist. It attempts to provide a well-defined framework within which the psychotherapist may engage in a therapeutic conversation with the patient, and has also been manualized (expressed in the form of a series of operationalized steps to guide therapeutic work) so that it can be used as a standardized form of psychological treatment in research studies. However, certain things which are central to psychotherapy are difficult if not impossible to operationalize, and Hobson accepts that this includes much of the non-verbal interaction between the participants.

Specific concepts underlying the Conversational Model

A conversation

The concept of a therapeutic conversation lies at the heart of the Conversational Model. The term 'conversation' has a literal meaning of intercourse, talk or discourse. But here a conversation is much more than a verbal dialogue: a more profound meeting between people is implied, which is not confined to verbal language but includes all aspects of the relationship as potentially understandable communication. This involves a mutual process of getting-to-know the other person, of understanding his words, his speech, his bodily gestures and movements, his fantasies and the metaphors he uses to convey feelings, wishes, fantasies and experiences; and to recognize these ways of thinking, feeling and expressing as uniquely his.

This mutual knowing and understanding can lead to new development; the creation of new ways of relating which are more satisfying and adaptive, and which can be generalized to relationships outside of the therapy. The aim is to experience feelings in the therapeutic relationship and to *talk with* rather than *talk about* feelings: the latter risks making them objects of study rather than belonging to a living subject and keeps them at a distance. The conversation concerns the patient and his experience in relation to the therapist, the other people in his life now and those in his past. The therapist's own feelings and thoughts in relation to this are important but are only thought about in regard to, and not talked about with, the patient.

Symbols

Hobson takes a Jungian approach to symbols. He defines a symbol as something known which hints at, or may reveal, if regarded with an open-minded, expectant attitude, something that is not yet known. These he terms 'living symbols' and a 'symbolical attitude'. A symbolical attitude requires that the therapist uses his capacity for imagination, and is actively receptive to what is conveyed to him by the patient. Symbols are seen as crucially involved in the process of managing transition and transformation in human life, particularly the important and intimate processes of separation, loss, reincorporation, disorganization and reorganization. Symbolic communication may be contained in words, looks, gestures and actions.

Symbols embody meaning, and the therapist's interventions are aimed towards encouraging amplification of the symbol. By this is meant that possible meanings of the symbol are explored and expanded, rather than reduced to a stereotyped or imposed meaning. Amplification allows the patient to elaborate associations to material which bring it to life and give it subjective value. Symbols are important in the process of creating new meaning in the psychotherapeutic relationship, representing and communicating aspects of new feelings, experiences and relationships discovered or developed in the course of therapy.

Metaphor

Hobson (1985) uses 'living metaphor' to denote the 'creative relationship' between two ideas which brings about a new meaning or understanding of an experience. Metaphor is seen not only as an important individual way of expressing feelings, thoughts and experiences but also as a potential vehicle for the creation of a joint language between patient and therapist which can help to create and to express a new and developing relationship. Metaphor can allow us to understand at least part of another person's experience, and to communicate that understanding. By associating an idea, feeling or experience with a vivid image, metaphor may illuminate it. However Hobson suggests that psychological symptoms can sometimes be conceptualized as 'dead' or incomplete metaphors. The therapist's own imaginative use of metaphor might also be used carefully in trying to convey understanding of the patient, helping to create a shared metaphor and feeling-language.

Meta-communication

This is defined as communication about communication and concerns the way in which interventions in psychotherapy are made. In contrast to a systemic view of meta-communication, where a communication about a communication between two members of a system is used to break the system's rules of dysfunctional communication, Hobson uses the concept to examine in minute detail cues giving feedback about how the therapist's interventions have been received. This allows patient and therapist to attune to each other more successfully and develop a mutual language in which ideas and feelings can be expressed and shared. Hobson considers that the manner of communication (how something is said) is even more important than the content of an interpretation (what is said).

Feeling-language

This is a term used to denote a personal way of understanding and communicating feelings and the associated thoughts and experiences. It is a language which intimates an essence of that person to another.

In the course of developing a therapeutic relationship, the therapist must first discover and learn the patient's feeling-language of verbal and non-verbal symbols. He conveys his wish to do so in the hope that this will help the patient to move towards sharing the therapist's own partly personal and partly professional feeling-language. All psychotherapists give subtle clues as to what language they would prefer their patients to speak and so, in this sense, all therapy is directive, but the psychotherapist should not be coercive. Hobson suggests that the psychotherapist should not say, 'You don't mean that, you really mean this'. Instead he should say, 'You certainly mean that but maybe you also mean something more' (Meares and Hobson, 1977).

Fantasy and imagination

Fantasy and imagination are important in the Conversational Model. Three levels of imaginative activity are defined:
- *Passive fantasy*: for example, a dream or unwilled fantasy.
- *Active fantasy*: encouraged by being intuitive and having a willingness to allow images or fantasies to emerge.
- *Imaginative activity*: in which fantasizing is the focus of concentrated attention.

The Conversational Model aims to encourage a progression in the course of psychotherapy from passive to active fantasy and into imaginative activity where fantasies and images are actively explored by the patient in-relation-with the therapist. Conscious thought is directed towards understanding and elaborating fantasy resulting in what Samuel Taylor Coleridge described as 'a union of deep feeling with profound thought' (Hobson, 1974). This use of imagination to examine and modify the internal world and to address problems of relating with other people and the world outside the self might be termed 'serious play', of which Winnicott's Squiggle Game is an example (1971).

Aloneness–togetherness

There is a rhythm of intimacy and distance in any relationship. Hobson suggests that an ideal in this respect might be to aim at a state of aloneness–togetherness. This means that a person has the capacity to be alone, that is, separate from others, at the same time as he has the ability to be together with another person, that is, able to have an intimate relationship. He suggests that these capacities are linked. A person can only be together with an other, as opposed to seeking a fantasy of fusion, in so far as he has achieved the capacity to be alone or separate, and can only be alone in company, as opposed to cut off and isolated, in so far as he has achieved the capacity for intimate togetherness. However, states of loneliness and fusion also play a part in any relationship. They are problematic when they are the only states that a person can achieve, or are obligatory.

Aims of therapy

The Conversational Model asks why a person cannot express his feelings directly, and questions what the fear or anxiety is that prevents a feeling from being expressed. Anxiety resulting from traumas and failures in past relationships are the most important reasons for the difficulties which cause people to seek psychotherapy. Anxiety also blocks exploration in the patient (and in the therapist), and crippling avoidance mechanisms develop to avert painful feelings. These mechanisms are linked to painful past experiences and become repeated patterns.

Therapeutic intervention is therefore aimed at reducing the fear which is blocking further exploration. The therapist tries to maintain an optimal level of anxiety and arousal in the therapy sessions, and encourages a pattern of feeling, thought, experience, fantasy and behaviour to be repeated in the therapeutic relationship, which can then be explored. The therapist should point out the distortions in the patient's perceptions and expectations of himself and others, based on picking up cues from both the patient and his own response to the conversation.

It can be difficult to achieve a truly mutual conversation. Some individuals may find that relating to another person in this way is too painful to tolerate, or may have withdrawn from contact with other people. This is why the therapeutic conversation is seen as being a setting for creating more satisfactory modes of intimate relationship, and not just a vehicle with which to explore re-enactment in the transference. Significant problems in the patient's life may come to be seen in a new way by this process and reformulated. New ways of relating to other people, which were previously blocked by anxiety, may be learned. There is an ongoing process of reciprocal adjustment in the conversation, in which insight and new meaning are reached.

Principles of practice

Active focusing on immediate experience

The therapist tries to help the patient to stay with immediate experiences even when these are uncomfortable or unpleasant. This immediate experience of feeling can connect past events and relationships to the present in the here and now of a psychotherapy session, bringing alive a thought or a memory. The model sees neurotic difficulties in terms of a maladaptive response to, and avoidance of, experience in relation to other people. By encouraging the patient to stay with, and think about, immediate experience, the therapist encourages thoughts and feelings to become integrated. In this way, the therapist encourages avoidance mechanisms to be discarded, and actively promotes the emergence of possible new solutions to feared internal and external experiences.

Picking up cues

Interventions are based, as far as possible, on cues; that is, on immediately present communications, conscious or unconscious, which can be recognized by the therapist. These may be verbal, in the form of the words the patient speaks; non-verbal, for instance in the emotionally laden tone of the patient's voice; or non-vocal, for example a gesture or an involuntary movement. The therapist's aim is to discover what is meaningful for this particular patient in this particular conversation with him. Interventions need to be correctly timed and made when the patient can be receptive to them. They must also be made in response to a meaningful communication at a time when there is evidence of optimal arousal and anxiety in both patient and therapist.

Maintaining an optimum level of arousal

If a patient is too anxious, he may be unable to reflect on or talk about his thoughts, feelings and experiences, and exploration within therapy may become blocked. The therapist needs to be able to recognize the signs of over-anxiety or over-arousal in his patients. There may be characteristic verbal, vocal and non-verbal signs (such as the use of a certain word or phrase, a tone of voice) or bodily manifestations (such as muscular tension or loss of eye contact). Through an 'understanding hypothesis', the therapist tries to clarify why the anxiety should arise now, and what is being blocked by it. The therapist will therefore try to relate the patient's immediate feeling to some aspect of the relationship with him. This may in part be transferred from another, internalized relationship, such as that with a parent.

Conversely, some patients may be under-aroused and not sufficiently anxious to motivate their exploration – particularly those who habitually use some form of mental retreat to avoid anxieties, such as a withdrawal into fantasy. Here it will be necessary to draw the patient's attention to whatever defence is being used against experiencing anxiety and, if there is evidence for doing so, suggesting what feelings may be blocked from consciousness and to what situations these might be linked (including the therapeutic encounter).

Making statements: not asking questions

The therapist who asks too many questions of the patient, particularly closed questions, will increase anxiety and close down the patient's capacity for thought about what is happening. Direct questions in particular tend to invite closed-down answers. The patient can feel intruded upon and interrogated, and thus less likely to offer feelings and associations to the therapist. Some patients may feel that their views and experiences are being devalued, and a persecutory spiral may develop with adverse effects for the therapy (Meares and Hobson, 1977). Hobson also suggests that therapists are particularly likely to ask questions when their own anxiety is raised.

The Conversational Model advocates following the patient's material carefully and the offering of a statement which tentatively expresses understanding (e.g. 'I wonder if you are feeling . . .'). The statement should be owned by the therapist as his own opinion, and not the definitive view of the situation, which allows for correction if necessary and further exploration within the relationship. The therapist frames interventions as 'an invitation to a mutual exploration' (Meares and Hobson, 1977).

The patient may at times ask direct questions of the therapist, and may feel in need of a direct answer. Whilst the therapist should convey a wish to understand why the question has been asked, to clarify what sort of response is appropriate, Hobson suggests that the therapist should, at times, be willing to share a feeling of his own, or to reveal something of what he is like as a person as without some indication of the real person of the therapist, the patient can never test out his fantasies against reality. Although achieving an appropriate balance may prove difficult for the inexperienced therapist, being selectively 'transparent' may at times prove therapeutically advantageous.

Using 'I' and 'we'

Using the first person pronouns 'I' and 'we' emphasizes involvement in the mutual, dialectical psychotherapeutic process, and suggests that each participant is prepared to own what he feels, thinks and says as his. Hobson advocates framing interventions with a phrase such as 'I wonder . . .', so as to emphasize both that the therapist owns the speculation, and that it is open to correction. Hobson also emphasizes the 'I–Thou' quality of the therapeutic relationship, a relationship in which each participant strives to know, as opposed to know about, the other.

Hypotheses

These are statements used by the therapist in an attempt to convey understanding of the patient's words, feelings, fantasies, experiences or actions. Hypotheses are designed to promote exploration of the patient's feelings, and to suggest meaning for them. They are intended to be modified by the patient's responses, and are tested within the session. Systemic therapy uses hypothesizing in a not dissimilar way; an initial hypothesis is made on the basis of what is known about the family or system, and is modified in the light of confirming or disconfirming evidence. Many of the operations involved in making and communicating hypotheses about what is happening in the session are similar to those involved in the process of making a psychoanalytic interpretation. Conversational Model interventions try to avoid being an external imposition of the therapist's view upon the patient, but aim instead to arise in a collaborative fashion from the dialogue and interaction between the two.

The understanding hypothesis

Understanding hypotheses are tentative formulations of the therapist's guess about how the patient may be feeling. It is the least complex form of interpretative intervention in the model, and is based on how the therapist imagines the patient to be feeling. As far as possible, this is guided by cues picked up from the patient. These cues may be *verbal* (based on what the patient actually says), *vocal* (based on how the patient says it) or *non-verbal* (based on gestures, bodily movements and involuntary movements).

The therapist does not aim for total accuracy in this (e.g. 'I guess it feels as if things will never change, something like that . . .'), instead leaving room for negotiation and adjustment, although the understanding hypothesis should be conveyed in such a way as to suggest a wish to understand even if it is wrong. This may lead to a modification of the hypothesis; and perhaps a new one which fits the evidence better or extension of the hypothesis leading to further exploration. Both of these developments are more useful than simple agreement on the patient's part with the therapist's interpretation or hypothesis. The monitoring of the patient's response to an intervention is a crucial part of this model. Understanding hypotheses could be compared to interpretation aimed at Malan's (1979) 'Triangle of Conflict'.

The linking hypothesis

Linking hypotheses are hypotheses about what the feeling may be linked with – in relation to whom or what. The hypothesis tries to connect feelings which are present in the session with other feelings, both within the present therapeutic relationship and outside it. Linking hypotheses attempt to make sense of experiences by linking feelings from different situations (e.g. 'I think you're feeling very frustrated here with me today and I guess it's a bit like when you and your father . . .'). The linking hypothesis does not attempt to explain the feelings, even though the therapist may have done so in his own thoughts. Linking hypotheses could be compared to interpretations aimed at Malan's (1979) 'triangle of person'.

The explanatory hypothesis
Explanatory hypotheses are hypotheses about why the patient may be feeling the way he does. In this form of intervention, the therapist looks for possible reasons underlying feelings, thoughts or behaviours. He bases this on what he has previously known of the patient; on previous under-standing and linking hypotheses, and the patient's response to these. Explanatory hypotheses will usually be given about repeating patterns of behaviour which take place either within the therapeutic relationship, outside it, or both. It is an attempt to suggest a reason for this pattern. (e.g. 'I think you feel that I don't care, that I'm abandoning you at a point where you need me, and I think you feel I'm doing that because I prefer to see to the needs of other people, as you felt your parents did with your sisters'). The therapist is also trying to identify an underlying pattern of conflict which may underlie the behaviour, and to relate it to feelings which are present at that moment. Explanatory hypotheses can therefore be compared to full transference interpretations.

How does the conversational model differ from other psychotherapies?

The study by Goldberg *et al.* (1984) examined predictions about behaviours expected to distinguish Conversational Model therapists from other practitioners. Conversational Model therapy has been shown to be clearly differentiable from other therapies, a difference which patients also perceive.

Features specific to the conversational model
- Patients are given a clear framework, know what is expected of them and know what to expect of the therapist. The therapist gives clear information about who he is, why the patient is being seen, in what setting and for how long, resulting in a clear therapeutic contract at the end of the first session.
- The therapeutic focus is on the patient–therapist relationship.
- The therapist:
  - makes statements and avoids questions
  - expresses understanding in a tentative way that allows negotiation
  - emphasizes involvement in mutual process by using the words 'I' and 'we'
  - clearly recognizes and picks up verbal and non-verbal cues
  - clearly derives hypotheses from the patient's cues, rather than theory
  - makes understanding hypotheses and linking hypotheses appropriately.

Which patient and why?

Suitable patients

Conversational Model psychotherapy is a suitable treatment for people whose difficulties can be seen as having arisen from frustrations and difficulties in intimate relationships, or whose problems may potentially be resolved within an intimate relationship. In practice this means that those who are broadly suitable for a psychodynamic approach might benefit from Conversational Model therapy. This includes a broad variety of patients who suffer from difficulties in interpersonal relationships; social, educational and work difficulties; neurotic disturbance; sexual problems and paraphilias; eating disorders; and moderately severe personality disorder. With its emphasis on accommodating to the patient's emotional state, the therapy will tend to promote an idealized transference relationship in which it may be difficult to gain access to the patient's more persecutory or hostile feelings. It is therefore best suited to patients who very readily feel persecuted or overwhelmed by hostile feelings, and who require active containment of their feelings to keep them engaged in the therapeutic process (e.g. borderline personalities) although it is suitable for less disturbed patients as well.

The model is also useful for patients whose developmental disturbance is at a primitive or early level because it allows the therapist to help a 'conversation' into being with a patient who cannot, at first, think about experiences or feelings. The 'conversation' need not be a verbal one: a dialogue of gesture or actions may constitute a conversation; for instance, a patient who attends sessions but does not talk may be indicating that in some way he feels contained or understood by what goes on between himself and the therapist. The terms of the conversation can be adapted to suit the prevailing circumstances.

Some people seem, even under reasonable therapeutic conditions, not to be able to join in a mutual, unfolding relationship with a therapist in which a conversation takes place. This may be because of:

- Severe anxiety where mechanisms for anxiety avoidance may have become fixed and too rigid to change easily
- Insufficient basic trust in other people, where this interferes with a person's capacity to make dependent relationships on others
- Isolation from others, and being cut off from a person's own feelings, often because contact would cause intolerable pain or discomfort
- A tendency to habitually act on feelings in a dangerous way, if the person cannot be helped to think about and reflect on them instead

The aim of Conversational Model psychotherapy is to help people to be able to converse and so there are no absolute contraindications. People with difficulties of the sorts defined above may be helped to relate to other people in a more satisfactory way through therapy, even if only to a limited degree.

Assessment for psychotherapy

Assessment for Conversational Model psychotherapy is broadly similar to assessment for any other form of psychodynamic therapy, in that the therapist tries to reach a dynamic and also psychiatric formulation of the patient's difficulties whilst also trying to form an impression of the way this person relates to others, internalized relationships, impulses, defences, fantasies and so on. In this model, the therapist is particularly interested in finding out whether the prospective patient can converse in the sense outlined above, and the therapist uses the techniques of the model from the beginning of the first interview in an attempt to reach a shared, mutual dialogue.

Which therapist and why?

Background qualities and skills

These are not significantly different from those required to practise any form of exploratory psychotherapy. Hobson particularly advocates a wide literary and artistic background, but artistic feeling needs to be combined with an understanding of and sympathy with the rigour of scientific methods. The therapist needs to have a degree of self-awareness – knowledge of his inner self, understanding of himself in relationships and insight into the defences he uses. He requires the capacity to be truthful to himself and to others, and should have some ability to be spontaneous and to experience feelings in a direct way. The therapist also has to be able to gain sufficient detachment from that experience to think, to reflect and to talk about it. The therapist must be able to recognize subtle verbal, vocal and non-verbal cues from the patient, and must be able to listen to his own feelings, thoughts and responses, as well as to the conversation between them. He must also look for evidence that he is wrong in his hypotheses about the patient. This is not so that he can be right but rather so that he can show himself able to admit to being wrong, to be corrected, and to assimilate the new view into his picture of the patient and the conversation. In doing so, the therapist is providing for the patient a role model of learning to adjust and accommodate to another person.

Teaching and supervision of psychotherapy

The Conversational Model is an effective tool for teaching basic exploratory psychotherapy skills to trainee therapists because the desirable skills, attitudes and techniques have been defined and specified. Teaching videotapes and written teaching material have been developed to introduce the model to students, but this cannot be a substitute for direct personal experience. Supervised practice forms an important part of training and regular, usually once weekly, supervision is an integral part of the model. Trainees are encouraged to audiotape or videotape their own sessions for supervision purposes, so that they can examine what they actually do in clinical practice rather than what they think or say they do. This forms the basis for corrective feedback within the setting of a supervisory relationship, a parallel process to the Conversational Model therapy, so that the trainee can 'go on learning more about how to listen' (Hobson, 1985). Hobson also advocated the use of role playing in supervision and, more controversially, the viewing, or listening to, of taped sessions together with the patient as an aid to both therapy and therapist learning. Supervision is often carried out in small groups of two or three trainees together with a supervisor. Membership of the supervision group is kept relatively constant to generate cohesion and mutual trust, creating an atmosphere in which learning about psychotherapy can take place safely.

Training to be a psychotherapist

Instruction in the basic techniques of the Conversational Model will enable the trainee to begin to work with an exploratory form of psychotherapy, and skills can continue to be learnt and refined in supervised practice. In common with other models of psychodynamic psychotherapy, a more lengthy and rigorous training will be required for the practitioner who intends to work mainly or wholly as a psychotherapist. No specific advanced training course in the Conversational Model exists, but many of the skills and techniques of the model are compatible with other models of psychodynamic therapy. Where they are not, they provide instructive contrasts which must be thought about in the course of development as a psychotherapist. The Conversational Model provides useful ideas and techniques for therapists with training in other schools of psychotherapy.

Personal psychotherapy for the trainee – not necessarily Conversational Model therapy, but any psychotherapy that increases self-knowledge – is an essential part of training as the Conversational Model makes marked demands upon the therapist's self-knowledge and awareness. It is particularly important to be able to judge when a modification in the therapist's stance towards the patient, ostensibly in the service of better attunement, is being made for defensive reasons on the therapist's part, such as the avoidance of aggressive or sadistic feelings towards the patient, which would be better explored as potentially important countertransference experience.

Therapeutic setting

The physical settings of the psychotherapeutic encounter are 'vital features of the therapeutic language' (Hobson, 1985). By this is meant that the setting – the room, the decor, the furniture and so on – all convey something about the therapist's personality, how he regards his patients, and what he expects of them.

Conversational Model therapy is usually carried out using two identical chairs set at an angle to each other so that patient and therapist can quite naturally look at or away from each other. This is not, however, a rigid rule and an alternative arrangement might be made for a patient who required something different. Sessions generally follow the 'analytic hour' of fifty minutes, although some practitioners have habitually used slightly shorter or longer sessions: the important point is that this time boundary is adhered to and made the focus of attention when it is not. Patients are usually seen once-weekly, although the model's concepts and practices can readily be used in therapies where the sessions are more or less frequent. The regularity and reliability of the setting lend stability to the therapeutic work and security to the patient. There is no set duration of therapy in this model, which can be applied equally to very brief therapies and those lasting several years.

The therapist and patient will agree on a therapeutic contract at an early stage specifying details such as how long sessions are, when and where they will take place and the duration of therapy. The therapist gives clear information about likely experiences in therapy, about what will be expected of the patient, what the aims of the therapy will be and what might be the focus of future sessions. There is evidence that this has a positive effect on outcome in psychotherapy. Successful psychotherapy also requires an optimal psychological setting which is neither intrusive nor too distant. There must be respect for the patient's personal and private mental space.

Clinical example

Ann, a forty-seven-year-old woman working as a home help, presented to the psychotherapy clinic with a six-year history of depression which had not been responsive to treatment with antidepressant medication. She was married to Steven, an unemployed ex-soldier. They had four sons, now grown up but still living at home. Ann's depression began in the months following her elderly mother's death. Her mother was an angry and demanding woman who had suffered lifelong ill health. Ann nursed her unfailingly and without complaint for many years until her death.

In psychotherapy, Ann at first gave a detailed factual account of her difficult life and her mother's death, but she politely refused to talk about the impact of this on her, or any feelings which she might have. She hoped that the therapist would give her advice: tell her what to do to feel better and resolve her family's problems. The therapist, though, was able to focus on cues such as her quavering tone of voice and her shredding of paper hankies, and use empathic statements and negotiation to encourage the emergence of her feelings, particularly her hidden and guilty anger with both her mother and her family. The therapist used the words 'I' and 'we' in making her interventions, and Ann was helped to recognize the active and mutual involvement of both herself and her therapist in the process. She was encouraged by finding herself working together with another person who seemed not to need Ann to care for her, and she continued to explore her feelings, but remained wary of her therapist. She felt that the actual expression of negative feeling towards another person was unacceptable, and potentially dangerous to her.

Her therapist continued to adopt a warm, friendly and supportive stance whilst declining to be drawn into giving the advice and direction for which Ann increasingly pleaded. Ann now experienced her therapist as uncaring, even rejecting of her. By helping her to focus on and stay with these immediately present feelings, the therapist was gradually able to help Ann to voice her disappointment and anger, at first with her therapist. Then, gradually, through the therapist's use of linking and explanatory hypotheses, she could explore her disappointment and anger with her mother, father, husband and her sons. She began to realize that she might not need others to impose their advice or direction on her and that, in fact, she might be quite angry when people tried to do so. It was a revelation to her that she felt able to participate actively in her therapy, the first time in her life that she had felt able and encouraged to be anything but the passive recipient of other people's ideas. Increasingly, a collaborative working relationship developed.

> *Ann felt encouraged to use and develop a metaphor which helped her and her therapist to understand how she felt about the process: she had described herself as being on the banks of a fast-flowing and dangerous river which, in order to rid herself of the depression, she had to attempt to cross. She had hoped that she would be carried across without getting wet, or facing the dangers of the turbulent current, but she had begun to give up hope of this ever happening. Now she found that she had taken a step or two into the stream, which no longer seemed to be so vast or threatening, and was actually learning to swim. She started to be able to feel more sad about her mother's life and about her relationship with her. She felt less compelled to meet her family's expectations of her without thought, had negotiated some changes in her relationships with her husband and sons, and felt able to think creatively about what she wanted from her life in the present.*

Problems in therapy

One potentially problematic aspect of the Conversational Model is the potential for an idealized relationship to develop between patient and therapist as a result of the active attention given by the therapist to the feelings and the self-state of the patient, and to the process of attaining mutual adjustment. Farrell (1986), when reviewing Hobson's book *Forms of Feeling: The Heart of Psychotherapy* (1985), commented on its strictures against the therapist being persecutory and suggested that 'his method may be seriously defective at this place'. Hobson argues that some patients require such care to keep them engaged in therapy. He does not suggest that the therapist should shirk from being experienced as persecutory if that is how the patient finds him, but rather that therapists can, and do sometimes, act in ways that are actually persecutory and which threaten the viability of a therapy. None the less, there is in this model a danger of encouraging an unhelpful fantasy of magical, perfect caregiving with some patients. Equally, therapists who are more comfortable with an idealizing transference than a persecutory one may be attracted to this model of working.

A second criticism which has been made of the Conversational Model is that it is not truly psychodynamic, being 'essentially behavioural and directive' in style (Dick, 1990) and perhaps not allowing a truly free unfolding of the patient's internal world. It is true that the model is explicitly directive, in that the therapist works to establish certain conditions, encourages staying with feelings and so on. As the Conversational Model tends to emphasize and encourage the patient's potential for mutuality and adult functioning, there is also less likelihood of regression to more infantile states than with some other approaches to psychotherapy.

The model is essentially optimistic that a mutual conversation can occur, or be helped into being, between therapist and patient. Although it was developed as a response to very disturbed patients who found it very difficult or impossible to converse, and who are very difficult to understand, it may not be an appropriate framework for some people. Here mainstream psychoanalysis with its deep exploration of unconscious phantasy may offer views and thoughts which extend psychotherapeutic practice beyond what can be achieved with this model alone. None the less, the features of the

Conversational Model outlined here can form a useful basis for most psychotherapeutic conversations.

Evaluation of therapy

Hobson was a founder member of the United Kingdom chapter of the Society for Psychotherapy Research, and there is an emphasis in the Conversational Model on empirical testing and the integration of new knowledge from research studies. The Conversational Model lends itself to being used in empirical psychotherapy research studies of both the process and outcome types, because the conditions in which therapy takes place and the interventions used can be specified quite precisely. It has been demonstrated that whilst remaining a therapeutic method which has the person and interpersonal relationships as its focus, its 'treatment effects can be studied methodically and rigorously in a way more commonly associated with behavioural and cognitive treatment' (Margison and Shapiro, 1986).

Barkham and Hobson, in a research study published in 1990, used the Conversational Model as the basis for an extremely brief model of exploratory psychotherapy (two-plus-one sessions). Some of these studies, particularly those concerned with process research, have helped to refine aspects of the Conversational Model, without changing its original psychodynamic and interpersonal premises.

The Sheffield Psychotherapy Project has used a version of Conversational Model psychotherapy for its work on comparing psychological treatments for depression and anxiety. This form of exploratory therapy was shown to be effective in patients with depression and anxiety, although slightly less so than cognitive behavioural therapy (Shapiro and Firth, 1987). However, it has been suggested by some commentators that the research methodology used in this study may not adequately assess some of the less tangible effects of psychodynamic therapies.

In 1991, Guthrie *et al.* published a controlled trial of Conversational Model psychotherapy plus relaxation and standard medical treatment versus standard medical treatment alone for refractory irritable bowel syndrome. This showed significantly greater improvement for the group treated with psychotherapy, which was 'feasible and effective in two-thirds of these patients'.

Much of the research work on the Conversational Model, and the teaching material, has concerned brief forms of psychotherapy, sometimes delivered by quite inexperienced therapists. Whilst brief psychotherapy can be very effective, it should not be inferred that the Conversational Model is a brief and basic model of psychotherapy. Rather, the model suggests an attitude, a frame of reference which can be used by a therapist of any level of experience, to inform his work with any patient in any setting, including general psychiatric interventions. The financial implications of using such a model of psychotherapy in an NHS clinic are similar to any other psychodynamic model: therapists require training and supervision and therapies may be brief or longer depending on clinical need. Psychodynamic psychotherapy services may be expensive to set up and run but may deliver considerable benefits to the health of some groups of patients (McGrath and Lowson, 1986).

Alternatives to therapy

People with troublesome focal symptoms or a discrete symptom area (such as a specific phobia) are more likely to benefit from prescriptive therapies such as behavioural or cognitive therapy. So are some patients who for various reasons find it too difficult to work with an interpersonal focus, and who require focus on a task (such as a behavioural programme) in order for the therapeutic relationship to function at all.

Some other patients who cannot utilize a Conversational approach might benefit more from a purely supportive one. People whose difficulties have been precipitated by, or are maintained by, their problematic current relationships might benefit from a family or marital therapeutic approach.

In common with other psychodynamic approaches to therapy, Conversational Model therapy is not designed to be used concurrently with another psychotherapy because of the splitting of both the transferential and the actual therapeutic relationships which would ensue. Consecutive treatments with therapies from different models presents no special difficulty if proper attention is paid to working through the end of one therapy before another is started.

Drug treatment, e.g. for depression or even psychotic symptoms, should not be a bar to Conversational Model therapy. However, as for all psychotherapies, the concurrent use of drugs that seriously interfere with concentration and new learning, such as minor tranquillizers, would be discouraged.

Acknowledgements
My grateful thanks are due to Dr Robert Hobson for his support and encouragement in writing this chapter, for much conversation about psychotherapy, the Conversational Model and about my work on it; and for allowing me access to his unpublished material for talks given over the years. Thanks are also due to Dr Frank Margison for his help and encouragement, and to Dr Helen Barker and Dr Else Guthrie for the clinical vignette.

Further reading

Hobson, R.F. (1974) Loneliness. *Journal of Analytical Psychology*, **19**, 71–89.
Hobson, R.F. (1985) *Forms of Feeling: The Heart of Psychotherapy*. London: Tavistock.
Meares, R.A. and Hobson, R.F. (1977) The persecutory therapist. *British Journal of Medical Psychology*, **50**, 349–359.

Bibliography

Barkham, M. and Hobson, R.F. (1990) Exploratory therapy in two-plus-one sessions. II: A single case study. *British Journal of Psychotherapy*, **6**, 89–100.
Dick, B. (1990) Two-plus-one brief psychotherapy: a response to Michael Barkham and Bob Hobson. *British Journal of Psychotherapy*, **6**, 327–330.
Farrell, B.A. (1986) Book Review. *Psychological Medicine*, **16**, 933–935.

Goldberg, D.P., Hobson, R.F., Maguire, G.P. *et al.* (1984) The clarification and assessment of a method of psychotherapy. *British Journal of Psychiatry*, **144**, 567–575.

Guthrie, E., Creed, F., Dawson, D. and Tomenson, B. (1991) A controlled trial of psychological treatment for the irritable bowel syndrome. *Gastroenterology*, **100**, 450–457.

Hobson, R.F. (1973) The archetypes of the collective unconscious. In: M. Fordham, R. Gordon, J. Hubback *et al.* (eds), *Analytical Psychology: a Modern Science*. Library of Analytical Psychology. London: Academic Press.

Hobson, R.F. (1974) Loneliness. *Journal of Analytical Psychology*, **19**, 71–89.

Hobson, R.F. (1979) The Messianic Community. In: R.D. Hinshelwood and N. Manning (eds), *Therapeutic Communities: Reflections and Progress*. London: Routledge and Kegan Paul, pp. 231–244.

Hobson, R.F. (1985) *Forms of Feeling: The Heart of Psychotherapy*. London: Tavistock.

Malan, D.H. (1979) *Individual Psychotherapy and the Science of Psychodynamics*. London: Butterworth–Heinemann.

Margison, F.R. and Moss, S. (1994) Teaching psychotherapy skills to inexperienced psychiatry trainees using the Conversational Model. *Psychotherapy Research*, **4**, 141–148.

Margison, F.R. and Shapiro, D.A. (1986) Hobson's Conversational Model of psychotherapy – training and evaluation: discussion paper. *Journal of the Royal Society of Medicine*, **79**, 469–472.

McGrath, G. and Lowson, K. (1986) Assessing the benefits of psychotherapy: the Economic Approach. *British Journal of Psychiatry*, **150**, 65–71.

Meares, R.A. and Hobson, R.F. (1977) The persecutory therapist. *British Journal of Medical Psychology*, **50**, 349–359.

Shapiro, D.A. and Firth, J. (1987) Prescriptive versus exploratory psychotherapy: outcomes of the Sheffield Psychotherapy Project. *British Journal of Psychiatry*, **151**, 790–799.

Stern, D.N. (1985) *The Interpersonal World of the Infant*. New York: Basic Books.

Winnicott, D.W. (1971) *Playing and Reality*. London: Tavistock.

10

Cognitive Analytic Therapy

Chess Denman

Historical perspective and overview

Cognitive analytic therapy (CAT) is a brief focal dynamic psychotherapy developed by Dr Anthony Ryle over the past thirty years. It draws on a number of different traditions in psychotherapy. The first is psychoanalysis. CAT takes from psychoanalytic thinking an emphasis on the importance of internal and external object relations, an understanding of unconscious processes and a stress on the use of transference and countertransference in therapy. The second tradition which CAT draws on is cognitive therapy. From this tradition, CAT takes an appreciation of active methods for inducing change and an emphasis on the value of measurement in psychotherapy. Patients are evaluated before and after therapy using standard measures. During therapy patients are also involved in evaluating their own progress. Most recently CAT has included the work of Vygotsky and his followers who emphasize man's distinctive capacity to use tools and stress the value of higher mental functions such as language.

The main theoretical contributor to CAT has been Dr Ryle himself. His work is summed up in two volumes: *Cognitive Analytic Therapy: Active Participation in Change*, published in 1990, and five years later, *Cognitive Analytic Therapy: Developments in Theory and Practice*. The second volume contains contributions from most other significant workers in the field of cognitive analytic therapy.

Principles of theory and practice

Principles of theory

CAT theory analyses human behaviour and experience in terms of a concept called a *procedure*. Procedures are organized sequences of wishes, thoughts, actions, emotions and appraisals which are organized and deployed in order to achieve an aim (see Figure 10.1).

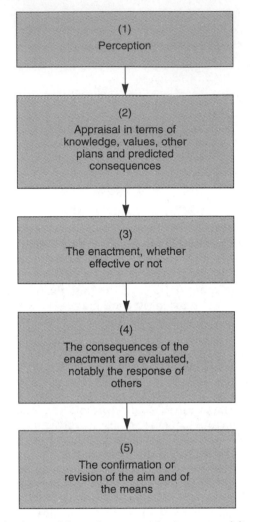

Figure 10.1   The fundamental form of any procedural sequence (after Ryle, 1995a, p. 2)

Vignette 1: A Very Simple Procedure

(1) Jane felt hungry, (2) so she went to the cupboard and inspected the contents. Several items looked tempting but Jane was also on a diet. (3) Consequently she selected an apple. (4) She felt less hungry but also a bit guilty about eating the last apple in the cupboard. (5) Although still rather hungry, being mindful of her diet, Jane went to distract herself by reading the paper.

Procedures are built up from experience. As the human infant develops, innate attachment and other instinctual behaviours are elaborated within the context of the infant's social and physical world into increasingly complex procedures. A crucial feature of this development is the use of signs which carry meaning and which culminate in language. Signs are not innate within the human infant, rather they are formed by interpersonal activities which use signs as mediators. Signs are first jointly developed as a result of communicative acts with emotionally significant others, and are later internalized with intrapersonal meaning. This theory of signs (Leiman, 1995) brings the influence of culture and the social world into the forefront of CAT's theory of the development of the individual, and into CAT's theory of the formation of those aims and intentions which drive procedural enactments.

Many procedures have little to do with interpersonal relationships, such as the procedure described in Vignette 1. However, the procedures which most people find problematic, and which bring them to the psychotherapist, are generally interpersonal or intrapersonal. CAT therapists are chiefly preoccupied with people, either the self or others, and CAT theorists describe inter- and intrapersonal procedures in the form of *reciprocal role relationships*. In each reciprocal role relationship, the self and the other (external or internal) take up complementary roles within a defining relationship. A benign example of a reciprocal role relationship would be that of one person providing care to another individual who wants to receive care. In contrast, an example of a malignant reciprocal role relationship would be an abusive interaction with reciprocal roles of abuser and abused. Reciprocal role relationships are stored as internalized templates but become apparent through the procedures by which individuals enact them in the world. Those procedures which enact reciprocal role relationships are called *reciprocal role procedures*. So individuals enact reciprocal role procedures in relation to others drawing on the template of their internalized role relationships which are aimed (successfully or not) at gratifying needs for various kinds of relatedness.

Vignette 2: Learning and Internalizing a Reciprocal Role Relationship

Paula is two, her mother scolds her for throwing food on the floor. Later she takes her doll and pretends it has thrown food on the floor. She scolds the doll. Later still Paula is clearly struggling with a wish to throw her food again. Aloud she says, 'No Paula don't do that.'

On the whole, children develop good internalized reciprocal role relationships and reciprocal role procedures if allowed to do so. Later, as adults, they may revise maladaptive procedures for the better by learning from experience. Fixed psychopathology is conceived of within CAT as being the result of the repetitive employment of maladaptive procedures. The theory therefore needs to explain why maladaptive procedures come into being, and why they continue to be repetitively employed and not revised when they do not work? In Ryle's (1994) view, the classical psychoanalytic theories of defence and conflict were insufficient explanations for the formation and perpetuation of procedural maladaptation. A more general theory of restrictions in procedural formation and revision was needed. In response, Ryle identified a range of reasons for procedural restriction and malformation.

Reasons for procedural restriction and malformation

Restrictions in life experience may result in limited repertoires of reciprocal role relationships, which are then kept narrow because they themselves result in procedures which limit further experience.

Vignette 3: Restricted Life Experience

Joe was brought up in a series of children's homes where he had numerous carers. Joe needed relationships and attention but, in the context of the children's home, attention had to be competed for from workers who kept moving on. Joe therefore developed methods of demanding attention, such as self abuse and the abuse of others and property. However, he was also careful never to get too close to any worker for they would surely move on. In later life, Joe employed the same procedures. He reacted to upsets in interpersonal relationships by making suicidal or violent threats, and he never let himself grow close to anyone. He sabotaged relationships whenever intimacy threatened. Sadly, the consequence of his behaviour was to alienate people he met and his adult life, like his childhood, was characterized by innumerable brief unsatisfactory relationships. His environment, by virtue of his procedures, was again restricted and offered no opportunities for new experience.

Self-reflection provides a vital way of revising procedures and enlarging procedural repertoires. However, it too is a learned procedure. In families where self-reflection is not encouraged, the child may fail to develop adequate tools for self-reflection. Without the benefit of adequate self-reflection, 'procedural maintenance and repair' cannot occur.

Two other ways in which consciousness and procedures can be restricted bear more resemblance to traditional psychodynamic defence mechanisms. One is the formation of erroneous beliefs about the cause of events which can lead to guilt. This results in avoidant or symptomatic procedures designed to overcome this guilt or to avoid a repeat of the (misattributed) events.

Vignette 4: Erroneous Beliefs

When John was 11, his father died suddenly of a heart attack. At the time, John and his father had been in conflict over various childhood issues. John formed the belief that these fights had caused his father's death. Henceforth, he was over-compliant in relation to male authority figures.

Another reason for procedural restriction is the abandonment of a desire or aim, because of guilty anxiety, in response to critical external or internalized voices. In this way, the individual avoids guilty and anxious thoughts and feelings.

Vignette 5: Abandoning an Aim Because of Critical Voices

Joan consulted a psychotherapist because of her extreme inhibition about sexual matters. She said she found the thought of sex consciously repellent. The attitude of Joan's parents towards sex was prudish and repressive, and It was clear that they had stifled any sexual exploration on her part. After some work, Joan became able to admit to some feelings of sexual arousal but they were soon extinguished. She said 'It's as though I hear my mother's voice saying "stop that – it's dirty."'

One particular restriction of self-reflection is extremely important in patients with borderline personality disorder. These patients display alarming and dramatic changes of emotional state. The reciprocal role procedures they adopt in each state vary but are mostly highly emotionally charged and have a tendency to exert unusually strong emotional reactions in others. CAT introduces the concept of a *state* to describe these patient's reactions. A state is a dominant view of the self and the world, often associated with a particular reciprocal role relationship. CAT hypothesizes that the patient's self-reflection is disjointed or fragmented because the different states they experience are simple, emotionally intense and discontinuously fluctuating. The unintegration which these patient's display is theorized in CAT as an expression of an early childhood experience in which the roles adopted by significant caregiving others were themselves highly discontinuous. Additionally, the narrative accounts given by caregivers for the differing experiences of the child, which can normally bridge discontinuities in experience and help to build stable and more complex states, were absent, misleading or disjointed.

Vignette 6: Fragmented Self-States

Tom came into therapy with a drink problem. He would binge drink, generally after a row with his partner, and could become violent towards him. Tom worked as an AIDS counsellor but his work was not going well. He found himself getting very over-involved with his clients, and feeling unaccountably guilty as though he was responsible for their difficulties. If they showed signs of recovering, or of not needing him, he would suddenly turn on them and refuse to visit them further. Tom's initial engagement in therapy was uncertain. He would turn up drunk to some sessions, and miss others with no explanation. Relatively early in therapy, Tom's therapist unaccountably forgot to attend a session. On the next occasion she apologized for her lapse and Tom spent a considerable amount of time trying to make her feel better about her lapse. Suddenly, in the middle of the session and for no apparent reason, Tom got up to leave saying that he could no longer stay in the session. The therapist was initially shocked by this turn of events, but then found herself oddly disinterested. She even found herself encouraging Tom to leave if he wanted to.

In supervision, Tom's symptoms and the variety of events in therapy were related to his early experience. Tom's mother was an alcoholic. She oscillated between maudlin remorse, drunken violence and ignoring Tom. Tom's reciprocal childhood responses to his mother were to adopt the positions of pseudo-adult comforter, battered victim and escapee. Once these discontinuous reciprocal roles were identified the therapist could see that she, Tom and his clients were all re-enacting one or another of the roles in the sequence of reciprocal role relationships. For example, when the therapist 'abused' Tom by 'drunkenly' forgetting a session, Tom responded by adopting the role of pseudo-adult comforter. Then, when Tom felt the therapist was better, he shifted into escapee role in order to avoid the risk that the therapist might ignore him and the therapist was in turn shifted into the position of an ignoring mother.

Aims of therapy

In general, CAT therapists draw on a wide range of distinctive techniques which have been built up as part of CAT. The timetable and the techniques of CAT all have in common the aim of helping the patient to understand and alter their maladaptive procedures. Although these techniques represent the collective experience of CAT therapists, each therapy is an individual event in which the therapist and patient collaborate creatively to find a way of working together. In relation to the techniques used by the therapist, CAT has many ideas and suggestions to offer but makes few demands. As long as what is being done in therapy is aimed at understanding and revising the maladaptive procedures which trouble the patient, and is suited to the patient's need rather than the therapist's preference, it is acceptable.

Principles of practice

Starting CAT – the first four sessions

Generally CAT therapies last sixteen sessions. In some cases of patients with borderline personality disorder, a twenty-four session treatment may be undertaken. On other occasions, a brief eight session version of CAT is used. The therapist uses the first four sessions to try to achieve a number of aims. These begin with the dual tasks common to all therapies of building a therapeutic alliance with the patient, and of gaining an initial perspective on the patient's problems and personal history. More distinctively to CAT, the therapist tries to agree a set of *target problems* with the patient. These represent a list of the main difficulties that the patient is experiencing, and include both those directly complained of by the patient and those not directly referred to or acknowledged but which the therapist has noticed.

Vignette 7: Target Problems

Jo complained of depression and anxiety, and also cut herself on a regular basis. These were easy target problems to agree. The therapist also noted, although Jo did not mention it, that her patient was significantly underweight and that she was also socially isolated. Jo's therapist therefore raised these two issues as possible further target problems.

The therapist also introduces the patient to two key elements of CAT. The first is the idea of joint working. Patient and therapist work together to create a space for mutual understanding and exploration between them. The second key element is that of self-monitoring. The mutual design of 'joint tools for self-reflection' which are used by the patient outside therapy sessions is an important element of CAT. Such tools enhance the patient's capacity for self-understanding, and provide useful information for patient and therapist alike. They can be very varied since they are fashioned by the patient and therapist jointly to serve the needs of the patient and of the problem being monitored. Many patients keep a diary during the week. This may be focused on target problems or be a more general record of feelings and problems. Some patients write their life story for the therapy, and very often the patient will fill in a document called the psychotherapy file. This document is a questionnaire which lists common problems and the maladaptive procedures which generate them. Its value lies in the way in which it describes procedures which may cause problems and, by reflecting on it, the patient may begin to move from a focus on problems to a focus on procedures.

Reformulation

As the first four sessions progress, the therapist tries to move from a problem focus to a procedural one. She will try out tentative procedural understandings with the patient in an attempt to *reformulate* the patient's problems. This activity assists the therapist in preparing a *reformulation letter* which is written to the patient, usually by the fourth session of the therapy. The letter contains two elements. It recapitulates the patient's story as told to the therapist which provides the patient with concrete evidence of having been heard. This is often a very powerful experience. The letter also tries to attribute the patient's difficulties to the operation of a small number of repetitive maladaptive procedures (called *target problem procedures* – TPPs) which cause them. A full description of these problematic procedures will often reveal their origins as attempts at adaptation in earlier life. It is helpful for the patient to see how these ways of reacting have a basic aim, and how the manner in which they fail results in problems.

The reformulation letter, given to the patient in the fourth session, often has a powerful effect on the patient. It provides them with the experience of being attended to, reflected on and hopefully understood. It should also incorporate the understandings that the patient has brought to the process, often using the patient's own words. The reformulation letter should not tell the patient what is wrong in the therapist's view – it should rather express the upshot of the four sessions the patient and therapist have spent together jointly exploring what might be going on. Consequently, the document may be open to modification as a result of negotiation between patient and therapist. During the fourth and, if necessary, subsequent sessions, the patient and therapist work to reach agreement in regard to the reformulation of the patient's difficulties.

Vignette 8: Part of a Reformulation Letter and its Impact

The therapist wrote: '. . . As a child it must have seemed to you that, after the death of your father, nothing in your world could ever be the same again. I think that you also felt responsible for his death because you had been told that you were a demanding and difficult child who would "be the death of your parents". You resolved to be a good and independent girl, and your mother's decline further thrust you into the role of a carer who had no one to rely on . . . Now you never ask for help and, if forced to, you fear that you may overwhelm your helper. It is as though you can adopt only two polarized positions: either you are a completely independent but isolated and secretly angry; or you risk becoming a dependent demanding person who will kill off those who offer help.' Jane, whose main problems were depression and social isolation, found the letter she received powerful and moving. Briefly she became tearful but then a look of terror overcame her and she pulled herself together. She began to quibble with parts of the letter and the therapist made some changes. But Jane's terror increased. The therapist said, 'I feel that you are letting yourself ask me for help, and are using me and the session time to work on the letter I have written you. But you also seem to be very frightened – I wonder if this could be because you fear that you are being demanding and may overwhelm me which, as I said in the letter, may be a particular problem for you.'

Initially the reformulation letter was entirely a text document. However, as the theory of object relations impacted on CAT, it became clear that for some patients with a more severe pathology a description of the states or groupings of their chief internal and external object relations (reciprocal role procedures from which interpersonal procedures emanated) was the most important task. These states interlock and succeed one another in sequences which may bewilder both patient and therapist. A description and naming of the states is therefore powerfully containing to both parties. For this purpose, a technical device called a *sequential diagrammatic reformulation* (SDR) was developed as a way of encapsulating the joint understanding of the patient's states. It resembles a computer flow diagram, or map, which shows the chief states in boxes and the ways that procedures emanate from them. Not every patient needs or benefits from the construction of an SDR but many, especially those with personality disorders which are characterized by considerable fragmentation and the experience of discontinuous self-states, find it extremely useful.

Vignette 9: Part of Tom's Sequential Diagrammatic Reformulation (SDR) showing the different Reciprocal Role Relationships

Above and below the boxes shown in Figure 10.2 (below) are descriptions of parts of Tom's therapy and life showing which state he and the others he interacts with are in.

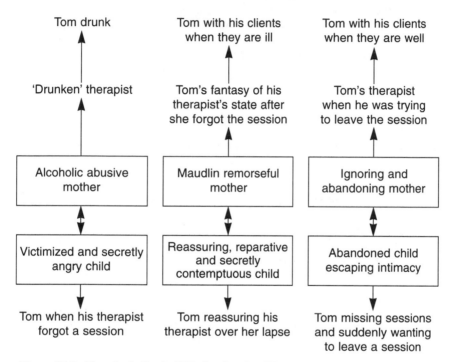

Figure 10.2   Vignette 9: Tom's SDR showing the different reciprocal role relationships

Addressing the target problem procedure (TPP)

Once the reformulation is agreed the middle phase of therapy can begin. In this phase the first aim is for the patient to become aware of the operation of their target problem procedures (TPPs) in daily life. There are a number of ways of achieving this which include self monitoring (which in the middle phase of therapy moves from a focus on problems to a focus on procedures) and discussion of the week's events with the therapist. Another crucial arena for becoming aware of the operation of TPPs is the therapy relationship itself. For example, if the patient's problematic procedures involve issues such as self care, dependency, feeding, new learning and envy; they are very likely to become active in the therapy setting because they are issues intrinsic to therapy. By monitoring both the patient's transference to the therapist and the therapist's countertransference responses, maladaptive as well as adaptive procedures can be seen in operation. Transference descriptions are particularly important because patient and therapist can start to disentangle the operation of problematic procedures in the therapy itself, within (it is to be hoped) a safe setting. From a learning theory perspective, transference descriptions also become potent occasions for learning.

The insights and new self-understanding generated by the first stage of therapy are often powerfully effective in helping the patient. The second stage of therapy, which is equally vital, helps the patient to acknowledge these insights and to apply them to life. In the third stage of therapy, once the patient has become able to identify the operation of the procedures in various settings, it is possible to try out different ways of proceeding which may be less damaging. The therapist needs to be particularly skilful here. There is always a temptation to tell the patient how to do things differently but this is rarely effective. The aim of the therapist in this phase of CAT is to stimulate the patient's creativity in devising exits from the problematic procedures, and then trying them out in various arenas. The therapy relationship can provide a relatively safe setting in which the patient may try different ways of being and acting.

Vignette 10: Trying New Ways of Being and Acting

Jane's main way of being was fierce independence (Vignette 8) and, whenever she gave up this stance, she feared becoming destructively demanding. Midway through her course of therapy, she discovered a breast lump and sessions had to be cancelled for a biopsy. She and the therapist explored whether it would be possible for Jane to telephone the therapist from hospital during her session time if she felt especially distressed. Jane felt that such a call would be both over-demanding and uselessly insufficient. However she did telephone and was able later to say that she had experienced the call as helpful and not too frightening.

Often the patient and the therapist may identify a number of different problematic procedures and wonder which ones to concentrate on. If nothing forces the therapist's hand it is obviously sensible to go for the TPPs causing the most difficulty or for those which the patient has latched on to most strongly. But one situation does force the therapist's hand. This is when a TPP acts within therapy to threaten, spoil or damage the process of therapy itself. In this situation the therapist and patient must try to attend to this TPP first or else no other work will be possible. As a result of the powerful nature of the therapeutic situation which both activates feelings to do with dependency and stimulates new learning, the TPPs which become active within therapy are often central to the patient's difficulties. They therefore need dealing with before their operation can destroy the therapy. Therapists who struggle with this situation in CAT frequently need considerable supervision and support.

Vignette 11: A Target Problem Procedure Threatens or
Damages Therapy

*As a child, Philip seems to have felt at the mercy of his mother's
whim. If she was in a good mood she fed, clothed and played
with him. If she was in a bad mood she ignored, belittled and
rejected him. He responded to her with anger and resentment.
Even her good actions were experienced by him as tantalizing
glimpses of a good life seemingly designed to torture him by
letting him taste happiness only to capriciously withdraw it.
Philip cut his losses and treated everything she offered as
worthless. By this move he also deprived her of the capacity to
tantalize and torture him. In therapy, nothing Philip's therapist
offered him was experienced by him as any good. Indeed the
therapist noticed that the extent to which Philip rubbished what
she offered was often proportionate to her sense that she might
have got things right. She came to see that Philip's TPP with his
mother was operating in therapy as well. Sharing this perspective
with Philip helped him to acknowledge that he often turned
things down because accepting them would be painful,
tantalizing and give the other the power to withdraw them.*

Ending therapy

By about session ten or eleven, the end of therapy is in sight. In truth, as
in any time-limited therapy, termination has been in view from before the
start of therapy. Consequently it is a feature of CAT practice that termination
should be explicitly discussed as soon as possible and that the therapist
should keep on raising it with the patient. One way of beginning to do this
is to count down the number of sessions with the patient. Dealing with
ending is important because all people have interpersonal procedures for
dealing with loss and separation, and for many patients these are maladaptive
or problematic and constitute part of their difficulties. Thus CAT therapists
focus on TPPs which are likely to cause problems in ending therapy in the
same way that they focus on the operation of any maladaptive procedure
in therapy. Negative feelings around ending need to be acknowledged, and
the recall and reworking of past losses is also important.

The joint work of the therapist and the patient is summarized in another
CAT document – the 'goodbye letter' – which is written by the therapist
and given to the patient at the penultimate session. This letter summarizes
the work that the patient and the therapist have done together, the
understandings they have reached and the changes which have been achieved.
It also acknowledges areas which have not been explored adequately and
tries to ensure that negative feelings about the end of therapy are brought
into the open. Sometimes the patient is also able to write the therapist a
goodbye letter.

Vignette 12: Part of a 'Goodbye Letter'

Dear Sara, When you first came to therapy you were complaining of depression and anxiety. You told me that you had spent much of your childhood anxiously hiding from a violent father and propping up a weak mother. We looked together at your life and began to see that you had never really allowed yourself to develop ways of getting your own needs met but instead had compulsively met the needs of others ... During therapy you have worked on all your problems and have come to quite a considerable degree of insight. You have tried out asking for things that you need in your marriage, and found that sometimes your needs can be met. Now, as we come to the end of therapy, we have talked together about your feeling that my attention is turning elsewhere. You didn't at first feel able to say to me that you had not had enough therapy or help, and instead you concentrated on telling me how tired and exhausted I looked. More recently, you have felt able to challenge me and to worry about how you will cope when therapy ends. We have been able to acknowledge together that you have made some changes in therapy but that you still risk, as you put it, 'slipping back into your old ways'. I have also tried to show you that focusing on a possible extension of your therapy, which is not an available option, may be a way of avoiding having to ask your husband and those around you for the things that you can have. I hope that you do manage to ask for your needs to be met.

In general, CAT therapists work to a fairly structured timetable within therapy. While elements of the timetable of therapy can be abandoned if good procedural and pragmatic reasons make it advisable, often the desire to alter the framework of therapy results from the countertransference pull of the patient's reciprocal role procedures on the therapist. Consequently urges to alter the timetable need careful inspection by the therapist and the patient, and also need to be discussed in supervision to see if they are manifestations of the countertransference before action is taken.

While ending may have a variety of meanings for the patient, it also has meanings for the therapist and these need acknowledgement and review in supervision. The therapist may have regrets about bringing to an end a longstanding and intense emotional relationship. Therapists may experience failures of growth in their patients as challenges to their sense of therapeutic skill and prevent this by saying that they needed more time with the patient. Other endings are experienced as a relief, and there may be considerable guilt on the therapist's part over this.

Follow-up

All patients are offered a review session about three months after the end of therapy. In this session, therapist and patient can look back over the experience of therapy and take stock. The therapist will also need to consider whether further intervention may be needed. Broadly speaking, there are three outcomes. Some patients seem to have taken in the experience of therapy and used it constructively. There is evidence of change in their life, and they do not want or need further input. Other patients say they have derived nothing of tangible value from their therapy. If this is truly the case, there may be legitimate questions about the value of psychological interventions for some of these individuals. A third group show evidence of partial benefit in various areas but have other areas which have remained problematic. For this group further interventions of various sorts, including a repeat of CAT, may be indicated.

How does CAT differ from other therapies?

Any integrative therapy may be subject to criticism from the groups it is trying to integrate. Criticisms of CAT from various quarters, and the responses that CAT has made to them, have helped to mark CAT off from its 'neighbours'.

Many psychodynamically oriented therapists see CAT as a variant of cognitive behavioural therapy. However CAT has a strong focus on object relations, both internal and external, and on the experience in the therapy setting of the phenomena of transference and countertransference. Nevertheless, CAT principles also contrast significantly with many aspects of psychoanalytic therapy. For example, it views the analytic relationship as an imbalance in power which is likely to induce regressions which are not necessarily therapeutic. CAT therapists have also expressed concerns regarding the lack of integration of modern psychology, psychiatry and child development into psychoanalytic thought, as well as being unhappy with the focus on negativity which characterizes certain strands of psychoanalytic thought (Ryle, 1992, 1993, 1995a, 1995b). CAT is openly educative and the therapist freely shares insight and knowledge with the patient and, as such, CAT distinguishes itself from the more reserved neutral approach in psychoanalysis. In its developmental theorizing, CAT stresses the impact of the environment on the developing child, and views maladaptive and self-defeating procedures as immature attempts by the patient to cope with early environmental situations which, as a child, they perceived to be hostile or barren.

Some cognitive behavioural therapists criticize CAT because it is unduly psychodynamic in its approach. For them CAT, in common with other psychodynamic therapies, imports theoretical complications which are unjustified by the experimental evidence. The most cogent replies to these criticisms have been formulated by Marzillier and Butler (1995) and Young (1990), who argue that there are many points of similarity between cognitive analytic therapy and recent advances in cognitive behavioural therapy (CBT). In this respect, CAT resembles the growing rapprochement between cognitive psychology and psychoanalytic theory currently evident in the United States of America – for example Horowitz (1991), Luborsky et al. (1992) and Safran (1990a, 1990b). However, the contribution that the theory of object relations makes to CAT remains a distinctive feature that responds to criticisms of a cognitivist bias in American ego-psychology.

Which patient and why?

As with all therapies, there is at present little firm evidence linking differential efficacy to particular patient groups in CAT. However, the therapy has been used extensively in National Health Service (NHS) settings and has been tried on a great variety of patients. From this experience a body of practical wisdom has grown up. CAT has been found to be a useful intervention in a very wide range of cases (Ryle, 1990). Even where long-term therapy seems to be necessary, patients are able to use CAT effectively and derive considerable benefit from it.

A second group of patients who derive greater than expected benefit from CAT are those with severe personality disorders and particularly chaotic borderline personality disorders (Marlowe, 1994). These patients benefit from the structure and the limited nature of therapy. They also benefit from its particular capacity to understand their personality fragmentation, and to help them to understand what are often experienced as bewildering discontinuous changes in experience. CAT's beneficial effect with this group of patients is important because they are often considered inappropriate for long-term analytic therapy while cognitive behavioural techniques may fail to address the developmental and psychodynamic issues which are important in their psychopathology.

The brief focal nature of CAT also makes it an extremely useful first intervention in a wide variety of cases. It can be used in effect as a 'trial of therapy' where the outcome is instructive. Some patients may recover entirely and need no further treatment. However, others may show only partial responses and require further therapeutic interventions – either additional CAT or a more appropriate patient-specific alternative. The remaining group of patients disappointingly show no benefit at all from their CAT and an alternative treatment option needs serious consideration.

Which therapist and why?

Different therapists choose to practise different kinds of therapy. The best CAT therapists are those who find it a congenial way of working. Therapists from cognitive, psychoanalytic and humanistic backgrounds have all trained in CAT. Some therapists also try their hand at CAT and dislike it. Therapists from cognitive backgrounds may find the psychodynamic and object relations aspects of CAT vague or unnecessary. Therapists from a humanistic background may find the theoretical restrictiveness of CAT, and its tight theoretical boundaries and requirements, harsh and potentially lacking in heart. Psychodynamically oriented therapists may find CAT prescriptive, dogmatic and superficial in relation to the internal world. Although CAT has engaged with all these criticisms theoretically and practically, the important point here is that therapists who find CAT uncongenial are likely to practise it sub-optimally and should instead pursue an alternative therapy which is better suited to their personality, belief systems and clinical practice.

CAT is a relatively easy therapy to teach because it builds on existing therapy skills at any level. It provides the trainee with a very clear set of activities to undertake in therapy, which beginners experience as supportive and reassuring. Later, as therapists grow in skill and confidence, they can modify their more formal practice of CAT and apply it more flexibly. However, there are different levels of experience as a CAT therapist, and those with a deeper understanding of the underlying theoretical constructs are likely to be most successful clinically.

Therapeutic setting

CAT's requirements in terms of setting differ little from other individual therapies – a private constant location free from interruptions. In the context of service provision, CAT has found its greatest use in NHS settings. Here its special value derives from the time-limited nature of the therapy and its focus on those kinds of patients who are frequently found in NHS practice. These patients often arouse considerable anxieties in their carers and the containment provided by the physical setting and proximity to general psychiatric services is often vital in ensuring that therapy can be safely undertaken. The therapist needs to spend considerable amounts of time outside the therapy room thinking about the patient and preparing documents. During sessions the therapist is required to think actively whilst staying in touch at a feeling level too. For all these reasons therapists should not carry too many CAT cases at a time. They will also need appropriate practical and emotional support during this time, and supervision needs to be regular and intensive.

Problems in therapy

Patients with weak or ambivalent motivation present a serious challenge to all kinds of therapy. In so far as successful CAT presumes a working alliance with the patient, these individuals can cause significant problems to the therapist. However, CAT theory has engaged vigorously with the technical problems that these patients present. CAT stresses that even patients who appear to derive significant pleasure from spoiling and damaging therapy are able, if managed correctly, to alter their procedural repertoire and improve their motivation and capacity for engagement in therapy.

The structure and format of CAT make it particularly likely that certain maladaptive procedures will, if they are present, be aroused during therapy. Unless they are dealt with accurately they can intersect negatively with therapy. Both the intensity of CAT, and its focus on homework, make it likely to arouse transferences based on previous experiences of learning. Patients with maladaptive procedures in this area may find CAT a difficult therapy to engage in. CAT's response to these issues is to argue that work on maladaptive procedures for learning is very likely to be of vital importance to the patient's capacity to learn from experience in life. Consequently CAT therapists try to be vigilant for these issues, and to engage with them early as any problems which threaten therapy are a priority. However, these difficulties are dealt with in the same way that CAT deals with all maladaptive procedures – by joint description, elaboration and trials of change.

Further problems with CAT as a therapy arise from a variety of misconceptions about its nature on the part both of its supporters and its critics. Some supporters and critics of CAT see it as a prescriptive therapy. By this they mean that the therapist more or less baldly tells the patient what to do. In fact, prescriptive advice is not part of CAT. If the therapist gets drawn into telling the patient what to do then they lose the focus on joint elaboration and exploration of problems and solutions which CAT conceptualizes as vital to the process of learning.

Yet others see CAT as an eclectic therapy: this may be conceived of as an advantage or a drawback depending on the standpoint of the commentator. CAT however refuses the label of eclecticism in favour of a focus on integration. Eclecticism is seen as drawing from different approaches what ever seems useful on a pragmatic basis without necessarily being based upon a sharp theoretical rationale. In contrast, CAT achieves an integrated approach by being theoretically strict but practically permissive. It licences a wide range of techniques and interventions as long as these are locked on to a clear procedural understanding of the patient's difficulties and as long as the interventions foster joint working between patient and therapist.

Overenthusiasm for CAT is another problem which can bedevil CAT therapists. Those who are charged with containing the costs of providing psychotherapy services often seize on CAT because it seems an easy therapy for trainees and junior staff to undertake. CAT is in fact a taxing form of therapy. It requires considerable training to do well and also considerable motivation to continue to do it well. In general, CAT practitioners at all levels need supervision and support.

As with all psychotherapies, some patients will not benefit from CAT and, while CAT may be an effective intervention in many cases, it is definitely not 'the answer to everything'.

Evaluation of therapy

Compared to other psychotherapies, CAT is relatively well researched. Much of the available work is summarized by Ryle, who in his 1995 book cites many studies that demonstrate the efficacy of CAT in regard to a variety of clinical conditions and in different treatment settings. These include deliberate self-harm, survivors of childhood sexual abuse, patients in a forensic setting and patients with anorexia and bulimia nervosa. Recently interest among CAT researchers has centred on the efficacy of CAT in the case of borderline personality disorder. A number of descriptive studies relating to its value in this group of patients have documented a growing interest in the necessary theoretical and practical innovations required to treat such individuals.

Research in CAT has also concentrated on the growing need to provide a relatively brief and inexpensive, yet efficacious, form of psychotherapy within the public sector. The comparative study of CAT versus brief dynamic therapy by Brockman et al. (1987) is an example of this kind of work. While neither therapeutic modality showed a clear advantage over the other, both were effective in resolving patients' difficulties according to standard measures such as the Beck Depression Inventory (BDI). A large scale audit of CAT in a naturalistic setting has also been carried out (Denman, 1995), which shows its general efficacy in both optimal and less-than-optimal settings.

Glossary of terms specific to cognitive analytic therapy

Procedure/procedural sequence: A sequence of mental functions deployed in order to achieve a goal. Procedures involve the following elements: perception, appraisal, enactment, evaluation and confirmation or revision of the aim and/or of the means.

Reciprocal role procedure (RRP): A procedure which establishes and maintains a particular reciprocal role in relation to the self or to others. A reciprocal role relationship is the aim of a special kind of procedure called a reciprocal role procedure.

Reciprocal role relationship: A pair of social or interpersonal roles such as caregiver and care-receiver united by a dominant relationship theme. Reciprocal role relationships are learned as part of early development and then enacted by the deployment of procedural sequences for achieving them. Such sequences are called reciprocal role procedures.

Reformulation: This term refers both to a process and to a document. The process of reformulation refers to the joint activity of the therapist and patient in generating a new understanding of the patient's problems in terms of maladaptive procedural sequences. The reformulation document embodies those understandings in the form of a letter to the patient from the therapist which is then jointly agreed by the patient and the therapist and forms the basis for future work.

State: A relatively stable (or at least repetitively experienced) psychic configuration that incorporates a particular emotional tone, attitude to self and attitude to others. It is founded on a dominant reciprocal role procedure. Some abnormal personality organizations are characterized by a bewildering succession of discontinuous states which are often emotionally intense and interpersonally crude.

Sequential diagrammatic reformulation (SDR): A diagram which describes both the successive internal states experienced by a patient and the procedural sequences which modulate changes between those states. In patients who suffer from bewildering state changes the diagram provides a valuable device for the therapist (and patient) to understand these changes, as they occur in and out of sessions.

Target problems (TPs): The patient's target problems are those difficulties which the patient and therapist jointly identify as the main symptomatic elements of their life which therapy will aim at altering beneficially.

Target problem procedures (TPPs): These are those procedures which result in the target problems. Consequently, they are the procedures that will need to be altered in order to alter the target problems. Because the target problems are problems that do not go away, the procedures which generate them must be in some way faulty or inadequate.

Further reading

Ryle, A. (1990) *Cognitive Analytic Therapy: Active Participation in Change.* Chichester: John Wiley.
    This is the fundamental 'how to do it' book. It sets out the theory and practice of cognitive analytic therapy.

Ryle, A. (1995a) *Cognitive Analytic Therapy: Developments in Theory and Practice.* Chichester: John Wiley.
    This book takes up from where the 1990 text left off. In it, Ryle and his collaborators outline the major lines of thought that have since been developed in CAT.

Bibliography

Brockman, B., Poynton, A., Ryle, A. and Watson, J.P. (1987) Effectiveness of time-limited therapy carried out by trainees: comparison of two methods. *British Journal of Psychiatry*, **151**, 602–609.

Denman, C. (1995) Auditing CAT. In: A. Ryle (ed.), *Cognitive Analytic Therapy: Developments in Theory and Practice*. Chichester: John Wiley, pp. 165–174.

Horowitz, M.J. (1991) Person schemas. In: M.J. Horowitz (ed.), *Person Schemas and Maladaptive Interpersonal Patterns*. Chicago: Chicago University Press, pp. 13–32.

Leiman, M. (1995) Early development. In: A. Ryle (ed.), *Cognitive Analytic Therapy: Developments in Theory and Practice*. Chichester: John Wiley, pp. 103–120.

Luborsky, L., Barber, J.P. and Diguer, L. (1992) The meanings of narratives told during psychotherapy: the fruits of a new observational unit. *Psychotherapy Research*, **2**, 277–290.

Marlowe, M.J. (1994) Cognitive analytic therapy and borderline personality disorder: reciprocal role repertoires and sub-personality organisation. *International Journal of Short Term Psychotherapy*, **9**, 161–169.

Marzillier, J. and Butler, J. (1995) CAT in relation to cognitive therapy. In: A. Ryle (ed.), *Cognitive Analytic Therapy: Developments in Theory and Practice*, Chichester: John Wiley, pp. 121–138.

Ryle, A. (1990) *Cognitive Analytic Therapy: Active Participation in Change*. Chichester: John Wiley.

Ryle, A. (1992) Critique of a Kleinian case presentation. *British Journal of Medical Psychology*, **65**, 309–317.

Ryle, A. (1993) Addiction to the death instinct? A critical review of Joseph's paper 'Addiction to near death', *British Journal of Psychotherapy*, **10**, 88–92.

Ryle, A. (1994) Consciousness and psychotherapy. *British Journal of Medical Psychology*, **67**, 115–124.

Ryle, A. (1995a) *Cognitive Analytic Therapy: Developments in Theory and Practice*. Chichester: John Wiley.

Ryle, A. (1995b) Defensive organisations or collusive interpretations? A further critique of Kleinian theory and practice. *British Journal of Psychotherapy*, **12**, 60–69.

Safran, J.D. (1990a) Towards a refinement of cognitive behavioural therapy in the light of interpersonal theory: theory. *Clinical Psychology Review*, **10**, 87–105.

Safran, J.D. (1990b) Towards a refinement of cognitive behavioural therapy in the light of interpersonal theory: practice. *Clinical Psychology Review*, **10**, 107–121.

Young, J.E. (1990) *Cognitive Therapy for Personality Disorders: a Schema-Focused Approach*. Sarasota, FL: Professional Resource Exchange Inc.

11

Cognitive Behavioural Therapy

Phil Davison and Jennifer Stein

Historical perspective

In the late 1950s and early 1960s, Aaron T. Beck, a psychiatrist and psychoanalyst based in Philadelphia, noticed during the treatment of depressed patients that emotions were accompanied by a stream of thoughts of which patients were initially unaware (Beck, 1976; Beck *et al.*, 1979). The thoughts were gloomy and pessimistic, and Beck postulated that they made the original problem of low mood even worse. Patients seemed to enter a cycle of low mood, resulting in negative automatic thoughts, which then led to low mood and further negative automatic thoughts.

Similar observations had been made by Albert Ellis (1962), who went on to develop Rational Emotive Therapy (1984). Although developed independently of Ellis' method, Beck's analyses are similar to it in some ways. For example, Beck suggests that depressed people are likely to consider themselves totally inept and incompetent if they make a mistake. This can be considered an extension of one of Ellis' irrational beliefs, that the individual must be competent in all things in order to be a worthwhile person.

Whereas Ellis appeals to reason and deduction in addressing the irrationality of thoughts, Beck takes a more traditional scientific approach. He taught patients to recognize their negative automatic thoughts and then to evaluate on what evidence they had based these thoughts. He found that when depressed patients were able to change their negative automatic thoughts, a change in their feelings followed and their mood improved. Both Beck and Ellis tried directly to change cognitive processes in order to relieve psychological distress.

Behavioural experiments were then added to the therapy, based on the premise that learning is maximized through experience. However, unlike behaviour therapy, which tries to alter behaviour without necessarily understanding the underlying cognitions, cognitive therapy sets up experimental hypotheses about a patient's cognitions which are then 'tested out' in behavioural experiments. Cognitive behavioural therapy relies on the principle that our feelings and behaviour are determined by how we view the world. According to the Greek philosopher Epicvetus, 'men are disturbed not by things, but by the views they take of them'.

Since Beck's early work with depressive illness, cognitive therapy has been adapted to treat most mental health problems, including neurotic disorders, personality disorders and also psychotic disorders.

More recently Beck's work has been developed in its clinical application by Persons (1989) and by Padesky (1994). Jaqueline Persons has focused on the therapeutic relationship, as well as on techniques of cognitive therapy, and she provides a conceptual framework for understanding the patient as a human being, and not just as a cluster of symptoms. Padesky (1994) and Young (1987) have also extended theory and practice in the understanding of schemas, or core beliefs. Schemas were first introduced to cognitive therapy by Beck who credited Piaget with the origin of the word. Young proposed a primary emphasis on what he saw as the deepest level of cognition, the Early Maladaptive Schema, which often forms the core of an individual's self concept and conception of the environment.

Principles of theory and practice

Principles of theory

Cognitive therapy is based on a model which explains how thoughts and feelings relate to each other. The synchronous relationship between cognitions, behaviour and mood suggests that a change in any one component is likely to produce changes in the others. The notion that changes in cognition can produce changes in mood is central to Beck's model of cognitive therapy. The idea that behavioural changes can also produce changes in mood has been used by Beck but is central to the model developed by Levinsohn in 1973 (Persons, 1989). Treatment aimed specifically at changes in mood or emotional change is characteristic of psychodynamic approaches.

Beck and his followers emphasize the underlying cognitions or beliefs in an individual's overt difficulties. The patient and the therapist together describe a formulation of the overall problem which consists of an extensive problem list and possible underlying and precipitating factors. Cognitive therapy is therefore a treatment aimed at understanding primarily cognitive structures in an individual's problems, and devising intervention strategies aimed at changing, but initially challenging, underlying irrational beliefs.

Both the problem list and the case formulation help the therapist to guide the patient towards a suitable solution. The choice of treatment modality by the therapist relies heavily on a good understanding of the relationship between cognition, behaviour and mood in any individual. Through modelling by the therapist and the use of educational and challenging verbal techniques, aimed at helping the patient to think about his problem and make the various links between symptoms and vulnerability factors, cognitive therapy guides the patient to a greater understanding of his problems.

The model states that in the presence of emotional disturbance there will be:

- Negative automatic thoughts
- Patterns of regularly occurring errors
- Core beliefs and dysfunctional assumptions

Negative automatic thoughts

It is postulated that negative automatic thoughts amplify the prevailing affect and cause further negative automatic thoughts (Figure 11.1). In Beck's

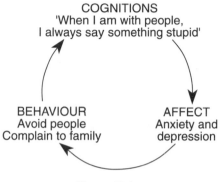

Figure 11.1

theory of depression, negative automatic thoughts are characterized by 'the cognitive triad'. There seemed to be three types of negative automatic thoughts that accompanied low mood: (i) negative views about oneself; (ii) negative views of the world; and (iii) negative views about the future.

Negative automatic thoughts	
A negative view of oneself:	'I know I am going to act stupid' 'I will fail' 'I am hopeless'
Negative automatic thoughts about the world:	'If there's someone whose going to have bad luck it will be me' 'Everything in my world is terrible' 'Things have a knack of going badly for me'
Negative automatic thoughts about the future:	'There's no point in trying, nothing will get better in the future' 'The future is hopeless' 'There is no point in going on'

A pattern of regularly occurring thinking errors

With time and practice, the patient and therapist come to recognize that negative automatic thoughts fall into patterns. These regularly occurring patterns are called thinking errors. Patients predominantly use two or three characteristic types of thinking errors. Common examples are:

- *Arbitrary inference* or jumping to conclusions: e.g. Because my boss did not come over and say hello at lunch the other day he must hate me and will therefore write me a bad reference.
- *Over-generalization*: e.g. Because I couldn't understand the first chapter in the book, I am therefore going to fail every part of the examination.
- *Dichotomous reasoning* or all-or-nothing/black-and-white thinking: e.g. As I'm not the best in the class, I must be useless.
- *Emotional reasoning* or using feelings as a basis for judgements and ignoring other factors: e.g. I feel it, so it must be true.
- *Personalization* or assuming of excessive responsibility: e.g. The children didn't enjoy the party – it must be my fault – I'm a bad mother.
- *Discounting the positive*: e.g. He's only saying that to be kind.
- *Shoulds*: e.g. I should be over this by now.
- *Global judgements (labelling)* or assuming that the value of a person can be equated with a single action: e.g. He's lost his job, he must be a total failure as a person.

Core beliefs and dysfunctional assumptions

Core beliefs are beliefs, which an individual holds to be 'the truth', about oneself, other people and the world. These core beliefs are also called schemas by some authors. For example: 'I am worthless', 'I am always wrong'. These core beliefs are formed from, and are understandable in terms of, the patient's life. Therefore, if a patient is continually physically abused

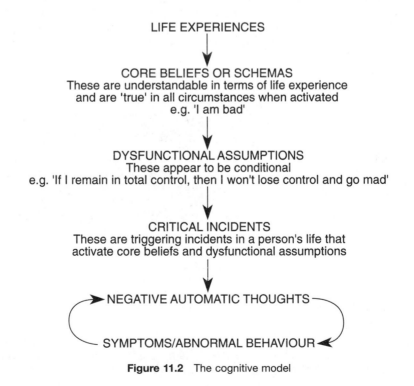

Figure 11.2   The cognitive model

throughout their childhood they may develop the core belief 'I must have deserved it, therefore I am bad'. If a patient did not receive love and affection as a child, they may develop the core belief 'I am unlovable'.

Dysfunctional assumptions differ from core beliefs in that they are dependent upon specific conditions, and often contain the words 'if' and 'then'. For example: 'if I remain in total control, then I won't lose control and go mad' or 'if I keep myself top of the class, then no one will notice that I am actually stupid'.

Core beliefs and dysfunctional assumptions influence thinking, mood and behaviour when triggered. They may be activated by a *'critical incident'* – when depressed, when rejected socially or when there is understandable and realistic fear. These beliefs and dysfunctional assumptioms appear to be almost permanently operative in individuals with personality disorders.

The three features of the cognitive model are shown diagrammatically in Figure 11.2.

The conceptualization or formulation

On the basis of the cognitive model a conceptualization or formulation is developed for each patient, and is a crucial aspect of cognitive therapy. It is a shared 'map' of a patient's problem (see Figure 11.3). The conceptualization or formulation is therefore a working hypothesis, generated by the patient and therapist, as to the cause of the patient's problem and the possible factors which maintain it. The formulation can be drawn out on paper, either by the therapist or the patient, in a way that the patient finds useful. This diagram or 'map' guides patient and therapist

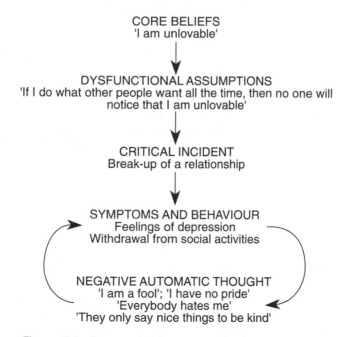

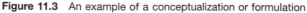

Figure 11.3 An example of a conceptualization or formulation

when they take the next steps towards resolving the patient's problem. To draw the map, information is obtained from the patient's history, the therapeutic relationship, a record of negative automatic thoughts (dysfunctional thought record), homework assignments, behavioural experiments and the cognitive model. It must be stressed that the conceptualization is only a current working hypothesis. It may be entirely correct or totally incorrect at first drawing, although this is highly unusual. It is more likely to represent only one aspect of a larger problem, or be only partially correct. In therapy all cognitive and behavioural interventions are based on this shared working hypothesis or conceptualization.

Persons' case formulation model emphasizes the underlying psychological mechanisms which are reflected in the overt difficulties. The interdependence of the cognitive, behavioural and mood aspects of problems is established through the therapist's and patient's efforts in arriving at a comprehensive problem list. The case formulation ties together all of the patient's problems and provides a hypothesis about the nature of the psychological difficulty underlying them. Persons also discusses cases where 'cognitive sense' does not make 'emotional sense' and how the therapeutic relationship can be used as a route to understanding.

Aims of therapy

• **Early decrease in symptoms**: An early aim is the relief of symptoms by challenging negative automatic thoughts as early success in the therapy builds confidence in the therapeutic techniques. These techniques can again be used if acute symptoms re-occur later in the therapy.

• **Exploration of vulnerability factors**: The second aim in therapy is to explore and solve factors in a patient's life that have made them vulnerable to developing mental health problems.

• **For patients to become their own cognitive therapist**: The final aim in therapy is for patients to become sufficiently skilled in cognitive therapeutic techniques to solve successfully problems that may arise in future without needing the therapist to be present.

Principles of practice

Structuring therapy

At the outset, patients discuss their aims for therapy. The appropriate aims are then recorded as realistic goals. These goals are regularly referred to as the therapy progresses, and can be changed at any time to meet changing therapeutic needs. In a similarly collaborative manner, an agenda is set at the start of each session which allows a structure for the session and makes effective use of the available time.

Introducing patients to the cognitive model

Patients will be introduced to the cognitive model at the first opportunity. The aim is for patients to understand that thoughts, feelings, behaviour and bodily sensation are linked, and that a change in one causes a change in the others (Figure 11.4). They are also shown how a change in the environment may cause a change in all of the above. However, it will be clarified at the earliest opportunity that the therapist will be focusing on thoughts and cognitions rather than on feelings, behaviour and bodily sensations.

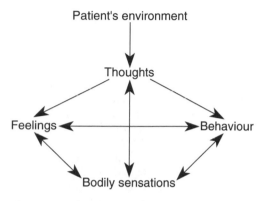

Figure 11.4   Interacting systems (modified from model developed by Padesky and Mooney, 1990)

A good way of educating patients about the model is to use an example that they bring up themselves early in the therapy. Another way may be to ask them how they felt whilst in the waiting room, and what was going through their mind, to demonstrate that anxiety, thoughts and bodily sensations are linked.

There is the danger that the therapist may adopt an over-didactic approach whilst trying to educate the patient about therapy. This should be avoided as the patient may not yet feel comfortable enough to question the therapist about aspects which they do not understand. As part of the educative process, written material about cognitive therapy and the methods it uses can be given to patients at regular intervals.

Therapist style

This should be warm, genuine and empathic. Decisions about therapy should be made collaboratively, based on the current conceptualization, which will have been shared with the patient at the earliest opportunity. The therapist is most likely to be sitting alongside the patient so that they can both study written material, such as the 'map' of the conceptualization when it has been drawn out. The therapist considers himself to be on the same team as the patient, and they jointly try to work out how they are going to solve the patient's problem. As part of the collaborative style, the therapist regularly summarizes the patient's account. This ensures that the therapist has understood the patient, and it gives the patient an experience of feeling understood. This deepens rapport. In addition, the summary provides a structure for understanding the patient's symptoms. It enables therapist and patient to focus down on the problem and to explore issues in a systematic way. The therapist uses a style of questioning called *guided discovery* which encourages the patients to try to find new perspectives for themselves.

Guided discovery

Guided discovery is a key feature of cognitive therapy. The therapist gives the patient as little direction as possible when asking questions. This encourages patients to question themselves about their problem, and come up with their own answers. The therapist's questions are open-ended, as opposed to closed-ended, so that answers of 'yes' or 'no' cannot be given. The questions usually start with the words 'what' or 'how'.

- 'What would be so bad about that if it were to occur as you suggest?'
- 'What would that say about you as a person?'
- 'What do you think other people will think of you?'
- 'How do you know they think that way?'
- 'What is your evidence, and how could we gather some more evidence?'

In addition, questions will be asked that translate vague and abstract difficulties into clearly defined problems that can be measured. For example, self confidence would be difficult to measure. If a patient was asked what it would mean to them if they were self confident, they may suggest that they could invite friends round for a drink, go to the shops alone and take up their old hobby of painting again. These aspects of behaviour could be readily measured by the patient and could therefore be incorporated into targets for therapy. In guided discovery, the therapist is also guided by the patient's answers both in his next question and formulation.

If a therapist and patient identify a negative automatic thought, guided discovery may occur in the following manner:

- What evidence have you got to support that thought?
- What makes you think your thoughts are true or valid?
- What is the evidence against your current thinking?
- Are there any other ways you could look at the situation?
- How might another person feel in the same position?
- How does thinking this way make you feel?
- Are there any advantages or disadvantages to feeling this way?
- What are your thinking errors?
- On the basis of the discussion above can you come to any conclusions that might be helpful?
- Can we draw up an action plan?

Diaries and record keeping

The patient is gradually taught the difference between thoughts and feelings, and taught how to recognize negative automatic thoughts which usually occur when there is change in emotion. A diary is kept of thoughts and feelings throughout the day in a 'dysfunctional thought record'. Keeping a dysfunctional thought record may be one part of the homework assignment allocated to the patient during a previous session or as part of the therapeutic programme. An example of a diary is given in Figure 11.5.

Date/Day/Time:	11 June, Monday, 0900
Stuation/Event:	Got up late again
Emotion:	Feeling down
Percentage score of emotion: (0–100%)	100%
Negative automatic thought:	'I am totally useless'
Belief in negative automatic thought: (0–100%)	95%

Figure 11.5 Example of a diary of thoughts and feelings

As therapy progresses, further columns are added and the patient learns to challenge their thoughts and substitute alternatives. They then re-rate their score for prevailing mood to see if challenging the cognitions has affected their mood (see Figure 11.6).

Date/Day/Time:	2 June, Friday, 0900
Situation? Event:	Late for work again
Emotion:	Feeling down
Percentage score of emotion: (0–100%)	95%
Negative automatic thought:	'I am totally useless'
Belief in negative automatic thought: (0–100%)	99%
Thinking error:	Over-generalization
Rational response:	First day late this week, an improvement
Belief in negative automatic thought following rational response: (0–100%)	45%
Percentage score of emotion following rational response: (0–100%)	Still feeling down, but only 50%
Effect on mood:	Positive, helpful

Figure 11.6 Example of a dysfunctional thought record

In normal clinical practice, the headings are arranged horizontally across the page to allow easy comparison of data, entered on separate occasions, within vertical columns.

Behavioural interventions

These are used frequently, both within the session and in homework assignments. The aim is to test out behaviourally predictions that are based on negative automatic thoughts, dysfunctional assumptions and core beliefs. They are also used to translate new ideas and perspectives into action in the real world, to examine the validity of the new ideas and consolidate change. For example:

- Vague thoughts are broken down into testable items, e.g. I will faint if I don't take regular and deep breaths during a panic attack.
- Patient is asked how much they believe this thought on a scale from 0 to 100%. This value is recorded, e.g. I believe 95% that I will faint in the following breathing experiment.
- Behavioural experiment takes place, proving to a patient that they do not faint when they breathe in a different and unusual manner for them in the session.
- A second percentage score is obtained for the original thought, 'I will faint', after the experiment, e.g. I believe 35% that I will faint if the experiment is repeated.

In many cases negative automatic thoughts are treated first and then, if appropriate, core beliefs are treated. This ensures that patients have already experienced some success in solving their problems and have confidence in the methods that are used, before potentially disturbing issues such as core beliefs are explored. Depending on the particular patient, treating core beliefs can require further sessions and involves an examination of problems in more detail.

Some patients may need the therapist to address their core beliefs at an earlier stage in the therapy. If this does not happen, it may lead patients to believe their therapist does not understand them.

Dysfunctional assumptions and core beliefs may be treated in the same manner as negative automatic thoughts, although assumptions and beliefs are now the subject of challenges as opposed to thoughts.

Schema-focused cognitive therapy

Jeffrey Young (1987) has developed the principles and practice of cognitive therapy to make it more useful in personality disordered and other difficult patients. He proposes an emphasis on the deepest level of cognition, the Early Maladaptive Schema (EMS). Beck et al. (1979) have referred to the importance of schemas but have offered few treatment guidelines. Young sees the EMS as a stable and enduring pattern of thinking that develops during childhood and is elaborated on throughout life. It consists of unconditional beliefs about oneself in relation to the environment which are experienced as a priori truths.

The EMS is resistant to change and individuals often engage in cognitive manoeuvres in order to maintain the schemas intact. Young (1987) reports that 'Once individuals acquire a system of expectancies they respond with increasing alertness to similar elements in their life situation ... The importance of expectancies, sensitivities and language habits lies in the fact that they tend to be distortions of objective realities.' The point is also made that EMS seem to be the result of dysfunctional experiences with parents and peers during the first few years of life.

Young has identified a number of EMSs which he sees as falling into four general areas of functioning: (a) autonomy, (b) connectedness, (c) worthiness and (d) limits and standards. Schema-focused therapy seems to uncover or elucidate this level of cognitive functioning and requires the therapist to be more intensely involved with the patient. This development in cognitive therapy has many similarities with dynamic theory and practice.

Safety behaviours

In spite of their name, 'safety behaviours' may intensify the patient's symptoms instead of actually keeping the patient safe. The patient comes to believe that they only just manage to save themselves from catastrophe by performing the safety behaviour, which in fact serves to perpetuate the cycle of ever-increasing anxiety and avoidance. These behaviours are also more likely to draw attention to the patient as they appear odd to other people. The patient should therefore have their need to keep these behaviours challenged.

Structure of the session

Each session will have a similar structure:
- Ask how the patient is feeling/review the week.
- Explore the reaction to the last session.
- The agenda is collaboratively set. Time is allocated depending on the perceived importance of agenda items.
- The agenda is worked through, this will include a review of homework set in the previous session.
- New homework is agreed.
- The session is summarized.
- Feedback on the session.
- The session ends.

Ending therapy

The end-point of therapy is not when the patient is symptom-free, but when they have learnt enough cognitive skills to cope with their current problem and also problems that could arise in future. Prior to ending therapy, time will be spent on 'relapse prevention' in which a contingency plan to manage future difficulties and setbacks is established.

A useful adjunct to ending treatment is a therapy blueprint. This usually consists of one A4 sheet of paper and summarizes what has been learned in therapy. It clarifies on paper what the patient can do if they feel close to relapse.

Therapy blueprint
  - I hold the belief:
  - It is understandable that I hold this belief because:
  - The belief is unreasonable because:
  - It is unhelpful because:
  - A more helpful belief would be:
  - Given that I have had this belief for a long time, it will take a long time to change it. What I need to do is:

Which patient and why?

Cognitive therapy is being successfully used to treat a wide variety of mental health problems.

Indications

Cognitive therapy was initially a treatment for depression. Following this, it was successfully used to treat anxiety, obsessional symptoms, phobic conditions and other types of neurotic disorders. More recently, cognitive therapy has been used to treat personality disorders and some features of schizophrenia such as auditory hallucinations and delusions. Cognitive therapy was initially meant to be a short-term therapy lasting, for example, up to sixteen sessions. More recently, longer treatment periods, of up to two years, have been used to treat personality disordered patients. Cognitive therapy may be used in conjunction with medication or ECT in severely depressed patients.

Assessment

Assessment should achieve a number of aims:
  - To obtain sufficiently detailed information about factors causing and maintaining the problem, and to start to design a treatment plan
  - To agree a formulation of the target problems and underlying factors with the patient
  - To start educating the patient from the outset about the cognitive model and, if possible, to provide some symptom relief in the first session using a cognitive technique
  - To start to build rapport and a therapeutic working relationship, where the patient feels safe to disclose important and often distressing information

The therapist must obtain details regarding the patient's thoughts, feelings and behaviour, as well as information about triggers that cause problems, factors that moderate and maintain the problem, and ways a patient has coped in the past. Whilst a full psychiatric history is often useful, it is not essential.

It is also important to explore the patient's understanding and willingness to work within a cognitive model and to enquire about their motivation to do the extensive homework that is required.

Self-monitoring may be a useful aspect of the assessment, and questionnaires, such as the Beck Depression Inventory and the Beck Anxiety Inventory, can be completed. These questionnaires provide useful measures of mood and anxiety. Alternatively, a diary can be maintained to monitor the patient's symptoms, feelings, thoughts and behaviours.

Behavioural tasks can be planned to obtain further information. For example, a patient with agoraphobia may be given, as homework, the task of recording their feelings and thoughts as they enter a crowded supermarket.

Contraindications

There are few absolute contraindications to cognitive therapy. Relative contraindications might be low motivation (because homework and behavioural experimentation are integral aspects of therapy) and an intellectual or emotional inability to understand the cognitive model. The use of drugs and alcohol would significantly impair the individual's ability to benefit from this treatment, especially if they arrive at the sessions intoxicated.

Which therapist and why?

Training

Rigorous training in cognitive therapy from established practitioners is considered essential and there are a number of approved training courses that now offer Diploma and Certificate courses. Unlike some other therapies, personal analysis is not considered essential. This is because interpersonal features such as transference and countertransference are not usually used as therapeutic vehicles.

Supervision

Supervision is essential when learning cognitive therapy. For trainees, a weekly supervision session is thought appropriate. Supervision is also considered essential for experienced therapists when working with difficult patients, for example when treating personality disordered patients where interpersonal issues may be important.

Supervision can take place either in groups or individually. In both form and content, the supervision is similar to cognitive therapy itself. Goals are agreed at the start of a period of supervision. A formulation is also collaboratively drawn up between supervisor and supervisee, which is a shared understanding of how goals can be achieved in the time available. At the start of every supervision session, an agenda is compiled to ensure efficient use of time and to ensure that key areas are focused on in the session. Cognitive techniques, such as Socratic questions, can be utilized within the supervision process. The supervisor may wish to review homework assignments or other behavioural experiments that were set during previous supervision sessions. Selected passages of therapy tapes can also be listened to and discussed.

The therapeutic setting

The majority of treatment takes place in a comfortable office located either in a clinic or hospital setting, or in a private residence. Most cognitive therapy takes place in a one-to-one setting although in certain conditions (e.g. agoraphobia), group cognitive therapy is used. In order to emphasize the collaborative nature of the treatment, the patient and therapist will sit in similar chairs either facing or at a slight angle to each other. The aim of the setting is to provide a working environment for the patient and therapist which helps in the development of rapport between them but also highlights the task to be undertaken. Sessions will normally be at agreed times, for the same duration on each occasion unless arranged differently by consensus.

Therapy sessions are often tape-recorded and the tape may be used by either the therapist or the patient to help them independently revise what happened in the session, or it may be used in a following session as a joint reminder of a particular part of a session. Consent for audio-recording is sought from the patient before therapy is begun. The patient will be given various questionnaires and forms on which they record their thoughts, feelings and beliefs between sessions. This 'homework' is looked at jointly in the following session.

The cognitive therapist will draw up an agenda for each session in collaboration with the patient. At the end of the session, this is reviewed and patients are encouraged to provide feedback on the session. It has been found that the development of empathy and rapport is facilitated by these techniques.

A cognitive therapist will influence the setting of the therapy by his manner, which aims to be confident and professional, but also relaxed. The therapist is sometimes directive and imposes structure, especially at the beginning of treatment, and this is more readily accepted by the patient if the therapist maintains professionalism.

In some cases, experimentation will become part of a session and may involve behavioural challenges and exposure to feared stimuli. It is often possible to conduct the experiments in the therapy room; however it may be necessary to take a patient to other settings. More often a patient will be given behavioural tasks between therapy sessions, and will be asked to report on them.

A cognitive therapist usually does not concern himself with 'transference' and will often be more revealing of himself. This may show itself in the setting by the use of an office that contains evidence of the therapist's personal (e.g. photographs) or professional (e.g. notes, textbooks) life. Therapists will vary in this regard, but at all times the professional nature of the relationship is held in mind, even though the therapy is collaborative in nature.

Clinical example

A 35-year-old divorced woman presented with symptoms of anxiety. The critical incident was her sister's imminent emigration to Australia. The patient had previously been sexually and physically abused as a child, and had also suffered a depressive illness ten years earlier. This episode was successfully treated with anti-depressant medication. At assessment, a clinical diagnosis of depressive disorder with associated symptoms of anxiety and panic was made. She also fulfilled DSM-IV diagnostic criteria for a panic disorder with agoraphobic avoidance.

At the start of therapy her scores on pre-therapy questionnaires were:

Beck Anxiety Inventory	Beck Depression Inventory
48	35

These scores confirmed that she had moderately severe depressive symptoms, with associated anxiety.

Sessions 1–8 *consisted of socializing her to the model, teaching her how to recognize negative automatic thoughts and behaviourally challenging some of her thoughts. For example: 'If I don't rush out of the concert when one of these panics comes on, I will go mad and end up screaming'; 'everyone can see that I am panicking and is staring at me going red and sweating'; 'I must hold my programme close to my chest at a precise angle to control my tendency of over-breathing, otherwise I will lose control and scream'. Holding her programme in such a bizarre manner is a good example of a safety behaviour (see Figure 11.7).*

The experiments set up were to count how many people were staring at her in the concert hall in a defined time, initially when using safety behaviours and then without.

Number of people that stared when using safety behaviours	Number of people that stared when safety behaviour dropped
4	0

This experiment proved to her that people were not paying attention to her, either with or without safety behaviours. If they were paying attention to her, it was more likely to happen when she was using her safety behaviours.

We also agreed that she would stay in the concert 'come what may', and rated her maladaptive belief before entering the concert hall. Afterwards, we asked her to rate her belief should she re-enter the concert hall.

Belief that I will scream if I force myself to stay in the concert	Belief that I will scream on next occasion I keep myself in the concert
95%	10%

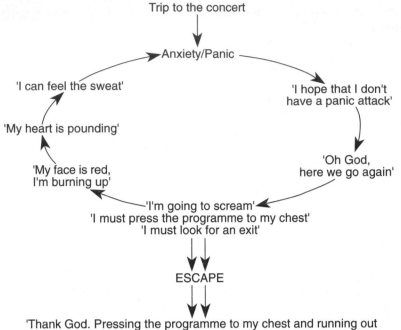

Figure 11.7

Sessions 8–16: *After initial symptom relief, much of the later sessions concentrated on her early life experiences and core beliefs. One of her beliefs was 'I am bad'. This belief was tackled in a number of ways: first, she was greatly helped by a conceptualization which helped her understand that early life problems were not her fault. Secondly, she developed an ability to rapidly recognize when the belief 'I am bad' entered her mind and she then immediately started challenging the belief in the ways which she had learned in the therapy. Thirdly, she carefully defined behaviour that she would consider as 'good', and then kept a diary of these occasions (sometimes called a positive data log). By doing this, she could reflect on, and have something concrete to remind her, that she was 'good' when she was feeling low. Fourthly, we noticed during therapy that she had a tendency to think in black-and-white terms and thought that she was either all bad or all good. She suffered corresponding feelings of intense happiness or extreme depression. Within the therapy, she learnt how to place her feelings of depression on a continuum scale, which ranged from 0 to 100%. She carried the simple scale around with her, so that she could score her mood at any time.*

Depression continuum scale		
0%	50%	100%
I feel OK	Feelings equivalent to being lonely and having no one to talk to	Feelings equivalent to what I would experience if my father died

At the outset she specified what level of feelings should be present to obtain any particular score. For example, if her father died she imagined she would feel depressed 100%. When feelings of depression arose, she marked the scale with a cross to score her level of depression at that time. This simple experiment helped her realize that she did not often feel 100% depressed, as she had initially thought. Finally, during the relapse prevention stage of therapy, we identified behavioural tactics that she could re-introduce when she felt depressed in the future, such as forcing herself to go for a swim, or for a run.

By the end of therapy, she had a greater understanding of her problems and had started to address them in cognitive therapeutic terms. In addition, her symptoms of depression, panic and agoraphobia had largely abated. Although it will take her many years until the belief 'I am bad' stops entering her mind, she left therapy having learned the principles of cognitive therapy which will allow her to help herself in future when these thoughts occur.

At the termination of her therapy, the patient's post-therapy questionnaires scored as follows:

Beck Anxiety Inventory	Beck Depression Inventory
12	7

The patient's therapy blueprint read as follows:

- **I hold the belief:** *that I am bad.*
- **It is understandable that I hold this belief because:** *for no good reason I was physically abused as a child.*
- **The belief is unreasonable because:** *there is no evidence to support it.*
- **It is unhelpful because:** *for no logical reason I feel I am hurting people and it makes me feel depressed.*
- **A more helpful belief would be:** *I am just as good as anybody else.*
- **Given that I have had this belief for a long time, it will take a long time to change it. What I need to do is:**
  - *keep doing my positive data log*
  - *keep my relapse prevention plan accessible and refer to it when I experience any symptoms which indicate an early stage of relapse*
  - *be especially careful when entering vulnerable situations*
  - *monitor myself for negative automatic thoughts, core beliefs and symptoms of anxiety*
  - *and commence challenging negative automatic thoughts or core beliefs immediately*

Problems in therapy

Pitfalls

- Dynamically trained therapists offering interpretations, as opposed to using guided discovery and other cognitive therapy techniques.
- Evidence for the negative automatic thought may not be successfully challenged. As a result, there is no change in emotions when negative automatic thoughts are confronted.

- The therapists may become absorbed into the patient's distress. Being unable to see the problem objectively enough to help challenge the evidence, the situation may then begin to seem hopeless to the therapist as well.
- Important interpersonal issues may be overlooked, especially when working with difficult patients.
- Over-intellectualization may be used as a method of avoiding change in some patients. Caution may need to be exercised as cognitive therapy lends itself to this avoidant approach.

Mistakes

Mistakes by the therapist may be turned to the patient's advantage because of the nature of the therapeutic relationship. When a mistake is made, an apology can be offered by the therapist and the mistake shared with the patient. This is a powerful modelling experience for many patients who often set unrealistically high standards for themselves. Mistakes show that the therapist is human and that it is human to make mistakes.

Misconceptions

- Cognitive therapy does not take into account early childhood experiences.
- The therapeutic relationship is unimportant.
- Cognitive therapy only treats symptoms and not the cause of symptoms.
- Cognitive therapy requires only a limited training by the therapist.

Evaluation of therapy

Cognitive and developmental therapies have claimed a sound scientific basis for their method (Gelder, 1997). This has been based on a tradition of attention to accepted scientific method and modern theory. However, it has been pointed out that evaluation, particularly when it is based on the findings of experimental psychological studies, may not be readily generalizable to clinical work. Beck bypassed this problem by basing the premises of his theory and clinical practice on the use of measures of thoughts, feelings and behaviours. In this way, he integrated scientific evaluation with clinical method.

Cognitive behaviour therapy has been evaluated in the following psychiatric illnesses using controlled trials. (These studies are all described in detail by Clark and Fairburn, 1997.)

- Depression (Beck, 1964)
- Anxiety (Beck, 1976)
- Personality disorder (Beck, 1990)
- Panic disorder (Clark, 1984)
- Hypochondriasis (Salkovskis and Clark, 1993)
- Eating disorders (Fairburn, 1981)
- Obsessive–compulsive disorder (Salkovskis, 1985)
- Chronic fatigue (Sharpe et al., 1996)
- Post-traumatic stress disorder (Foa et al., 1989)

Since cognitive interventions are often aimed at underlying beliefs and attitudes, it is possible to evaluate the impact these may have on treatment effectiveness. Various aspects of cognition have been addressed in the studies described above, including:

- Thinking
- Attention
- Memory
- Visual imagery
- Worry
- Meta-cognition

Experimental methods have been generated from clinical observations of the above and provide feedback into clinical techniques. In this way, the evaluation provides an audit loop which is relatively easy to demonstrate and which can be used to modify practice. Studies can both identify cognitive abnormalities in psychiatric disorder and suggest ways of changing them. The role of safety behaviours, in social phobia for example, has been shown to maintain fearful cognitions and, similarly, the suppression of distressing intrusive thoughts may help maintain post-traumatic stress disorder.

In addition to the routine incorporations of evaluative methods into the treatment model of CBT, specific research areas have been developed from the practice of cognitive therapy. These include the schema work of Young and the studies on the inter-relationship between cognition and emotion by Teasdale (Clark and Fairburn, 1997). The latter work has looked at the state-dependent effects of mood on cognition and memory. This has led to a greater refinement and sophistication of the ideas underpinning cognitive therapy. The work of both Young and Teasdale has begun to integrate cognitive and psychodymanic theory and practice.

The comparative effectiveness of cognitive behaviour therapy and pharmacological drug treatment of psychiatric illness has had only limited evaluation. Studies of depression, social phobia and panic disorder seem to suggest that CBT and pharmacotherapeutic treatments have equal effectiveness and, in some cases, may enhance each other. CBT has been shown to reduce relapse as compared to drug treatment alone.

Clark and Fairburn (1997) consider that the resistance of policy-makers to allow research findings on the effectiveness of CBT to influence service provision is linked to accessibility. CBT often requires the services of highly skilled therapists. Studies have shown that treatment outcome is linked to the therapist's competency, and that the delivery of psychological therapies, such as CBT, requires sophisticated skills. Many mental health providers are not at present investing in the provision of sufficient numbers of well-trained therapists.

Cognitive behaviour therapy lends itself more easily to manualized treatments than does dynamic therapy, and there is some evidence to show that briefer, more structured interventions, which are more easily taught and require less experience and skill, may be effective with certain patients if delivered early enough. Such interventions would be very cost-effective.

Although cognitive behaviour therapy is usually a relatively short treatment, and therefore cheaper to provide, the work described by Young and Teasdale often requires treatment of longer duration with expert therapists. This type of work is likely to be required for more seriously compromised patients or for those with more chronic and intractable problems which are often linked to personality disorder.

Key principles of cognitive therapy

- Cognitive therapy is based on a model which shapes a conceptualization for each patient in regard to their problem.
- The problem is formulated in terms of negative automatic thoughts, dysfunctional assumptions and core beliefs.
- Therapists are encouraged to be warm, genuine and empathic.
- Patient and therapist share a collaborative, non-hierarchical journey of guided discovery.
- Questions are based on the premise that patients adopt new perspectives more readily if they can come to their own conclusions (Socratic questions).
- The therapist is a guide, not an expert.
- All interventions are made explicit by the therapist.
- The therapist ensures that the patient understands by regularly asking for feedback.
- Therapist guides the patient to examine evidence that contradicts negative automatic thoughts, or dysfunctional beliefs.
- The therapist guides the patient to gather new information by testing hypotheses.
- Behavioural interventions are used to test out hypotheses.
- Diaries and other homework assignments may be used to monitor progress.
- The patient leaves therapy with a range of cognitive and behavioural skills for coping with problems and for preventing a relapse in the future.

Further reading

Beck, A.T. (1976) *Cognitive Therapy and the Emotional Disorders*. New York: International Universities Press.
Beck, A.T., Rush, A.J., Shaw, B.F. and Emery, G. (1979) *Cognitive Therapy of Depression*. New York: Guilford Press.
Hawton, K., Salkovskis, P.M., Kirk, J. and Clark, D.M. (1989) *Cognitive Behaviour Therapy for Psychiatric Problems: a Practical Guide*. Oxford: Oxford Medical Publications.
Padesky, C.A. and Mooney, K.A. (1990) Presenting the cognitive model to clients. *International Cognitive Therapy Newsletter* (Center for Cognitive Therapy, Newport Beach), **6**, 13–14.

Bibliography

Beck, A.T. (1976) *Cognitive Therapy and the Emotional Disorders*. New York: International Universities Press.
Beck, A.T., Rush, A.J., Shaw, B.F. and Emery, G. (1979) *Cognitive Therapy of Depression*. New York: Guilford Press.
Burns, D.D. (1988) *The Feeling Good Handbook*. New York: Morrow.
Butler, G. (1989) Issues in the application of cognitive and behavioural strategies for the treatment of social phobia. *Clinical Psychology Review*, **9**, 91–106.
Butler, G., Fennell, M., Robson, P. and Gelder, M. (1991) A comparison of behaviour therapy and cognitive behaviour therapy in the treatment of generalised anxiety disorder. *Journal of Consulting and Clinical Psychology*, **59**, 167–175.
Chadwick, P.D.J. and Lowe, C.F. (1994) A cognitive approach to measuring and modifying delusions. *Behaviour Research and Therapy*, **32**, 355–367.
Clark, D.M. and Ehlers, A. (1993) An overview of the cognitive theory and treatment of panic disorder. *Applied and Preventive Psychology*, **2**, 131–139.
Clark, D.M. and Fairburn, C.G. (eds) (1997) *Science and Practice of Cognitive Behaviour Therapy*. Oxford: Oxford University Press.
Ellis, A. (1962) *Reason and Emotion in Psychotherapy*. New York: Lyle Stuart.
Ellis, A. (1984) Rational Emotive Therapy. In: R.J. Corsini (ed.), *Current Psychotherapies*, 3rd edn. Itasca, IL: Peacock Press.
Gelder, M.G. (1997) The scientific foundations of cognitive behaviour therapy. In: D.M. Clark and C.G. Fairbairn (eds), *Science and Practice of Cognitive Behaviour Therapy*. Oxford: Oxford University Press, pp. 27–46.
Greenberger, D. and Padesky, C.A. (1995) *Mind Over Mood: a Cognitive Therapy Treatment Manual for Clients*. London: Guilford Press.
Miller, W.R. and Rollnick, S. (1991) *Motivational Interviewing*. New York: Guilford.
Padesky, C. (1994) Schema change processes in cognitive therapy. *Clinical Psychology and Psychotherapy*, **1**, 267–278.
Padesky, C.A. and Mooney, K.A. (1990) Presenting the cognitive model to clients. *International Cognitive Therapy Newsletter* (Center for Cognitive Therapy, Newport Beach), **6**, 13–14.
Persons, J.B. (1989) *Cognitive Therapy in Practice: a Case Formulation Approach*. New York: Norton and Co.
Safran, J.D. and Segal, Z.V. (1990) *Interpersonal Process in Cognitive Therapy*. New York: Basic Books.
Salkovskis, P. (1991) The importance of behaviour in the maintenance of anxiety and panic: a cognitive account. *Behavioural Psychotherapy*, **19**, 6–19.
Young, J.E. (1987) Schema-Focused Cognitive Therapy for Personality Disorders and Difficult Patients. Unpublished Manuscript, Cognitive Center of New York, 111W 88 St, New York, NY 10024.
Young, J.E. and Klosko, J.S. (1993) *Reinventing Your Life*. New York: Plume Books.

12

Child Psychotherapy

Gerry Byrne

Historical perspective

Child psychotherapy is a twentieth-century phenomenon. It was conceived through the combination of European concepts of the child and the theory and practice of psychoanalysis. Child psychotherapy is concerned with the psychodynamic assessment and psychotherapeutic treatment of emotional disturbance in children and adolescents. In earlier centuries infanticide went largely unpunished, child labour was widespread and infant mortality was very high. It was not until the end of the nineteenth century that the Society for the Prevention of Cruelty to Children was established in London (de Mause, 1974; Radbill, 1987) and there was a move towards a more empathic response to children. In the years after the First World War, both in the fields of medicine and education, there was considerable concern expressed about the welfare of infants, children and their mothers. Medicine began to concentrate more on the early detection and prevention of illness.

Margaret Lowenfeld, a doctor and later a child psychiatrist, worked for a time at the battlefront of the Russo-Polish war and later became passionately interested in working with children. In the 1920s she conducted research on rheumatic children, maternal lactation and infant feeding. Her observations of children within a research context and her experiences with refugee children in the war led her to establish the Clinic for Nervous and Difficult Children in 1928 (Urwin and Hood-Williams, 1988). Lowenfeld developed a particular approach to working therapeutically with children which aimed to enable children to express their ideas and fantasies through play, and to facilitate insight into their own personalities, difficulties or conflicts.

Education underwent radical reforms, emphasizing the importance of fostering emotional as well as intellectual growth. Many of the developments in education drew on psychoanalytic theories. By 1927, the first Child Guidance Clinic was operating and the National Child Guidance Council had been established with psychoanalytic ideas informing the approach adopted by the clinics.

Principles of theory and practice

Theoretical principles

Child psychotherapy is the application of psychoanalytic understanding to the treatment of children with problems of emotional development. As such, it draws on the analytic theories which concentrate significantly on childhood experience; notably those of Sigmund Freud, Anna Freud, Melanie Klein, John Bowlby, Donald Winnicott, Wilfred Bion, Selma Fraiberg and Daniel Stern.

Sigmund Freud

Freud based his contributions to the study of normal child development and developmental psychopathology on three key areas of observation: (a) his work with the psychopathology of adult patients; (b) his observations of his own children and grandchildren, and reports from friends on observations of their own children; and (c) his self-analysis. Child psychotherapy trainings, historically and currently, have these three key areas of investigation at their core.

It is generally accepted that the origins of child psychotherapy lie in Freud's (1909) account of the psychoanalytic treatment of Little Hans. Freud did not analyse Little Hans directly but treated him through the agency of the boy's father. Under Freud's direction, Hans' father encouraged his son to talk about his fantasies and dreams. With Freud's help, he gained an understanding of Hans' conflicts and conveyed this to Hans who appeared to respond by relinquishing his symptoms. Freud discovered what he considered to be a critical stage in early development, the Oedipus complex, in which the child aged three to five desires the parent of the opposite sex and becomes a rival of the parent of the same sex whom he hates but also loves. Thus the child experiences guilt, and fears punishment. Freud believed that the resolution of this dilemma was essential for healthy emotional development. Failure to resolve this early conflict would result in an 'infantile neurosis'. Although repressed in childhood, the infantile neurosis would reappear later in the adult's neurotic symptoms.

Anna Freud

Anna Freud, adhering faithfully to her father's theories, held that neurotic conflicts in children arose from their failure to resolve the Oedipus complex. It was the task of the analyst to help the child resolve these conflicts. Like her father, Anna Freud viewed the normal development of children as progressing through sequential stages identified as oral, anal and genital. Difficulties could arise for the child at any of these stages, and the child might pathologically defend against the attendant anxieties and respond by becoming stuck in that stage or by retreating to a former stage.

Melanie Klein

Melanie Klein started with the observation of a normal child and, with Karl Abraham's encouragement, began analysing very young children in 1919. She developed her 'play technique', in which she provided toys and play materials and treated the child's play as the equivalent of free association in an adult analysis. Play was seen as a symbolic expression of the child's unconscious conflicts (Klein, 1955). Klein discovered, through her analysis of a two-year-old girl, that even very young children develop a transference to the therapist (Klein, 1932). She placed great emphasis on the emotional development of infants in the first year of life, and how the infant's earliest relationship with his mother (an 'object relation') centred on the breast. Klein analysed children and adults in much the same way, seeking to interpret their deepest anxieties and speaking to the child in a direct way using the child's own special words for parts of the body and bodily functions.

Melanie Klein suggested that the neonate is born with both an unconscious awareness of the 'good breast', and with persecutory anxiety which is aroused by the process of birth. The infant splits his feelings and experiences into good and bad, and feels that he relates to two mothers, a good breast/mother who reassures and feeds him, and a bad breast/mother who persecutes him. The infant's bad, aggressive and destructive feelings are projected out into the 'bad breast' and experienced as persecutory for the infant perceives such feelings not as originating in him but as coming in from outside. Similarly, the infant's loving impulses are projected outwards and attributed to the 'good breast'. By introjection, a good and bad breast are established in the internal world of the infant as 'internal objects'. Klein described this way of relating as the 'paranoid–schizoid position', prevalent up to 3 or 4 months of age. Gradually the infant realizes that the mother who frustrates him and whom he hates is the same mother who comforts him and whom he loves. This realization creates feelings of guilt and 'depressive concern' for his loved object which are described by Klein as the 'depressive position', occurring typically at the age of three to six months.

Melanie Klein's theories of child development, pathology and child analysis are rooted in classical Freudian theory and she viewed them as faithful extensions of the same. However, Klein's and Anna Freud's respective theories evolved along divergent lines, resulting in important differences of technique and emphasis. For example, Anna Freud believed that a preparatory phase was necessary for the child before commencing analysis to build a positive and trusting relationship between therapist and child. Anna Freud also attached less importance to the role of transference in child analysis, feeling that the negative transference would actually be unhelpful. In contrast with Melanie Klein, Anna Freud believed that the psychoanalyst was not just the receptacle for the child's projections but also existed as a real person for the child and even had an educational role with the child. These differences led to a period of extended and sometimes bitter conflict between those psychoanalysts who favoured the Kleinian school and those favouring the Freudian. A series of meetings termed the 'Controversial Discusssions' (1941–4) in the British Psycho-Analytical Society were held after Freud's death in which these differences were aired.

John Bowlby and attachment theory

John Bowlby, who was a qualified psychoanalyst at the time of the Controversial Discussions, felt that psychoanalysis neglected the role of the child's environment. He believed that it was essential for psychoanalysts to focus not only on the internal phantasy of the child but also on the nature of the mother–child relationship. Bowlby, who was trained in developmental psychology and psychiatry in addition to psychoanalysis, also felt that psychoanalysis overlooked the importance of accurate scientific observation (Daws, 1987). Bowlby studied juvenile delinquents and noted that some of these children had suffered maternal deprivation and separations. He linked these experiences to some of the boy's affectionless characters (Bowlby, 1944). Bowlby became interested principally in the impact of the mother's inadequacies and absences on the development of the child's self. He stressed the vital importance of a secure base for the child's healthy emotional development (Bowlby, 1991). His work with James Robertson, filming children separated from their mothers in hospital, demonstrated the profound impact of separation on infants and young children, and explored the grief process manifested by children enduring such losses (Bowlby et al., 1952; Bowlby and Robertson, 1952a, 1952b). It had considerable impact in changing paediatric practice.

Mary Ainsworth, a psychologist, joined Bowlby at the Tavistock Clinic in London where she admired the naturalistic observations of Robertson and was fascinated by the children's patterns of responses to separation from their parents. Ainsworth studied the process of infant–mother attachment and observed a relationship between infant security, maternal sensitivity and the amount of holding the infant received from his mother. This supported Bowlby's emphasis on the importance of a secure base. Ainsworth developed the 'Strange Situation' to study the interplay between attachment behaviour and exploratory behaviour (Ainsworth et al., 1978). She initially described three major patterns of attachment behaviour: secure (B), insecure–avoidant (A) and insecure–resistant (C). Mary Main and Ruth Solomon (1988) later added a fourth category, anxious disorganized (D). The Strange Situation has been statistically validated and has been used in studies involving normal and maltreated samples of children.

Donald Winnicott

Winnicott, a paediatrician and a psychoanalyst, was able to combine both disciplines in a way that added a new dimension to child analysis. He believed that, for psychoanalytic purposes, infant and mother should be regarded not as individuals but as a 'nursing couple'. Winnicott did not see the infant as 'object-related' from birth, but as undifferentiated from his mother and therefore unable to perceive himself and his mother as separate objects until a later stage. He emphasized the importance of the 'facilitating environment' and the process of maturation within the child himself. He saw 'holding' as both a physical and emotional process by which the 'good-enough mother' facilitates healthy development in her infant. He described the state of mind of the mother engrossed in the care of her infant as one of 'primary maternal preoccupation'.

In the matter of technique, Winnicott had a remarkable intuition and capacity to empathize with the child. He was imaginative and innovative in his approach to the analysis of children, one example being his invention of the 'squiggle' game. In this, he would draw a squiggle on a sheet of paper and invite the child to complete the picture. The child would also be encouraged to make the initial squiggle and Winnicott would intuitively respond to the unconscious communication and comment on the possible meanings of the drawings. Winnicott did not establish his own school of thought or training yet there are psychotherapists who would describe themselves as 'Winnicottian' in orientation.

Selma Fraiberg

Selma Fraiberg, an American child psychoanalyst, made significant contributions both to developmental theory and clinical practice. Fraiberg described pathological defences in infants between three and eighteen months of age who experienced extreme danger in their environment, including deprivation. Fraiberg saw these defensive patterns, which include avoidance, freezing, fighting, transformation of affect and the turning of aggression against the self, as based on the biological 'fight–flight' response. They have as their aim the removal of pain from consciousness. Fraiberg emphasized the importance of the child's environment, and developed a model of parent–infant psychotherapy which aimed to free the infant from parental neurosis. Fraiberg wrote eloquently of this in her seminal paper, 'Ghosts in the Nursery' (Fraiberg et al., 1975), in which she described the influence of the parents' past experiences of parenting on their capacity to parent their own children appropriately.

Daniel Stern

There has been a wealth of research in child development in the past thirty years, and a number of writers have attempted to link developmental and psychoanalytic theories. Daniel Stern, a developmental psychologist and psychoanalyst, has attempted to bring together the infant as 'observed' by developmental research and the infant as 'reconstructed' in psychoanalysis. In describing the emergence of the infant's sense of self, Stern has enriched our understanding of infant experience and how the infant relates to others.

In his review of parent–infant psychotherapies, Stern speaks of 'the motherhood constellation', a term referring to the unique psychic organization into which the mother enters with the birth of her baby (Stern, 1995). These insights influence the way in which child psychotherapists work therapeutically. Stern urges clinicians working with mothers and infants to adopt a therapeutic alliance and treatment plan based on the mother–infant dyad.

Aims of therapy

Psychoanalysis originated in Sigmund Freud's attempts to relieve his adult patients of their neurotic symptoms. He realized that many symptoms had roots in the patient's infancy and childhood, and that some symptoms indicated a block in the normal developmental process. Some symptoms would be resistant to change unless the patient was helped to reach certain emotional milestones, such as the resolution of the oedipal conflict. Melanie Klein was, early on, very enthusiastic about the potential widespread provision of child analysis to promote healthy emotional development in children. Many child psychotherapists today would still hold that the primary aim of child psychotherapy is the promotion of emotional growth and the relief of mental suffering. If this is carried out judiciously and appropriately, later problems, such as disturbance in adulthood, can potentially be avoided. Almost invariably, it will be accompanied by symptom relief and (usually desirable) behaviour change.

These changes are brought about by the gradual introjection and internalization of a capacity for thought. This is based on the child's experiences of the therapist as able to contain their feelings and anxieties, and later to interpret them. The sense of self is strengthened and changes occur in the child's internal world. Improved relationships to people in the external world follow improvements in internal object relationships. A common aim to all approaches is to increase self-esteem in the child.

However, child psychotherapists often do not have the opportunity to see children in long-term intensive psychotherapy. Those practising within the National Health Service (NHS) will be under pressure to provide short-term therapies with more specific aims. These treatments may have as their primary aim symptom relief or behaviour change. For instance, therapy may aim to bring about improvements in the child's social competence and his capacity for intimacy.

Principles of practice

Child psychotherapists of all orientations are trained in theories of child development and developmental psychopathology. They take into consideration the changes which individuals, families and communities undergo over time. Child psychotherapy also recognizes that the child's development is determined at several levels; from the genetic and constitutional, through physical and psychological influences, to influences emanating from the family, neighbourhood and cultural spheres of life. Therefore childhood symptomatology and disorders are more likely to be perceived as developmental deviations than as childhood illnesses.

Psychoanalytic and developmental thinkers such as Anna Freud and Sroufe (1996) have described how dissimilar disturbed pathways in children can arrive at similar destinations in terms of psychopathology and, conversely, how similar pathways can have quite dissimilar destinations. 'The developmental outcome is determined not by the environmental interference per se, but by its interaction with the inborn and acquired resources of the child' (A. Freud, 1926–7). In other words, it is not the environmental experience by itself which determines the impact upon the child, but the internal response to it and how it is interpreted by the child. Psychological illness is both the product of and an indicator of significant failure by the individual psyche to deal adequately with internal conflict (Reeves, 1977).

Child psychotherapy is not strictly concerned with the external functioning of the child, such as practical, familial and social behaviours. However, this is not to say that it discounts familial and social factors as significant contributory causes or even as the main cause of the child's difficulties. Instead, because it gives priority to the presence and influence of the unconscious in the child's conflicts, child psychotherapy places the internal world of the child at the heart of treatment.

There are several core principles common to all schools and approaches to child psychotherapy:
- The importance of play as a means of communication
- The concept of containment of anxieties
- The transference relationship between the patient and the therapist
- The use of interpretation to promote insight into the patient's inner world
- The constancy of the setting of the therapy

The importance of play as a means of communication

Sigmund Freud observed a small child at play with a cotton reel, reeling it in and reeling it out again. He understood this to be symbolic of the repeated but temporary loss of his mother, which the small child was attempting to master through play. In this observation he affirmed play as a very serious business indeed. Melanie Klein developed her play technique and provided toys for the child in therapy not 'to reassure the child or to give him a joyous time, or to provide a creative or an abreactive outlet – although they may function for him in all these ways. Primarily they are there to provide the child with a vocabulary. They are a means of facilitating the expression of his thoughts and feelings and clarifying their exploration.' Klein considered that the child's play could be understood and interpreted in very much the same way as the psychoanalyst interprets adult dreams.

Containment of anxieties

The reliable and regular presence of the child psychotherapist in a familiar and safe setting, and his deep attentiveness to the child in all aspects of his inner world as shown through play, is reminiscent of what Bion (1962) called 'maternal reverie'. Bion described the mother–infant relationship in terms of containment. The infant projects intolerable feelings into the mother who acts as a container for these feelings; a container strong enough not only to absorb and bear these feelings but also to digest them and then feed them back to the infant in a more tolerable form. By introjecting the concept of a containing and understanding mother, the infant begins to build up his ego. The child psychotherapist is similarly available to the child as a container. This is communicated through the attitude of attentiveness, interest in the child's feelings and state of mind, and a willingness to tolerate and understand painful communications from the child.

The transference relationship

Through the child psychotherapist's availability as a container of the child's projections, the transference relationship develops. Transference describes the ways in which the child interacts with the therapist and the therapeutic setting as an expression of the relationship to internal objects in an inner world. Thus, in exploring the transference and countertransference relationship, the child psychotherapist aims to explore the internal world of the child, including their phantasies, their wishes and their understanding of the external world.

The use of interpretation to promote insight

It is a central idea to psychotherapy that interpreting and naming what is going on in a child's internal world brings relief, facilitating insight and creating room for change. The process is one of 'reflecting the patient's view of the world back to them, but with more light let in' (Wallace, 1997). Interpretations are offered in simple words, appropriate to the child's capacity to understand. The child can increase his capacity to think something through, and to see the choices that might be available, having had the opportunity to thoughtfully negotiate difficulties rather than impulsively act them out. This can further protect the child from the adverse impact of later life events.

Which patient and why?

Child psychotherapy is not widely available and therefore treatment is usually reserved for the more disturbed child. Broadly speaking, psychotherapy is appropriate for children in whom confusion and conflict in their internal world effects their adaptation to the external world. The following list includes many of the difficulties manifested by children which are amenable to psychotherapeutic treatment. The role of child psychotherapy in the treatment of psychotic and autistic conditions has been comprehensively discussed by Alvarez (1992) and Tustin (1988).

Referral process

Child psychotherapists work both within health care services and privately, and referrals may come via a number of different routes. In the private sector, parents who are concerned for their child and who may be acting on advice from other health care professionals are the most frequent referrers. Otherwise, referral for psychotherapy may be made by professionals who, following their own assessment and (often) treatment of the child and family,

Problems amenable to child psychotherapy treatment
- Enuresis
- Encopresis
- Eating disorders
- Withdrawal and depression
- Attachment difficulties
- School refusal
- Poor social skills
- Excessive masturbation
- Excessive retreat into fantasy
- Hyperactivity
- Sleep disturbances
- Conduct disorders
- Psychosis
- Autism
- Children who are suffering sequelae of sexual, physical or emotional abuse
- Children who are struggling to cope with major life events such as bereavement, divorce, chronic illness in self or family member, physical or mental handicap

may wish for a psychodynamic assessment of the child in his own right. In the public sector, referrals are most often received from primary health care teams including general practitioners, paediatricians, community nurses and health visitors. For those children who manifest difficulties in coping at school, concerns by teachers and educational social workers may prompt a referral for assessment. In all referrals, permission and cooperation from the parents or main carers is essential.

Assessment

The therapist meets with the parents and child, initially to outline the treatment offered and the commitment needed. He may also invite the child and parents to describe current difficulties, and gather some information about the early development of the child. It can be very helpful in the course of a therapy to have obtained the parents' view of their child as a baby, including pregnancy, birth, the nature and quality of the early attachment relationship, how the baby slept, how the feeding relationship was negotiated and so on. In some cases it may be necessary to have a separate meeting with the parents who may need to express some of their concerns and give sensitive historical details which they feel might be harmful for the child to hear.

The boundaries of the child's therapy, including the issue of confidentiality, are addressed. Generally this is specified as absolute unless the therapist becomes concerned for the child's (or another child's) safety. In such an event, the parents are reassured that the therapist will inform them and any appropriate authority of his concerns in order that action can be taken to protect the child in question. In common with all psychotherapy, assessment of suitability includes commitment to the process. With young children there is the added difficulty that the parents' or carers' commitment to the therapy must be firmly established.

Following the initial meeting or meetings, the child is seen individually for a small number of sessions during which time it is usually possible to ascertain whether psychotherapy is appropriate for the child. The therapist attends very carefully to the child's play and, where possible, explores the child's views on his difficulties and his understanding of what is happening around him. In these exploratory sessions it is important for the therapist to pose 'trial interpretations' to obtain some idea of the child's receptivity and responsiveness to the insights offered. These interpretations are kept at a general level, for instance talking about the patterns of the child's relationships with family members and others external to the therapy.

Additional meetings with the parents may be necessary at this stage to feed back progress without breaching confidentiality. This is an opportunity for the therapist to outline his concerns and recommendations and, if proposing to proceed with therapy, to emphasize the boundaries of the therapy and to establish commitment. If all agree to proceed, the therapy commences and the therapist begins to 'gather in the transference' (Meltzer, 1967). It is accepted that the child's life is full of transference processes, and internal object relationships are externalized and acted out upon other people, pets and toys. As Meltzer describes, toys break, pets flee and generally speaking parents and other adults (at least occasionally) revolt against being the object of a tyrannical, restrictive transference. The child's transference processes are therefore forced to seek new objects. The child experiences relief of anxiety by the provision of repeated, reliable, attentive contact and understanding by the adult child psychotherapist. The tendency is for transference processes to find expression in such places. Thus, over the first weeks of therapy, transference processes tend to gather on the therapeutic situation. This is facilitated or 'gathered in' by the therapist's interpretation of anxieties manifest in the material.

If the decision is not to proceed then it is important to have one further session with the child to separate and say goodbye. At this point it may be appropriate to explain that at some future point in time the child may benefit from psychotherapy but not now.

In the initial interviews with the parents, the therapist should be at pains to acknowledge the willingness and generosity of the parents to allow the therapist to treat their child. He should attempt to reassure the parents that he is concerned primarily with the internal world of the child and that he will not be attempting to interfere in the child's external relationship with the parents. However, it is important to stress that they may see changes in this over time.

It follows then that one contraindiction to commencing therapy is a lack of commitment shown in the assessment period by the parents, carers or agencies involved in the child's care. This must be stressed, as it can be damaging to the child's development and trust if therapy is terminated through a breakdown in a parent's commitment. When considering a child for referral for psychotherapy, the referrer should outline the commitment needed very clearly and advise that there is often a period in therapy when the child's symptoms may get worse before getting better. In conduct-disordered boys, for example, this can lead to family breakdown. It is useful also to explain that the child may often idealize or denigrate the therapy and therapist, straining the parents' commitment to the treatment.

In many cases it is essential that another clinician offers the parents regular appointments to help them with their own difficulties and with any questions that arise during treatment. Many therapists find it best if their contact with parents is kept to an absolute mimimum and any meetings should preferably be conducted in front of the child. This can be enormously helpful in allowing the therapist and child to do the work necessary whilst unhindered by outside information and anxieties. However, not all therapists work in this way, and some only do so with certain children and families. A therapeutic approach which includes regular meetings with the family or parents can be more effective, particularly if one aim of therapy is to effect direct change in the interactions between family members. In some individual therapies, the therapist may review progress with parents or carers at regular intervals. Towards the end of therapy it is usually necessary for the therapist or a colleague to meet with the parents to review progress and discuss issues that may arise in the future.

Which therapist and why?

The first centre to offer training in the psychotherapeutic treatment of children, the Institute of Child Psychology (since discontinued), was set up in London by Margaret Lowenfeld in 1933. In 1947 the Hampstead Child Therapy Course and Clinic (now the Anna Freud Centre) was inaugurated thanks to Anna Freud and her work in the war nurseries. The following year saw the founding by John Bowlby and Esther Bick of the Child Psychotherapy Training at the Tavistock Clinic based on the teachings of Melanie Klein. In 1973, a Jungian training in child psychotherapy was set up by the Society of Analytical Psychology.

The British Association of Psychotherapists, founded in 1949, currently approve five child psychotherapy trainings. All the major theoretical approaches in psychoanalysis are represented including Freudian and Contemporary Freudian, Kleinian and Post-Kleinian, Jungian and the British Independent School of Object Relations. All trainees require an honours degree in social science, medicine or nursing, or an honours degree with additional qualifications in a related and relevant field. They are expected to have some professional experience of working with children, and are assessed for suitability and aptitude for psychotherapeutic work with children.

All of the trainings have an initial twelve or twenty-four month period which constitutes the pre-clinical training. This usually includes an infant observation, work discussion and theoretical seminars on child development and psychoanalytic thinking. During this period it is not a requirement to receive individual therapy. However, once accepted onto any of the child psychotherapy clinical trainings, the trainee has to undergo a personal analysis, usually at a mimimum rate of three times weekly. Their analysts must be approved by the training establishment, and by the Association of Child Psychotherapists. Clinical experience is closely supervised, both individually and in small groups, throughout the training.

Qualities desirable in a trainee child psychotherapist are not easy to define, difficult to assess effectively and even harder to quantify. Applicants are interviewed individually, references are sought from tutors and employers, and group procedures may also be used as part of the selection process. A capacity to attend to children and adults with great sensitivity, especially to the subtle nuances of communication, is necessary in order for a meaningful contact between therapist and patient to take place. Equally essential is the capacity to tolerate one's own and others' painful mental states in order to provide the necessary containment or holding a patient requires.

The therapist must also be capable of tolerating 'not knowing' and of delaying his own gratification or desire for success as this will adversely affect the patient. Very important is the capacity to learn from experience. The therapist will need a capacity to bring all experiences, both internal and external, from his own life to bear on the material from the patient and, equally, a willingness to re-evaluate his own experiences in the light of information from his clinical work. It is also essential that a therapist has the capacity to apply scientific principles in describing and studying both his patients' and his own internal worlds.

At the core of the clinical training lie three intensive individual psychotherapeutic treatment cases; one child under five, one latency child and one adolescent. The trainee sees these patients at least three times weekly, receiving weekly individual supervision for each case, for a minimum of one year for two patients and two years for one patient. The trainee sees a wide range of other cases less intensively for short-, medium- and long-term psychotherapy. In addition, child psychotherapists are trained in assessment, consultation and supervision. They also have opportunities to experience mother–infant therapy, couple therapy, therapy with parents, family therapy, group work and other therapeutic approaches.

Therapeutic setting

The function of the setting is to provide the child with some personal space in which there is a minimum of interference from external and internal distractions. The total setting includes the external realities of the room, the toys, the timing of the therapy and the mental receptivity of the therapist. Consistency and reliability are essential to enable the transference to be 'gathered in' by the therapist and to help create an atmosphere of physical and emotional containment. It also makes the therapist's task easier in detecting changes in the child's play and communications which arise from his internal world rather than in response to external factors. For example, the therapist's lateness may accentuate the child's anxiety of abandonment.

In a 'good-enough' setting, the room should be simply furnished, have nothing which is indicative of the therapist's private life (like photographs of spouse and children) and ideally have access to water. Drawings or work by other children are not displayed as this may provoke envy. The session should occur at the same times and on the same days and any breaks, such as holidays, should be prepared for well in advance.

Toys and drawing materials are necessary and many therapists prefer to provide a box or drawer of toys exclusively for each child. These include small human figures, wild and domestic animals, fences, building blocks, small cars and other transport vehicles, a ball, string, paper, Plasticine, Sellotape, glue, scissors and crayons or colour pencils. Others prefer to provide a communal box of toys which is available to all patients who come into the room, although difficulties can arise with this arrangement; it may be impossible to differentiate between the changes in a child's behaviour which are a response to his encountering evidence of other children's use of the toys and those which indicate a change in the child's state of mind from one session to the next. Communal toys cannot be safely left from one session to the next in a particular arrangement or construction as subsequent children may rearrange them. This can, at times, be an inhibition to the degree to which the child feels free to play. Some therapists provide a combination of a number of toys or play materials communally available and a separate box of toys exclusive to each child and, as the distinction is clear to the child, this causes less problems.

While many psychotherapists work privately, many also work as part of a multi-disciplinary team in various settings, including paediatric and child mental health units. This has many advantages as there is potential for rich discussion about particular children and their families, drawing on the differing theoretical and experiential frameworks of each professional. It allows scope for the therapy to be well supported by other team members, particularly those cases in which family therapy or support for the child's parents is needed. Psychotherapists contribute greatly in the areas of staff supervision, providing opportunities to look in depth from a psychodynamic perspective at clinical cases, their impact on individual staff members and their impact on the team as a whole.

Clinical example

Eight-year-old Peter was referred with recurring nightmares and aggressive behaviour at home and school. Peter's father had committed suicide three months earlier. His father had suffered with depression and had planned to kill his family also, but finally shot himself in the family car outside the home. Peter had heard the shot and accounts differed as to whether he had seen his father's body clearly. Peter had made comments that indicated he sometimes blamed himself and sometimes his mother for his father's death.

In the initial meeting with his mother and siblings his mother talked about the suicide and its effect upon the family, while Peter said he needed to draw a picture which he later left with me.

He drew a bright yellow sun in the top left hand corner over a blue sea. Under the sun he drew a line horizontally across the page, and above this signified heaven. He drew his father as a stick figure lying down in heaven. He then added a glider flying under heaven with his father lying down inside the glider, a smile drifting off the side of his face, one eye obscured by his hair and his left arm unconnected to his body. Peter said the glider was taking his father up to heaven. He then drew a shark leaping up out of the water trying to bite the glider from behind. He drew a fish to the right of this, also out of water, and this fish, Peter explained, the shark would catch as he re-entered the water. The fish had already been bitten and Peter drew blood gushing out of the fish and spreading all over the water. More fishes were drawn in the water and four clouds in the sky. Orange lightning came out of each cloud and two struck the glider, one striking his father inside, and another striking the shark and the water. Peter then drew a big circle below heaven and asked me how to spell 'Bang'. He carefully wrote 'BANG' inside the circle. He drew a similar circle in heaven and again wrote 'BANG' inside. Finally he drew a lot of rain falling from the clouds. Before he finished the picture, Peter told me he had nightmares of witches chasing him. He thought his daddy was in heaven, at least his skin was in heaven, his bones were in the ground.

Peter was struggling to make sense of his feelings following the sudden and traumatic death of his father. He was troubled by images of his dead father in the car and in subsequent sessions continued to draw pictures with lots of blood, saying that red was his favourite colour because it reminded him of his father's blood. Peter was in the habit of biting his fingernails until they bled and said he enjoyed drinking the blood. The shark in his first picture may have represented both his angry and hateful feelings towards his previously depressed daddy, including the feeling that he contributed to his death and also his angry feelings towards his now absent daddy. The four clouds appeared to stand for the four remaining members of the family: Peter continued to draw clouds throughout his therapy. Often clouds stood for the stored up grief and dark feelings hanging overhead.

In this very first meeting Peter appeared to have rapidly become attached to me. This immediate positive transference was in part due to the relief he experienced on expressing his feelings through the picture, but was also an indication that he possessed a rich inner world which could be transferred onto me and which would permit him to experience containment in his sessions. Thereafter, he ran eagerly to his sessions. On one occasion he and his mother appeared breathless in the waiting area and she explained that it was not that they were late but that he was so keen to come he ran all the way. Peter was not in need of long-term therapy and his therapy lasted six months with two holiday breaks. A task of the therapy was to facilitate an understanding of his father's death with the threat to kill his family, and permit Peter to mourn.

The following extract from one session illustrates his capacity to use me and the space to explore his feelings and to process the loss.

After the first holiday break Peter's mother reported that he had cried one night for two and a half hours for his daddy. Although she was pleased that he was now able to do this, his behaviour had got worse. In this first session after the break Peter spoke of missing his father and for the first time used 'babytalk': 'Me can't do it, me need help.' In the transference I was a father figure to whom he could bring his very helpless and babyish feelings.

Peter recalled accompanying his father to work on a building site and being allowed to pretend to drive a mechanical digger. He then made a very large card and with felt-tips drew two diggers on the front, a very big one with his daddy driving with someone on his knee and a second smaller one on a big mound of earth which Peter was driving. The big digger had fierce teeth facing forward and the little digger could not quite reach the ground. Peter wrote 'TODAY' above the diggers. As I talked about a part of him missing his daddy Peter painted over the letter 'Y' and replaced it with 'DDY' and now the card read 'TO DADDY'. Inside the card he wrote, 'To Daddy, we miss you, love Pete'. He then used black paint to draw two heavy black clouds in the sky *above the diggers and nodded when I spoke about his heavy, sad feelings and his worry that his daddy was also sad.*

Peter spoke of how his father had been often angry and of how he would see his mummy and daddy shouting at each other. I wondered if there was a feeling that daddy might be angry with him, and Peter said he did not know if his daddy was happy in heaven. 'Me went to the funeral. Me not allowed to put flowers into grave. Me wanted to jump in.' I said it must have felt awful for him, wanting to be with his daddy and his daddy's body going into the ground. Peter drew four hearts raining from the clouds onto the diggers and I wondered if these were the four remaining family members. Peter nodded and wrote everyone's name in a heart.

I spoke about loving and sad feelings and Peter drew, as I spoke, a large picture with two huge eyes and a huge nose that at first looked like holes in the head. I wondered if there was a question in his head as to what had happened to his father's face when he shot himself. Peter nodded. He then carefully drew in the eyes and drew a small body and thin legs, no arms. 'Big head, little body' he commented. He then drew the rest of his family all without arms and I wondered if there was a sense that there are no arms strong enough to hold him now: again he nodded.

Peter made a kite coloured red and dark blue and Sellotaped string to it. I wondered about kites reaching up to the sky, and perhaps finding a link between Peter on earth and daddy in heaven. Peter, in literally the last minute, drew another picture of his father's face. He drew a circle for the head and, using a large circle of wood which he asked me to hold in position for him, he drew three huge circles for the eyes and the nose in the centre of the face, almost filling all the space inside. He then drew hair on top of the head and a thin smile that began on the face and finished outside and a squiggle above this for his father's moustache. This time he did not fill in the holes but drew four clouds in the four quarters of the page around the head. Peter left before we could speak about this picture, and it appeared he had drawn the terrible image that often intruded into his mind – his daddy's face with huge holes. He left it with me to bear until his next session.

In subsequent sessions Peter continued to speak in a 'baby' voice and felt he needed my help with everything. On occasion he would play 'peepo' from behind his knees or through slatted fingers which hid his face. His mother reported that he was speaking almost exclusively in this 'baby voice' at home throughout this period and he often cried, missing his father. Peter found it difficult to go to bed, saying he was thinking about his daddy.

Peter asked in one session how the police knew his father was dead, and said there was a boy in his school who could die any minute because he 'has a blood vessel near his heart'. Peter nodded when I spoke about his anxieties about his own health and wondered what sense he made of his father wanting to kill all of his family before he died. Peter thought that his daddy wanted to take him and his family to heaven with him because he could not bear to leave them behind. I think that Peter was now feeling that his daddy did indeed love him and had not intended to harm him in an angry way but had found it very painful to leave him and his family.

Peter's behaviour at home and at school had substantially improved by the second break and he was no longer hitting out at others. His nightmares had also stopped and the 'baby voice' was used less and less at home. In his penultimate session, Peter made me a farewell card. He drew a sun, rain, a rainbow above a heart with his name on it and inside this heart another heart with my name on. He wrote 'Goodbye Gerry' on the front of the card and inside wrote, 'Thank you for helping me, I hope you have a good holiday'. I think my heart inside his heart stood for his internal daddy who was restored to good health and with whom he could now engage in meaningful dialogue.

Interestingly, he perhaps showed in his wish for me to have a good holiday that he was not yet ready to let me go completely but wished to hold on to me in his mind. In the final session Peter elected to leave all his drawings with me, anxious, I think, that I should hold on to the distressing images but also asking me to hold him in my mind and not forget him.

Problems in therapy

Seriousness of disturbance

A common misconception is that psychotherapy is only for very disturbed children, probably arising from the scarcity of child psychotherapists. In fact, psychotherapy is enormously helpful for any children who are struggling with major life events such as bereavement, diagnosis of chronic illness, separation and divorce. Similarly, many people believe that child psychotherapists are only interested in intensive long-term therapy. However, only when children at the severe end of the spectrum are referred is this indicated. Child psychotherapists are also trained and skilled in brief interventions and, where appropriate, these can have great benefits for the child and family.

Commitment

A common pitfall when working psychotherapeutically with children in acute child and family psychiatry is the failure to adhere to better judgement in taking on a child for treatment whose parents or carers have difficulty in giving full commitment to the therapy. The child may be in acute distress and a number of anxious and influential people within the service may urge the therapist to initiate treatment without the required guarantee of full commitment from the caregivers. It does not serve the child's best interests to begin treatment under these circumstances as abrupt termination by the parents or carers gives yet another disappointment to the child, and can be harmful if he has truly engaged in therapy. On the other hand, it is very difficult and not always appropriate for the therapist to be unswerving in his attitude about such cases. Also, it may happen that useful work is accomplished even in a therapy prematurely ended or if, surprisingly, the parents settle down and allow the child a good period in therapy.

Family support

Inadequate provision of support for the family or parents from another member of the team can contribute to premature termination. The parents may feel unable to bring their child against his will, or find this too difficult to bear if the child is punishing them whilst idealizing the therapist. They may then be tempted to take the child out of therapy. Good preparation at the beginning of treatment, ongoing support or the availability of support at difficult points in the therapy can pay great dividends.

Dysfunctional families

Psychotherapy may be contraindicated and should not be pursued in families characterized by deep enmeshment and splitting. It can prove impossible to gather in the transference with a child who is in a *'folie-à-deux'* type relationship with a mother. Similarly, children who are convinced that they have no influence on their internal world whatsoever, and who project all responsibility on to external events, can be very difficult to work with.

Evaluation of therapy

All psychosocial interventions, including child and adolescent psychotherapy, are under increasing pressure to prove themselves to be not only effective but also cost-effective. At any one time 20% of children and adolescents suffer from a psychiatric disorder, with only 10–15% of these being seen by psychiatric services (Roth and Fonagy, 1996). The long-term outcomes of these severe psychiatric disorders are poor as general anxiety disorder and obsessive–compulsive disorder show high levels of persistence, and there is increased risk of antisocial behaviour in adulthood for children with disruptive disorder in childhood. Roth and Fonagy conclude that an intervention at all stages of development is justified and, given that a much greater number of disruptive children than emotionally disordered children are referred for treatment, there is a need to educate caregivers to the possibility that distressed children under their care may not just 'grow out of it' and may need specialist help. A video by the Child Psychotherapy Trust called *Won't they just grow out of it?* makes just this point, and provides a good introduction to the work of the child psychotherapist for all caregivers.

Fonagy and Moran (1990) have outlined the major difficulties in evaluating psychological treatments of childhood disorders including:

- Difficulties in finding correlations between the informants of children's symptomatology
- The necessity to assess outcome in the context of the natural history of the disorder
- The necessity for support and cooperation from caregivers and professionals involved with a child for a therapy to be effective
- Co-morbidity
- The lack of well-standardized measures of symptomatic outcome
- The absence of long-term follow-up data

Despite these difficulties, careful reviews of child psychotherapy research since 1957 have shown that psychotherapy for children can bring about a high rate of improvement in symptomatology, thus demonstrating its effectiveness in promoting positive changes (Tuma and Sabotka, 1983; Casey and Berman, 1985; Kazdin, 1991; Gorin, 1993; Weiss and Weisz, 1993). Meta-analyses of child psychotherapy outcome studies have shown significant improvements in children following psychotherapy.

Evidence has not been available in relation to the full range of disorders but in the following conditions child psychotherapy was either shown to be effective or, in the absence of reliable studies, showed considerable promise:

- Depression
- Anxiety disorders
- Disorders associated with physiological disturbances
- Specific developmental disorders

In recent years the emphasis of the question has been changed from 'Is psychotherapy effective?' to 'What therapy, by whom, is most effective for this child with this specific problem, and under what circumstances?' (Phillips, 1987; Heinicke, 1989). Mary Boston and Dora Lush at the Tavistock Clinic have been researching a methodology of evaluating psychoanalytic psychotherapy with children for some years now (Boston, 1989). They attempt to address the difficulties in trying to measure not only outcome in terms of external change (symptoms) but also in terms of internal changes. They have devised a research tool using therapist questionnaires at the beginning and end of treatment. These forms are designed to measure therapists' predictions and assessment of change in their patients (Boston, 1989; Lush et al., 1991; Boston and Lush, 1994), and interfere little with actual clinical practice. Therapists have reported finding them useful in promoting thought and reflection on their work despite the inconvenience of regular form filling.

Fonagy and Moran (1990) have recommended that future research on outcome in child psychotherapy requires the development of standardized ways of measuring childhood functioning including symptomatology and developmental processes and will need to take into account the natural history of disorders in relation to the child's developmental age when evaluating change.

Alternatives to therapy

Play therapy

Play therapy may be considered as an alternative to child psychotherapy. In play therapy, the therapist is a facilitator who presides over the play of the child. Play therapy acknowledges a drive towards growth, maturity and fulfilment in the individual. It assumes that the individual has an ability within him to solve his own problems satisfactorily, and that his growth impulse will make mature behaviour more attractive and satisfying than immature behaviours (Axline, 1947). The child is perceived as having work that needs doing, and the therapist facilitates this work and provides the child with a language, through play, in which to do it (Newson, 1992). Play therapists do not work in the transference, and many do not see as their task the elucidation and interpretation of the child's internal world as the child psychotherapist does. Rather, the child is provided with opportunities to play out his accumulated feelings in the security of the playroom and the presence of the therapist. The child is offered the experience of being master over the therapist and the play (no hurting or breaking allowed). Play therapy is effective in treating children whose capacity to achieve resolution through play has not been compromised. Newson (1992) suggests two basic criteria in considering a child's suitability for play therapy: that the child is capable of symbolic play and does not lack boundaries between reality and fantasy.

Family therapy

Family therapy is indicated when the assessment shows that the child's symptomatology fulfils functions for other members of the family, and is less a result of confusion in his own internal world. Child psychotherapy does not discount familial and social factors as significant contributory causes, or even as the main cause. It is often the case that the child and family, or child and parents, are in need of therapy – and it may be impossible really to promote growth and change in the child's internal world unless there is a corresponding change in his external world. Family therapy may be the treatment of choice where psychotherapy is contraindicated, as in families with deep enmeshment and splitting.

Behaviour therapy

With circumscribed problems, or difficulties in obtaining the necessary commitment to an exploratory approach, behaviour therapy can have considerable benefit. Although specific positive effects are often generalized, improvement may not be sustained in the long term if structural problems underlie the presentation.

Therapy for parents and other family members

Problems with other members of the family often emerge during the process of a child's referral to psychotherapy. Appropriate referral of the adults for psychotherapy can often have significant benefit, and prevent relapse and the dysfunctional patterns which may maintain difficulties.

Acknowledgements
I am grateful to Andrea Watson, who supervised my work with Peter, and to Daphne Briggs, who provided useful guidance and advice in regard to the writing of this chapter.

Further reading

Boston, M. and Szur, R. (eds) (1988) *Psychotherapy with Severely Deprived Children*. London: Routledge.
Bowlby, J. and Robertson, J. (1952) A two-year old goes to hospital: a scientific film. *Proceedings of the Royal Society of Medicine*, **46**, 425–427.
Child Psychotherapy Trust video. *Won't they just grow out of it?* Star House, 104–108 Grafton Road, London NW5 4BD.
Freud, A. (1926–27) Introduction to the technique of child analysis. Reprinted in: *The Psychoanalytic Treatment of Children*. London: Imago, 1946.
Klein, M. (1932) The technique of early analysis. In: *The Writings of Melanie Klein*. London: Hogarth Press, pp. 16–24.
Stern, D.N. (1995) *The Motherhood Constellation: A Unified View of Parent–Infant Psychotherapy*. New York: Basic Books.
Winnicott, D.W. (1971) *Playing and Reality*. London: Tavistock.

Bibliography

Ainsworth, M.D.S., Blehar, M.C., Waters, E. and Wall, S. (1978) *Patterns of Attachment: A Psychological Study of the Strange Situation.* Hillsdale, NJ: Lawrence Erlbaum Associates.

Alvarez, A. (1992) *Live Company: Psycho-Analytic Psychotherapy with Autistic, Borderline, Deprived and Abused Children.* London: Routledge.

Axline, V. (1947) *Play Therapy.* London: Churchill Livingstone.

Bion, W.R. (1962) A theory of thinking. *International Journal of Psycho-Analysis*, **33**, 306–310.

Boston, M. (1989) In search of a methodology for evaluating psychoanalytic psychotherapy with children. *Journal of Child Psychotherapy*, **15**, 15–46.

Boston, M. and Lush, D. (1994) Further considerations of methodology for evaluating psychoanalytic psychotherapy with children: reflections in the light of research experience. *Journal of Child Psychotherapy*, **20**, 205–229.

Bowlby, J. (1944) Forty-four juvenile thieves: their characters and home life. *International Journal of Psycho-Analysis*, **25**, 1–57 and 207–228.

Bowlby, J. (1991) Ethological light on psychoanalytic problems. In: P. Bateson (ed.), *Development and Integration of Behaviour.* Cambridge: Cambridge University Press, pp. 315–329.

Bowlby, J. and Robertson, J. (1952a) A two-year old goes to hospital: a scientific film. *Proceedings of the Royal Society of Medicine*, **46**, 425–427.

Bowlby, J. and Robertson, J. (1952b) Responses of young children to separation from their mothers. *Courier, Centre International de L'Enfance*, **2**, 66–78 and 131–142.

Bowlby, J., Robertson, J. and Rosenbluth, D. (1952) A two-year old goes to hospital. *The Psychoanalytical Study of the Child*, **7**, 82–94.

Casey, R.J. and Berman, J.S. (1985) The outcome of psychotherapy with children. *Psychological Bulletin*, **98**, 388–400.

Child Psychotherapy Trust video. *Won't they just grow out of it?* Star House, 104–108 Grafton Road, London NW5 4BD.

Daws, D. (1987) 30 years of psychotherapy. *Association for Child Psychology and Psychiatry Newsletter*, **9**, 3–11.

Daws, D. (1989) *Through the Night: Helping Parents and Sleepless Infants.* London: Free Association Books.

Fonagy, P. and Moran, G.S. (1990) Studies on the efficacy of child psychoanalysis. *Journal of Consulting and Clinical Psychology*, **58**, 684–695.

Fraiberg, S., Adelson, E. and Shapiro, V. (1975) Ghosts in the nursery: a psychoanalytic approach to the problems of impaired infant–mother relationships. *Journal of the American Academy of Child Psychiatry*, **14**, 387–421.

Freud, A. (1926–27) Introduction to the technique of child analysis. Reprinted in: *The Psychoanalytic Treatment of Children.* London: Imago, 1946.

Freud, S. (1909) Analysis of a phobia in a 5-year-old child. In. *Standard Edition of the Complete Psychological Works of Sigmund Freud*, vol. 10. London: Hogarth Press.

Gorin, S.S. (1993) The prediction of child psychotherapy outcome: factors specific to treatment. *Psychotherapy*, **30**, 152–158.

Heinicke, C.M. (1989) *Psychodynamic Psychotherapy with Children: Current Status and Guidelines for Future Research.* New York: Plenum Press.

Kazdin, A.E. (1991) Effectiveness of psychotherapy with children and adolescents. *Journal of Consulting and Clinical Psychology*, **59**, 785–798.

Klein, M. (1955) The psycho-analytic play technique: its history and significance. In: *The Writings of Melanie Klein.* London: Hogarth Press, pp. 122–140.

Klein, M. (1932) *The Psychoanalysis of Children.* London: Hogarth Press.

Klein, M. (1932) The technique of early analysis. In: *The Writings of Melanie Klein.* London: Hogarth Press, pp. 16–24.

Lush, D., Boston, M. and Grainger, E. (1991) Evaluation of psychoanalytic psychotherapy with children: therapists' assessments and predictions. *Psychoanalytic Psychotherapy*, **5**, 191–234.

Main, M. and Solomon, J. (1988) Procedures for identifying infants as disorganized/disoriented during the Ainsworth Strange Situation. In: M. Greenberg, M. Cummings and B. Cicchetti (eds), *Attachment in the Preschool Years: Theory, Research, and Intervention*. Chicago: University of Chicago Press, pp. 121–160.

de Mause, L. (1974) *The History of Childhood*. London: Souvenir Press.

Meltzer, D. (1967) *The Psycho-Analytical Process*. Perthshire: Clunie Press.

Miller, L., Rustin, M. and Shuttleworth, J. (1989) *Closely Observed Infants*. London: Duckworth.

Newson, D. (1992) The barefoot play therapist: adapting skills for a time of need. In: D.A. Lane and A. Miller (eds), *Child and Adolescent Therapy: A Handbook*. Buckingham: Open University Press, pp. 89–107.

Phillips, R.D. (1987) A primer for conducting child psychotherapy outcome research. *Psychotherapy*, **24**, 178–185.

Radbill, S.X. (1987) Children in a world of violence: the history of child abuse. In: R.E. Helfer and R. Kempe (eds), *The Battered Child*. Chicago: The University of Chicago Press.

Reeves, A.C. (1977) *Freud and Child Psychotherapy*. London: Wildwood House.

Roth, A. and Fonagy, P. (1996) *What Works for Whom? A Critical Review of Psychotherapy Research*. New York and London: Guilford Press.

Sroufe, A. (1996) Psychopathology as Development: Implications of Attachment Theory and Research for Developmental Psychopathology. Conference paper presented at St George's Hospital, London.

Stern, D.N. (1995) *The Motherhood Constellation: A Unified View of Parent–Infant Psychotherapy*. New York: Basic Books.

Tuma, J.M. and Sobotka, K.R. (1983) Traditional therapies with children. In: T.H. Ollendick and M. Herson (eds), *Handbook of Child Psychopathology*. New York: Plenum Press, pp. 391–426.

Tustin F. (1988) Psychotherapy with children who cannot play. *International Review of Psycho-Analysis*, **15**, 93–106.

Urwin, C. and Hood-Williams, J. (1988) *Child Psychotherapy, War and the Normal Child. Selected Papers of Margaret Lowenfeld*. London: Free Association Books.

Wallace, W. (1997) Children on the couch: Is three the perfect age to meet your shrink? *The Independent*, 16 September 1997, p. 17.

Weiss, B. and Weisz, J.R. (1993) *The Effects of Psychotherapy with Children and Adolescents*. Newbury Park, CA: Sage.

13

Group Psychotherapy

Rex Haigh

Historical perspective

In 1907 Joseph Hersey Pratt, a physician from Boston, Massachusetts, wrote about the benefit of treating tuberculosis patients in a holistic way. As well as attending to their physical illness, he brought twenty-five of them together each week in the 'Emmanuel Church Tuberculosis Class' to discuss their symptoms and progress. He observed an improvement in morale and a reduction in symptoms of depression and isolation. This is probably the first description of a therapeutic group as we now understand it.

In the 1920s, Alfred Adler saw patients in groups. This was as part of his belief in the social construction of human suffering and his drive to bring humanity, compassion and care to the working classes. In 1925, Jacob Moreno (who first coined the term 'group therapy') introduced his ideas of psychodrama, although he had already been working with groups for some years. In the late 1920s, L.C. Marsh used a variety of group techniques, including lectures, open discussions and directed discussions, to treat a wide range of neurotic, psychotic and somatic complaints.

A few years later, Louis Wender started to treat psychiatric in-patients in groups of about twenty. He made psychoanalytic interpretations of individuals' psychopathology, and encouraged mutual exchanges and discussion. At about the same time, D. Schilder ran single sex groups of up to five out-patients who had already received extensive individual analysis from him. In these groups, case histories were discussed and interpreted with patients in turn. In the 1940s, Alexander Wolf ran thrice-weekly groups using individual psychoanalytic techniques such as the analysis of dreams, transference and resistance on each group member in turn. In addition to their sessions with Wolf, the groups frequently met to work by themselves.

Sigmund H. Fuchs was a German psychoanalyst who fled the Nazis and emigrated to England before the Second World War, taking the name Michael Foulkes. In the early 1940s he started an out-patient group in Exeter and went home to his wife declaring that 'a historical event has taken place in psychiatry today, but nobody knows about it'. He later refined and developed the technique of *group analysis*, as it is still known today.

The Northfield Experiments in Birmingham grew from the need to treat large numbers of battle-traumatized Second World War servicemen: the experiments with groups involved Wilfred Bion, and later Thomas Main, Harold Bridger and Michael Foulkes. It was here that Main coined the term 'therapeutic community'. After leaving the Army, Bion was employed at the Tavistock Clinic in London. Here he set up experimental groups, which were influenced by contemporary psychoanalytic theory and practice, which was predominantly Kleinian. These were put into clinical service by Henry Ezriel and others, but did not find much favour among clinicians or patients. Much of Bion's theory is still seen as essential in understanding groups, but the highly specialized techniques are now little used clinically.

An approach similar to J.H. Pratt's treatment of TB was being used by Maxwell Jones with soldiers suffering from effort dyspnoea at Mill Hill Hospital in London. After the war, Jones went on to set up the Henderson Hospital, the first intentionally organized therapeutic community. It spawned a multitude of similar group-based approaches in Britain and elsewhere in the following twenty years.

In the 1930s and 1940s in the United States of America, Trigant Burrow made intensive studies of the tensions that arise in groups, mainly between colleagues working closely together on the same American campus. He first used the term 'group analysis' but, apart from his anti-individualistic emphasis, it was not related to the 'group analysis' which later emerged in the United Kingdom. The *T-group* ('Training in Human Relations') movement started in Connecticut under Kurt Lewin, a non-clinical social psychologist. He developed complex group theory without reference to psychoanalytic ideas: for example, he introduced the term 'feedback' from electrical engineering. This developed, by the 1960s, into the *encounter group* movement. The educational element of T-groups had become 'therapy for normals'. Dividing lines were lost between training groups and treatment groups, normality and pathology, and therapy and personal growth. Group therapy and experiences of encounter groups had become a way of life for large numbers of Americans. Irvin D. Yalom went from this to describe *interpersonal group therapy,* which drew together many theoretical and practical strands of group therapy as it was being practised.

In the United Kingdom, after the War, Foulkes published *Therapeutic Group Analysis* and gathered a number of interested clinicians around him. The Institute of Group Analysis was founded in London in the 1970s to train clinicians and develop this way of working. As a result, it spread widely throughout Europe, including the establishment of professional training schemes in many countries, and the formation of a group analytic therapeutic community in Athens.

Brief focused group therapy, for example anger management, assertiveness training and groups for survivors of sexual abuse, became established as useful treatments. These are based on psycho-educational and cognitive principles, and use other therapeutic techniques in a group setting, rather than using the group itself as the primary therapeutic agent.

In the 1990s regulation and registration of psychotherapists is of increasing importance in the United Kingdom, with a number of different courses for training group therapists. Most of the early work with groups was done by psychiatrists, but now group psychotherapy is practised by therapists with a range of professional backgrounds – most, but not all, in mental health. The courses are based on humanistic/interpersonal or group analytic principles. The former include approaches such as Gestalt and psychodrama, as well as the type of groups Yalom describes. The latter are based on derivatives of Foulkes' work, and use more psychoanalytic concepts. The two approaches share many common principles, but describe them in different ways.

Principles of theory and practice

Principles of theory

It can be helpful to think of group therapy as therapy *in* the group, therapy *of* the group and therapy *by* the group. Some types of group therapy use a mixture of these three, and some aim to limit the technique to one of them.

Therapy in the group closely resembles the early experiments in which patients took turns to discuss their psychopathology and have interpretations made. These interpretations aimed to give insight and produce subsequent change. The model is a direct translation of early psychoanalytic theory, and it makes no reference to the psychological impact that group members make on each other. Most contemporary group therapy will include an element of this, although its prominence varies with different approaches.

Therapy of the group grew out of Bion's work, and is based on the notion that groups have definable modes of functioning. Bion (1961) described the two dominant patterns as *basic assumption* and *work groups*. When a group is 'in basic assumption mode', it is operating in an ineffective, defensive and pathological way. When it is a 'work group', it is functioning in a sophisticated and coherent way.

There are three types of basic assumption groups – *dependency* (for example, asking a group leader for answers), *fight-flight* (for example, hostile comments about the group or absences from it) and *pairing* (where two members or a subgroup of the whole group start a relationship exclusive of the rest of the group). Work groups are those in which trust and cohesion exist, and where personal and emotional material is freely discussed.

In therapy *of the group*, the therapist will only make group level interpretations aimed at elucidating the relationship between the group-as-a-whole and the therapist. Analysing the group in this way is seen as the therapeutic task. Techniques for doing so were refined by Ezriel and others at the Tavistock Clinic in the 1950s.

Another approach is to examine patients' *internal representation of the group*. The group functions as an *internal object* in relation to which patients are continually experiencing, exploring and changing their habitual emotional reactions – for example, how safe or criticized members feel in the group; these can be analysed either in reference to individual patients' previous experience or as a group level phenomenon.

A different approach puts these theoretical considerations into the background and sees the primary task as building and maintaining a safe *group culture* in which communication of deep underlying distress can take place in an intimate and supportive milieu.

Therapy by the group depends upon the network of relationships that constantly develops, changes and deepens between members of a group. In this aspect, the therapist is equal to the other participants: patients can have as much, or more, effect on each other. An example would be an exchange between patients who have been through similar trauma, who find deeper understanding and support from each other than would be possible from a therapist without that experience. There is also an important impact upon other group members who are not directly involved in any given event: they learn something directly about human relations between others, as well as deepening their relationships with others by being with them – perhaps as silent but attentive observers – through difficult, intense and emotional exchanges.

Therapy *by the group* refers to the discussion, interactions and communication between all members of the group – as discrete events which may be helpful or therapeutic in themselves, and also the summation to a collective and non-individual experience. This is a powerful and positive affective experience – sometimes described as a sense of deep belonging, intimate contact or 'koinonia'. It is a relaxed state, but of heightened awareness, and is akin to what has been called the 'oceanic feeling': it needs few words to communicate it. In occasional moments, it can be experienced by a whole group simultaneously but more often members are engaged in it to differing degrees.

The value of the network of relationships as a powerful therapeutic agent is recognized and acknowledged by most group therapists, and generally referred to as the *group matrix*. Some group therapies, particularly group analytic approaches, hold these processes to be central; others give them less prominence. The terminology and theoretical principles used to describe them differ.

Group analytic psychotherapy (group analysis)

Foulkes was a psychiatrist and psychoanalyst who was influenced by the Frankfurt School of Marxist sociology before moving to England. One of his main themes was the inseparability of an individual from his or her context. This makes it impossible to gain a meaningful understanding of a person, or their neurotic symptoms, in isolation from their social world. This is played out in the social context of the group, so disturbed and abnormal subjective experience can be examined and understood, with some new-found objectivity, in the relationships within the group.

In clinical theory, this principle of meaning being established through context gives the law that *the group constitutes the norm from which its members individually deviate*. It follows from this that the aggregated health in a group is sufficient to produce a healing environment, and individual pathology is diminished by making open and articulating what is unconscious and destructive. Foulkes saw the symptom as an isolated and incoherent expression of distress, which *'mumbles to itself, secretly hoping to be overheard'*. In this way, the therapeutic process is one of working towards an ever-more articulate form of communication. Then the symptom, as a marker of deep underlying disturbance, is freed of its destructive potential by understanding what lies beneath and giving it meaning in a social context. In this process, powerful affect is experienced and the individual's unconscious conflict loses much of its destructive charge (Foulkes, 1964).

This group analytic process can only happen in a group where it is safe: this is the task called *dynamic administration*. It establishes containment, and includes all the work that the therapist needs to do when he or she is not sitting with the group: arranging the practicalities of referrals and membership, the place and time (including its institutional setting) and communications outside the group itself. Through careful attention to these, a therapeutic milieu is established in which the communicative work can take place.

Four levels of communication are defined by Foulkes, of increasing depth and communality. The first, predominant in early stages of groups, is the *conscious level*: discussion of rational material in everyday awareness. The second is the *transference level*, where an individual can experience others as if they were emotionally important figures from the past. Next is the *projective level*, where more primitive, dissociated and inaccessible emotions will be re-experienced and explored in relation to others. The deepest, the *primordial level*, bears much similarity to Jung's collective unconscious and archetypal experience: the *foundation matrix* in group terms. They can be represented diagrammatically by individuals as islands, connected together deep beneath the surface of the sea (Figure 13.1). In the live situation of an analytic group, there is continual movement between these levels.

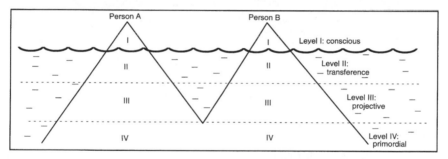

Figure 13.1   Levels of group process

Other important processes described in group analytic psychotherapy are translation, mirroring, resonance and socialization. *Translation* is somewhat different from interpretation as made in individual analytic psychotherapy. It is the process of helping a patient to articulate subjective distress and its meaning, and not necessarily seeking an objective cause or explanation. Most of this does not need to be performed by the therapist, but can equally well be done by other group members. *Mirroring* is seeing characteristics or attributes of oneself in another, and the process of working out the emotional response to that experience. *Resonance* is a form of 'live' empathic response to another, in which similar emotions are experienced by more than one person at a time. *Socialization* in therapeutic settings is the ability to abandon a habitual position of isolation: the realization that one is not alone with problematic symptoms, anxieties or impulses (Foulkes, 1964).

Interpersonal group therapy

Interpersonal group therapy and theory grew out of the American T-group and encounter group movement. Lewin's original work was research based, and he devised complex ideas, which he called 'field theories', to describe what happened in groups – with little reference to previous psychological work, and none to psychotherapy and psychoanalysis. As it rapidly attracted interest and became a 'movement', the theoretical basis became less prominent and the experiential 'here and now' nature of the groups dominated. They particularly encouraged interpersonal honesty, exploration, confrontation, heightened emotional expressiveness and self-disclosure.

Yalom became involved in researching encounter groups, and he is best known for describing twelve *therapeutic factors* (Yalom, 1985). These are derived from sixty items sorted by many of his patients who benefited from group therapy.

Yalom's twelve therapeutic factors
- Interpersonal input (learning the impression one makes on others)
- Catharsis (feeling and expressing powerful emotions)
- Cohesiveness (belonging, acceptance and loss of isolation)
- Self understanding (insight into previously unacknowledged parts of oneself)
- Interpersonal output (experience of successful relationships with others)
- Existential factors (facing death, meaninglessness, isolation and responsibility)
- Universality (not being alone in distress or problems)
- Installation of hope (seeing improvement in others)
- Altruism (being able to help others)
- Family re-enactment (understanding how childhood patterns are repeated)
- Guidance (didactic instruction and advice from group members or therapist)
- Identification (modelling behaviour on others)

A common theoretical basis

Primary emotional development is what happens to everybody as their psychosocial environment has an impact upon their developing personality; certain events such as trauma, abuse, deprivation and loss have an impact upon this development which can cause considerable damage. Of course, individuals are also born with differing needs and vulnerabilities. In groups, an environment for secondary emotional development is created: this is not as formative as the 'original experience', but it can make a considerable difference to behaviour, symptoms and somebody's concept of their personal identity core self.

A necessary sequence for both primary and secondary emotional development has been described in analytic terms (Haigh, 1996). This begins with attachment and containment, then moves through communication and involvement to an adult and autonomous position of agency. These stages all correspond to various aspects of Yalom's therapeutic factors, and could be seen to underpin the notion of 'non-specific therapeutic factors', often described as a contaminant in research. They are largely experienced unconsciously, and are the ways in which the therapeutic environment (including the therapist) affect the individual. They can also be construed as the 'culture' required for therapy to be effective: attachment corresponds to a culture of belonging; containment to a sense of safety; communication to a culture of openness or enquiry; involvement to inclusion or a living–learning experience; and agency and autonomy to a culture of empowerment. These factors can also be used to consider dynamics at levels of staff teams and institutions.

Aims of therapy

Group therapy aims to make patients more aware of themselves in relationship to others, to be better equipped to behave adaptively with others, and to gain more fulfilment in all human relationships. It has been said that individual therapy makes patients less neurotic but not necessarily any more mature, and that group therapy makes patients more mature but not necessarily any less neurotic. This indicates how difficult it is to define what the aims of group therapy are. Although research questionnaires can show that group therapy is effective in specific ways, they cannot accurately focus on the predominantly unconscious personality changes which group therapy hopes to achieve.

Patients asked to list problems that brought them into therapy usually amend the list as therapy progresses. Some of the initial problems become irrelevant as deeper underlying difficulties are exposed and some improve. New difficulties become evident as patients start to view their experience in different ways.

Group analytic psychotherapy is unusual amongst the analytically based psychotherapies in believing that change can come before insight. The task of understanding the meaning and dynamics of psychopathology in a rational way is less important than the experience of being part of a group in which a developmental process happens.

Principles of practice

Group psychotherapy requires a good flow of suitable referrals, facilities for seeing individuals for assessment and preparation, and for conducting the groups themselves. Although groups can be run successfully in independent private practice, it is generally easier for group therapists to be part of an organized professional network or a larger institution.

It is through scrupulous attention to detail about practical matters that much of the unconsciously perceived safety and belonging in a group will be secured. The therapist is responsible for preserving, protecting and maintaining the group setting as a space in which deep, intimate and mutative conversations can take place.

Referrals

Referrals will generally come from patients themselves, their general practitioners or mental health professionals. Most members of the public will have heard of group therapy, although the public image is probably closer to the original experiments than to current practice. Some will have a positive impression from friends or acquaintances who have benefited, but it is unlikely that individuals who seek therapy will think of a group as their first choice. This is in keeping with the wider individualistic rather than collective ethos which currently predominates.

General practitioners might be more aware of the benefits of group therapy, partly through awareness of group process used in general practice training. However, they are likely to be influenced by patients with defensive reasons for opposing referral for group therapy. If they know of good local services they may be better placed to recommend it for their patients. Practice counsellors may also be a good source of referrals; they will commonly have patients whose problems are too complex and deep-seated to deal with in the practice setting, yet who are well prepared for further therapeutic work.

Psychiatrists and other professionals in general mental health services may be a source of appropriate referrals. They will often have insufficient time and resources to explore the dynamics underlying the mental illness present in many of their patients. This will particularly be the case where there are marked disturbances in personality organization, which underlie a limited ability to cope with stress without becoming uncontainably symptomatic. A common example would be self-injury by cutting: often appropriately diagnosed as a depressive episode and successfully managed with physical treatment, the underlying psychopathology is rarely explored and understood enough to make a difference to the likelihood of subsequent episodes.

Group format

The most common format of out-patient groups is weekly sessions lasting for an hour and a half which start and finish punctually. A few therapists run more intensive treatment with twice-weekly groups: more than that is not practicable outside a specialist setting such as a therapeutic community. Out-patient groups are often timed to accommodate members' work or domestic obligations – in the evening, early morning or lunchtime. They normally have one or two therapists, and between six and ten members.

Groups may be *slow-open* or *closed*. A slow-open group runs continuously, often over many years, and has new members join as old ones leave. The length of stay can thus vary considerably according to the individual members' needs: a member would normally stay at least a year, and some may remain for three to five years or even longer. In a closed group, all the members start together and the group is set up to run for a specific time. Typically this would be eighteen months or two years. If there are early drop-outs, new members can be recruited after it has started – although late starters will receive a shorter period of therapy, and this needs to be considered when recruiting them. Both these types of groups will have breaks at holiday times – commonly two weeks at Christmas and Easter, and three or four weeks in the summer. There may be other breaks if the therapist needs to be away, or it may be negotiated for the group to meet without the therapist, or with a stand-in.

Newer and less common formats of groups include *block* and *termly* meetings. Block groups meet for intensive periods of group work which are widely spaced. For example, they might meet over a weekend to hold six ninety minute groups, and repeat this every two months. Termly groups have specific term dates, for example, four ten-week terms per year with gaps between. Members 'sign up' for one or a number of terms: those who feel ready to leave do so at the end of the terms, and new recruits join at the beginning of a term.

Communications outside the group

Patients need to understand professional confidentiality and routes of communication. This should be mentioned and explained to patients before they join a group. An example would be a telephone call to the therapist from a group member's general practitioner about a change of medication: it would reduce the therapist's effectiveness if he or she was expected by the patient to keep that sort of information confidential. Likewise, if a crisis develops, the group therapist might need to seek help from colleagues: such events are best treated in a spirit of collaboration, and discussed openly in the group. More complex confidentiality and boundary issues often arise, for example a group member whose children go to the same school as the therapist's children. In all cases they need to be handled with understanding and clarity: the boundaries must be understood by everybody, and difficulties cannot be ignored in the hope that they will go away.

There is usually no contact between the therapist and the group members outside the group. If there is any, it should be open for discussion within the group. Deliberate contact between patients outside of group time is strongly discouraged and needs to be addressed during the group. Usually, first names are used for everybody as this gives some degree of confidentiality.

There needs to be a reliable system for patients to inform the therapist about being late, unable to come or giving other messages in advance of groups. There may also be letters or phone calls from family members, friends or others – sometimes about a member who does not come to the group. Groups may also want to send messages or letters to absent members. It is up to the therapist to decide how to handle such issues, and how it is done will have an impact on the group.

Institutional considerations

If a group is being held in a building or institution which is not accustomed to having group therapy, explanation and preparation with various members of staff is worthwhile. The security and consistency of a group can be easily disturbed by very trivial practical events. Examples could include a previous user of the room who does not always finish on time, a receptionist who puts phone calls through, or a cleaner who vacuums the floor outside at the time the group is running. These can be minimized by time spent in thinking through likely problems beforehand, and explaining and discussing the requirements for running this type of group.

Which patient and why?

Referrals for group therapy need to be assessed for suitability for psychotherapy in general, and joining a group in particular. This is usually done as an individual appointment with a therapist. If the practical arrangements mean that the assessing therapist is not the group therapist, then it helps if the group therapist meets the patient individually at least once before starting in the group.

Ideal patients for out-patient group therapy are those with ego-dystonic personality traits, who see that those traits could be related to their symptoms, and which cause most problems in establishing and maintaining satisfactory relationships. Others to benefit include those who are more symptomatic: with anxiety in its many different forms, depression and other affective disturbance, somatic complaints without physical pathology, eating disorders, self-injurious behaviour and dependence on alcohol or drugs. However, patients with somatic complaints that are 'not negotiable' (i.e. fixed hypochondriasis) do not engage well in groups, and patients with active recent self-harm can be at risk of escalation unless this is appropriately addressed at assessment, with a clear contract if necessary. Some conditions, such as eating disorders, may be better treated in homogeneous groups where all the members have similar problems.

Patients who are likely to fare better in a group than in individual therapy are those for whom a number of different people to challenge established defences will prevent an impasse, and where involvement in a variety of relationships at different levels will be helpful. The former particularly includes patients who use intellectualization as a defence. The latter is useful where individual therapy would lead to an unmanageable transference – either dependent or hostile. The various relationships in a group will ensure that reality can be tested regularly and openly, so transferential expectations will always be open to challenge.

A reason sometimes given against group therapy is that a patient needs the individual attention, or is 'too fragile' to be able to tolerate joining a group. Many of these patients can be helped to join a group by a period of individual preparation, as two or more individual sessions. When anxieties about therapy are addressed and lessened in this way, clinical experience is usually that likelihood of subsequent drop-out is reduced. Shame and fear of compulsory exposure frequently need to be directly countered. Patients reluctant to join groups will often explain that they 'have enough troubles of their own, and do not want to take on others' problems as well'. This can be addressed with a discussion about the focus not being on problems, but on relationships in general – and how the experience of being able to help others is very often helpful in itself. Theoretically, this sort of unwillingness to accept a group is often a resistance which can be usefully explored, if done sensitively, and may add to the dynamic formulation.

Patients for whom out-patient group therapy is contraindicated are those who are not likely to benefit, who might become more disturbed by the therapy, or who might disrupt the group and stop it being beneficial for others. Diagnostically, there is good clinical consensus that this means acutely psychotic, actively addicted, sociopathic, hypochondriacal, paranoid or organically damaged patients. Acutely psychotic patients will not be able to engage in therapeutic relationships with the others, and their incomprehensibility is likely to be detrimental to cohesion and the necessary sense of safety for other members. Members actively addicted to alcohol or drugs are likely to be using the substances in a way that obscures and blunts their emotional availability for therapy, whether intoxicated or not during sessions. In the service of their addiction, they are also prone to deceit, secrecy and lying which are destructive processes for the whole group. Sociopathic members often at first appear engaging, lively and useful members of groups. However, when their fundamental inability to engage in empathic relationships is uncovered, very destructive consequences can occur. Predominant hypochondriacal symptoms are often suffered with such conviction that no psychological exploration of them is accepted: it can cause a great deal of frustration and wasted time in groups. Paranoid patients frequently suffer severe anxiety in groups, for which it is rarely possible to establish sufficient trust to explore or mitigate it. Brain damaged patients frequently lack the normal emotional responsiveness which is required to establish and use the type of relationships needed in group therapy.

Contraindications for heterogeneous group therapy
- Acute psychosis
- Active addiction to drugs or alcohol
- Sociopathic personality organization
- Severe hypochondriasis
- Paranoid personality organization
- Organic brain damage

Timing of group therapy is also important to consider in deeply depressed patients and those in the midst of life crises. Patients who have severe depression may well benefit from group therapy, but not at the time they are significantly retarded or actively suicidal. Retardation would mean that contact was very difficult to make, and discussion slow and frustrating. Although a group can be very helpful in safely containing some degree of suicidal feelings, frequent or severe expressions of suicidal intent cause considerable anxiety in other members, and can hamper the whole group. In such cases it may be more appropriate to start group therapy once antidepressant medication has started to improve mood, or when a course of medication has been completed.

In selecting group members, the mixture of patients must always be considered. In general, the more heterogeneous the better: age and gender should be as evenly balanced as possible, and a wide range of social, educational and occupational backgrounds is an advantage. In trying to achieve such a mix, care must be taken to avoid isolating single members – for example, one patient twenty years older than anybody else, or one member without any qualifications in a group of university graduates. For non-specialized out-patient group therapy, it is generally accepted that two patients with borderline personalities is the maximum that can be safely managed.

Which therapist and why?

All therapy requires a fundamental attitude of care, the capacity for empathy, and the ability to be affectively involved yet sufficiently detached to observe and think about what is happening. In group therapy, the therapist needs to be able to tolerate a high level of not understanding, and accept that too much goes on in groups for most of it to be directly addressed. Temptations for a therapist to impose his or her own solutions or understandings on the group need to be resisted. Therapists differ widely in their personal style: some speak more than others, some are charismatic and others quite authoritarian. 'Conductor' is a good word often applied to group therapists: one who has a view of the overall process and direction, and who uses that knowledge to help the others make their individual music fit into the overall composition.

For practitioners to conduct group therapy outside a training setting where close supervision is available, they should have undertaken an accreditable group therapy training. To be eligible for specialist accreditation, the therapist must have completed a training course with a recognized training institution. This includes supervised clinical practice, theoretical teaching and personal therapy in a group, over a minimum of three years. Fully trained and independent group therapists should also receive supervision for their work in some form.

In institutional settings, group therapy is often conducted by professional staff without specific group therapy training. Here, well-organized and regular supervision is obligatory, and other functions of the institution (examples include audit procedures, staff support, peer discussion, referral processes and in-patient facilities) will be in place.

A common way to introduce new therapists to groups is as the co-therapist with a more senior, trained therapist. This allows the trainee to be supported as much as necessary at first, but to have the scope to become more active and responsible as confidence and competence develop. Most psychotherapy services that use group therapy welcome motivated and competent trainees with appropriate professional backgrounds. It demands being sufficiently committed to regular and dependable attendance, for both the groups and for supervision. This can be quite an onerous commitment for busy professional staff, but it is often after this sort of clinical experience that potential therapists decide to undergo further training in groups.

Therapeutic setting

Group therapy in its widest sense takes place in numerous different settings. Examples include nurses organizing anxiety management groups in community mental health centres, probation officers running anger control courses for convicted offenders, psychologists taking cognitive behavioural groups for eating disorders, occupational therapists conducting skills groups, management trainers running personal development courses, psychiatrists running doctor–patient relationship seminars, staff from voluntary agencies setting up self-help groups, and many others. Although all these may have some general therapeutic effect, they do not constitute 'group psychotherapy' as a specific treatment in its own right, where experiencing and exploring relationships between the participants is the primary task.

A room for group therapy needs to be large enough to hold an evenly spaced circle of chairs, free from interruption, as quiet as possible and neither too hot nor cold. The chairs need to be comfortable enough to sit on for an hour and a half, but not so large and soft that group members are likely to fall asleep. They should all be a similar height, and there may be a small table in the middle of the circle. The room needs to appear constant from one session to the next, without major changes of decoration, furnishing or other features. Some group rooms are very plain and functional, and others have many items belonging to the therapist or which have been left by ex-members. Most therapists set up the circle before members arrive, and deliberately choose either to include or exclude chairs for members who have sent apologies.

Clinical example

Hilary was a 42-year-old single mother of two school age children. They had recently been in social services' care, and their father was her first husband, who left to remarry five years previously. She divorced her second husband after two years: he was alcoholic and violent. She was referred to the psychotherapy services by her community psychiatric nurse, six months after discharge from psychiatric hospital. She had a long history of depressive disorder, which was usually treated successfully as an out-patient with antidepressants. She had required one admission following the birth of her first child, when she needed ECT (electroconvulsive therapy) and was in hospital for five months. Her problems at referral were social isolation, slight agoraphobia and continuous low grade anxiety. She presented as mildly depressed and somewhat irritable. She took little care of her appearance and was dressed in old clothes.

Hilary was the last of three children, with two elder brothers. She had been a much-wanted girl, to 'complete' the family. Her father ran a small business and left the family when she was five to emigrate to Australia. Her mother received little financial support, and did not remarry or find another partner. She had a long admission to psychiatric hospital from when Hilary was seven: for this time, Hilary was separated from her brothers and stayed with a paternal aunt and uncle for eighteen months.

She remembered little of her childhood at the assessment appointment, apart from their standard of living dropping after father left, but thought it was 'fairly normal'. There were occasional visits from him. She did comment that there was no cuddling or physical affection in their household, and her mother was strict and expected high standards of her at school. The elder brothers were rather rebellious and were frequently in trouble. Hilary went to university and later qualified as a physiotherapist: she last worked in her late twenties, just before having her first child.

At initial assessment, she was frightened of the idea of a group and thought she would never be able to speak in it. The psychotherapist doing the assessment therefore arranged for her to have a number of individual sessions with the group therapist, Peter, before she started; they arranged three in the first case, but fitted in two more as she was not ready by then. The sessions were wide-ranging in content – initially about her current difficulties and failed marriages, then her specific concerns about talking in a group and later more general anxieties about being able to trust people at all, and ever being able to establish fulfilling intimate relationships. Peter was supportive, acted to avoid anxious silences, and was open about what group therapy entailed.

Hilary joined an established slow-open group; there were four other women, three men and Peter, the therapist. In her first group, she was attentive and silent for most of the session. She expressed some of her fears about exposure when gently prompted by Ann, a longstanding member of the group, about ten minutes before the end. For the next three months, she attended each week and sometimes contributed to the discussion of others' issues. She started to express doubts that the group could ever help her, and started to have practical difficulties in attending – she was often late and frequently phoned to apologize for being absent, in advance of the groups. After about four months, she missed a group without sending an apology and the other members expressed their concern, and irritation, that they did not know where she was or whether anything serious was wrong. At the next session, Peter commented that it seemed to be getting difficult for her to attend, and one of the others, Sarah, asked her how difficult it was for her to feel safe in the group, and trust the others enough for her to 'be herself' there. She became tearful, saying she did not know how to trust people and didn't know what 'being herself' was. After receiving some support from the others, she asked for the subject to be changed, and it was.

She did not attend the next group, and sent a letter to Peter explaining that her childcare arrangements had collapsed, and she wouldn't be able to come any more. She added that she had arranged for her GP to refer her to a psychiatrist for further treatment.

At the next meeting, the therapist gave the group the letter to read, and they discussed it. They were variously concerned, sad and angry. A decision was reached to write to Hilary, expressing concern and asking that she at least came back to 'say goodbye properly'. Peter agreed to get the letter typed and sent.

She returned the following week and spoke a great deal about how the psychiatrist she had seen in the meantime had offered her antidepressant medication and out-patient appointments, but suggested that she should really try to persevere with the psychotherapy. Over the next few weeks she spoke extensively about her disappointment with people in general, and particularly those in authority or with responsibility for her. She started to assert herself more strongly in discussions and was particularly firm when another new member talked about leaving prematurely: in fact he stayed. She spent time talking about what she began to see as her deprived childhood, and gave and took much support from others who had experienced similar upbringings.

When Hilary had been in the group about a year, one of the other members, Michael, formed a strong attachment to her. This caused problems when he started writing letters to her. After it had been going on for about six weeks, during which time she appeared sullen and unapproachable, she mentioned it in the group. The discussion led to the fact that they had met twice, and had sex on the second occasion; Michael wanted the relationship to continue, but Hilary was unsure. In a very difficult, tense group Michael decided to leave as he felt his feelings for Hilary were too overwhelming to be able to manage in the group: after a few months he joined another group.

Hilary started discussing a leaving date for herself, about eighteen months after she started: she planned it with three months' notice. Her life was better ordered, she had a much firmer and more coherent sense of self, and she had started in a job as a personal assistant to the chief executive of a small computer software company. She occasionally felt low and overwhelmed by the responsibility of bringing up her children, but had made one or two close friendships in which she could successfully ask for support.

In the last six weeks in the group, she divulged that she had been sexually abused several times by her uncle at the age of eight when her mother was in hospital, and it left her with great fears about ever managing to have a satisfactory sexual relationship with any man. Although she had never spoken of it to anybody beforehand, she spoke about it at some length. One of the other women in the group disclosed sexual abuse she suffered as a child, and Hilary postponed her leaving date by six weeks. By the time she left the group, she was a very important part of it. Her last session was a mixture of great sadness for the loss – both her of the others, and they of her – and excited anticipation that she would be much better able to cope with the stresses and traumas that her life would bring.

She was offered a follow-up appointment after three months but declined. She later remarried and was referred for couple therapy, to help with sexual difficulties, about two years after she finished in the group.

Problems in therapy

Unsuitable patients

However carefully they are assessed and selected, some unsuitable patients will find their way into groups. Some simply do not contribute or improve clinically, others find the group a strongly negative experience and some disrupt the useful processes of the group for its other members. There are various ways of categorizing these patients in terms of personality diagnosis, behaviour in the group or previous history, but these are always much clearer in retrospect than at assessment.

Some patients, such as borderline and narcissistic personalities, are referred for group therapy precisely because they are difficult. Others find the process of trusting people and being open about personal matters difficult. Within the group they may exhibit hostility, extreme quietness or defensive over-talking. These are routine matters for a well-functioning group to deal with and do not necessarily indicate that a patient should not be in a group.

However, some patients do turn out to be unsuitable. A member who becomes increasingly paranoid and suspicious of other members is likely to be harmed by staying in a group, however hard a diligent therapist or other members attempt to explore such suspicion, or demonstrate that it is groundless. Such a patient needs to leave the group, and although this is usually difficult and traumatic, it needs to be done. A patient who becomes increasingly depressed and unable to discuss this in a group is also likely to need other interventions – either medication or individual therapy. However, they may benefit from being 'held' by the group over a difficult time. Patients who undermine the safety and cohesiveness of a group in a way that cannot be openly scrutinized or modified must also be asked to leave as soon as possible. This includes obvious cases such as offensive or insensitive individuals who refuse to discuss their behaviour or see that it is unacceptable, and the much more subtle ways of undermining the group typical of charming, plausible and seductive individuals with marked antisocial personality structure.

Difficult group processes

'Basic assumption' processes, as described by Bion (1961), are inevitable stages of a group's life, and will usually come and go at different times, even in mature 'work' groups. Thus looking to the leader for the answers (dependency), attacking the way a group is functioning or being absent from it (fight–flight), and forming a degree of exclusivity within some member–member relationships (pairing) are processes which most groups will exhibit. If containment is well established by meticulous attention to all practical details, and the therapist is not made anxious by these perturbations, they can provide much useful material for the group to process – and transition to a work group culture will normally follow.

Two particularly difficult group processes which are less easy to manage well are *scapegoating* and *malignant mirroring*. Scapegoating is a projective process in which an individual is unconsciously invested with attributes and qualities that belong to the person who is disowning these qualities. In fact they are predominantly parts of their own personality which they find undesirable. If scapegoating goes unchecked, several members may round on one unfortunate in this way and, as the process is mostly out of conscious awareness, this person will be made to feel alienated (by projective identification) and may well leave. The therapist, and perhaps other members who sense that something 'odd' or unfair is going on out of conscious awareness, need to question, point out and explore what is happening. It is often most effective to openly 'share out' the negatively perceived qualities amongst all the members: everybody is then forced to look at the feelings they would rather disown. Also, the group therapist may be well placed effectively to draw negative feelings on to himself.

A similar process underlies malignant mirroring, but this is between two individuals. Each sees the other as behaving entirely unacceptably in some way, and they cannot be helped by support, interpretations, feedback or other interventions. No trust or depth of rapport can be established between them, and it can lead to splitting of the group into followers of each. Acceptance of the difficulty, time and patience can sometimes help to ameliorate malignant mirroring, but often one or both members need to leave that particular group.

Practical difficulties

Although there are therapist actions which will guarantee the demise of a group, there are none which will guarantee its survival. Particularly important is the safety which comes with meticulous attention to any issues concerning the boundaries around the therapy. Examples could include a member of a group seeking individual therapy without discussing it, or members giving each other lifts to and from groups which develop into social relationships. A well-functioning group will understand the need for the protection of the therapeutic space, and police itself. In a newer or more fragile group the therapist will need to take on this role in a more authoritative way: a group will often later reflect how useful such boundary-maintenance was. Unobtrusive attention to the physical space for the group, by making it comfortable and congenial, with satisfactory arrangements for members who arrive early or late and a regular routine for the therapist of joining and leaving the group on time, will help to prevent many practical difficulties.

Low membership is preventable in a slow-open group with a good source of referrals; new members can be introduced individually or in pairs until the group is a good size. In long-running slow-open groups with a good referral network, leavings and joinings can be co-ordinated so that the group remains at an optimum size. In a closed group, low membership is more problematic: members can drop out for several reasons, and the group can become unviable. It is not advisable to introduce new members for the last few months of a group, however small it has become, as they are unlikely to receive a satisfactory course of treatment.

Therapists differ in their views on the minimum acceptable number for conducting a group. Some cancel a group if less than three members attend, while others will consider the group is existing 'in mind' with a single member present. Groups differ, and some closed groups run satisfactorily to a planned ending with three members while others struggle considerably with five or six: adequately supervised clinical decisions need to be made about how to manage such situations.

Attendance of groups is often cyclical: there can be spells of weeks or months of full attendance, alternating with times during which there are many absences, often with good practical reasons given. Some therapists write standard letters after two missed sessions, and others make contact by telephone. Therapists will also vary in the balance between being supportive, directive or interpretative – a sensitive interpretation of difficulties in attending can lead to productive discussion and considerable improvement, as can a more directive statement to newer or less mature groups. Some patients will need more support, and these actions should be judged clinically with the particular patients in mind. Attendance is a particularly robust measure of how successfully a group is being conducted.

Misconceptions

Fears patients have of groups include forced exposure, unwelcome intimacy, their 'turn' coming round and not being taken seriously. In a well-conducted group, none of these things happens. It helps to explain to potential group members that the group 'becoming a safe place' is an important part of therapy itself, and taking turns, or being in 'the hot seat' or 'under the spotlight' is not how group psychotherapy works. Worries about not being taken seriously, and feeling shame or embarrassment about the reasons one is there can be helped by an accepting and empathic therapeutic demeanour, and a sufficient number of preparatory sessions.

New therapists often feel that they need to know exactly what is going on in the group at any moment, and to make accurate and helpful interpretations in order to earn their position as therapist. In truth, no group therapist knows 'exactly what is going on' at every moment of a group, and even if it were possible for one therapist to do so, another therapist is likely to have an equally valid but quite different understanding of the process. Interpretations are not the main tool of therapy, are often better coming from patients themselves or other group members than from the therapist, and should be used sparingly. It is a group analytic maxim that 'interpretations begin where analysis fails'.

Fallibility can often be helpful in working with patients' expectation of unrealistically high standards of themselves and others, although this should never include transgressing therapeutic boundaries. Most of what is discussed in therapy is serious and can frequently be upsetting – but there are lighter moments, and to experience a sense of playfulness (which can be light-heartedness, humour or gaiety) is often therapeutically helpful.

Evaluation of therapy

Research

Two notable British papers offer an interesting insight into different methods of conducting groups: Dick (1975) demonstrated the effectiveness of a group analytic approach using a variety of pragmatic outcome measures; Malan et al. (1976) discussed doubts and difficulties about the group methods developed from the work of Bion at the Tavistock Clinic.

Yalom is a prominent American researcher, and gives a very readable account of much of the work he has done (Yalom, 1985). Most notably, this includes the work which led to the development of the twelve therapeutic factors.

Bednar and Kaul (1994) provide a comprehensive overview of outcome and process research in groups, although their conclusions are somewhat circumspect. The only two robust inferences that they draw from an extensive literature review are:

- Group treatment is more effective than no treatment, placebo or non-specific treatments, but not all groups are uniformly beneficial.
- Evidence is insufficient to support any causal statements about the curative forces operating in the group context.

They suggest that methodological sophistication in the design of studies has exceeded the conceptual foundations upon which group therapy is based. These foundations will need to be considerably developed before satisfactory explanatory or causative processes are demonstrated. This will need much work with the elementary scientific methods of detailed and accurate observation and description.

Therapeutic outcome

The subjective outcome for patients, of a life with increased potential for satisfying relationships, and the experience of agency which underpins that, must be of central importance to clinicians and patients. These are not possible to measure directly, and any measured therapeutic outcome will be secondary to these changes.

The simplest psychotherapy research uses numerical questionnaires, which are validated instruments measuring observable or reportable variables. Examples include symptom ratings, interpersonal problems and self-esteem. The CORE (Clinical Outcomes in Routine Evaluation) is one of these measures, which uses a wide variety of clinically meaningful factors (Barkham *et al.*, 1998). Others use ideographic techniques, such as rating problems identified at referral, during and after therapy. Very pragmatic outcomes, for example employment status, are also used effectively.

Cost-offset studies are relevant for groups, and have been used in therapeutic community research. In these, the balance between the cost of treatment and the cost saved by treatment is examined. The costs saved can include primary health care time, accident and emergency attendances, psychiatric admissions, social services care for children, police, probation and prison costs, unemployment and use of other state benefits.

More direct measures of 'health care seeking behaviour', such as number of attendances at a general practitioner surgery before and after therapy, also have a strong theoretical foundation: such behaviour indicates an underlying attachment problem, concerned with the way in which care is sought, which is close to what group psychotherapy aims to modify and treat. Sophisticated clinical measures of attachment (the Adult Attachment Interview/AAI) have been developed and are used in some research centres to obtain a detailed assessment of problems of attachment, but no out-patient group research has yet been published using them.

Alternatives to therapy

If well prepared, most patients who are suitable for psychotherapy will benefit from group therapy. However, it is important not to assign patients to group psychotherapy who would be better served by a different approach.

For those unlikely to be well able to tolerate the increased anxiety that analytic therapy entails, a more directive group approach could be used. Examples are psychodrama, Gestalt, art therapy or symptom-directed treatments such as anxiety management, anger control or assertiveness training. Psychodrama, Gestalt and art therapy are all exploratory, but are more structured than interpersonal or group analytic psychotherapy. They are more suitable for patients who have difficulty in verbalizing their difficulties: they encourage symbolic representation or demonstration through action. The symptom-directed treatments do not pay direct heed to the dynamics underlying distress, and they focus on symptom resolution.

However, they will often also establish a therapeutic group milieu in which a reasonable degree of attachment, containment and communication can be experienced, to general therapeutic benefit.

Patients for whom group therapy is contraindicated will sometimes benefit from individual therapy. Certain diagnostic categories, such as active psychosis, could benefit from receiving group therapy in specific settings, such as in-patient groups. Others may benefit from a group approach at a later stage. The choice between individual and group psychotherapy will also depend on local availability of services. If an area is poorly served for groups, then few referrals will be made; if an area has a well-established group service but limited resources for individual psychotherapy, many patients will benefit from group therapy for whom it would not normally be considered the first line of treatment.

For those with a level of disturbance that is not manageable in an out-patient group, but would benefit from the general effects of group therapy, a more intensive treatment with a higher level of containment is indicated. This is particularly the case for patients with long and complex psychiatric histories, or those in whom the risk of impulsive or self-harming behaviour is high. It may be sufficient to run twice-weekly groups for such individuals, or to offer concurrent individual and group psychotherapy. Otherwise, the next 'level of intensity' of group therapy is a therapeutic community, where patients are immersed in a therapeutic milieu with groups for several hours each day, or are residential in such a setting. Such facilities provide a very high level of containment, challenge and support. Such containment could only be matched by acute psychiatric in-patient admission, the challenge by daily psychoanalysis, and the support by a close cohesive social network.

Further reading

Bion, W.R. (1961) *Experiences in Groups*. London: Tavistock.
Foulkes, S.H. (1964) *Therapeutic Group Analysis*. London: George Allen and Unwin.
Hinshelwood, R.D. (1987) *What Happens in Groups*. London: Free Association Books.
Pines, M. (1992) *Bion and Group Psychotherapy*. London: Routledge.
Yalom, I.D. (1985) *The Theory and Practice of Group Psychotherapy*, 3rd edn. New York: Basic Books.

Bibliography

Barkham, M., Evans, C. and Mellor-Clark, J. (1998) *CORE System Handbook*. University of Leeds: Psychological Treatments Research Centre.
Bednar, R.L. and Kaul, T. (1994) Experiential group research. In: A.E. Bergin and S.L. Garfield (eds), *Handbook of Psychotherapy and Behaviour Change*, 4th edn. New York: John Wiley, pp. 631–663.
Bion, W.R. (1961) *Experiences in Groups*. London: Tavistock.
Dick, B.M. (1975) A ten-year study of out-patient analytic group therapy. *British Journal of Psychiatry*, **127**, 365–375.

Foulkes, S.H. (1964) *Therapeutic Group Analysis*. London: George Allen and Unwin.

Haigh, R. (1996) The ghost in the machine: the matrix in the milieu. In: J. Georgas, M. Mantnovli, E. *et al.* (eds), *Contemporary Psychology in Europe: Theory, Research and Application*. Gottingen: Hogrefe and Huber.

Jones, M. (1968) *Social Psychiatry in Practice*. Harmondsworth: Penguin.

Main, T.F. (1983) The concept of the therapeutic community: variations and vicissitudes. In: M. Pines (ed.), *The Evolution of Group Analysis*. London: Routledge and Kegan Paul.

Malan, D., Balfour, F.H.G., Hood, V.G. and Shooter, A.M.N. (1976) Group psychotherapy. *Archives of General Psychiatry*, **33**, 1303–1315.

Pines, M. (1993) The world according to Kohut. *Group Analysis*, **26**, 47–63.

Yalom, I.D. (1985) *The Theory and Practice of Group Psychotherapy*, 3rd edn. New York: Basic Books.

14

Family Therapy

Steve Thwaites

Introduction

Contemporary family therapy is not one single model, but a number of different paradigms, approaches that may be used individually but which are increasingly used as an integrative, or combined, approach. As a consequence, therapists work with concepts and techniques drawn from different schools of family therapy. This chapter will focus on the three established methods: structural family therapy, strategic family therapy and Milan/post-Milan family therapy. For the sake of completeness it will also include a brief description of four further important approaches: brief/focused, behavioural, narrative and medical family therapy.

It is a common misunderstanding that family therapy has to involve the family, the whole family and nothing but the family. In reality family therapy can also be used with couples, individuals, parts of a family or even a wider network; in this chapter the term family will refer to all these different configurations.

Historical perspective

Although clinicians such as John Bowlby and J.L. Moreno had begun to involve families in therapy as early as the 1930s, it was only in the mid 1950s that the use of a family approach gained momentum. Its first applications were principally in the United States where psychiatrists started to involve family members in the treatment of psychotic patients. The significance of family dynamics was further developed by the findings of a Californian research group headed by Gregory Bateson, an anthropologist and philosopher. In 1956, this group introduced the theory of the 'double bind' as a central determinant of schizophrenia in children. A double bind is a communication where contradictory messages are delivered simultaneously through different levels of communication, such as verbal and non-verbal. Thus the recipient receives conflicting messages that they cannot logically disentangle.

From these early initiatives, two schools of family therapy evolved. In Palo Alto, California, the Mental Research Institute (MRI) developed the *strategic therapy* approach (particularly associated with Jay Haley and Chloe Madanes) and in Philadelphia, Salvador Minuchin established a *structural model* of family therapy. Both these models are described as 'first order' systemic approaches, because the therapist's position is one of an 'objective' observer positioned outside the processes of the family system.

In the 1970s, four Italian psychoanalysts (Selvini Palazzoli, Luigi Boscolo, Gianfranco Cecchin and Giuliana Prata) developed the *Milan systemic approach* from the earlier work of Bateson. It differed from preceding therapies by adopting a 'second order' systems perspective. Therapists were not seen as objective observers but as subjective participants of a 'therapy system'. It also looked beyond the presenting behaviours to understand the beliefs, rules and relationships influencing the functioning of the family system.

Since the introduction of the Milan approach, there have been two particular developments in family therapy that warrant inclusion. First, the field has been strongly influenced by feminism and a belief in anti-discriminatory and anti-oppressive practice. Therapy and therapists have concentrated upon redressing the effects of gender inequality, the abuse of power (including therapist power) and racial and cultural stereotyping. Secondly, the theoretical and ethical concerns of the therapist defining objective reality has stimulated a 'postmodern' movement which has developed the idea of '*post-Milan therapy*'. This model uses co-construction along with Milan therapy principles to produce therapy where problems are explored and developed jointly with the family and solutions are reached using the family's own strengths and strategies.

Principles of theory and practice

General principles of theory and practice

General systems

Family therapy can trace its roots back to General Systems Theory, a model that originates from biological and mechanical systems (von Bertalanffy, 1968). Principles from this theory have been continually developed in a form more commonly known as 'systemic thinking'. Systemic thinking can be applied to human behaviour and thought to develop therapy models that can address the complex and unique nature of human systems.

Human systems

A human system may involve an individual, a couple or any larger configuration. The principles that govern human systems determine that personal beliefs, actions and relationships are all interrelated. They too will influence the beliefs, behaviours and relationships of others, and will similarly be affected by others. Thus, as one part of a human system affects another, so that in turn will give feedback both to the originator and other parts of the system. It is not simply a case of cause and effect (linear action) but of complex interaction and feedback (systemic effect).

Interactive processes between beliefs, behaviours and relationships may be illustrated using an example of a poorly communicating family. Suppose a mother believes that a father is pushing their child too hard over schoolwork. She attempts to moderate the father's effect by protecting the child. If the father interprets her behaviour as holding the child back, he may push the child still harder. This may then be seen by the mother as further evidence that the father's over-zealous approach needs moderating. Subsequent action by each of them will feed into an escalating pattern. When two behaviours act to intensify each other (as with mother and father) the pattern can be said to be symmetrical. When an increase in one behaviour leads to a decrease in another the pattern is complementary.

Structural family therapy

Structural family therapy is inseparable from the charismatic approach of its prime originator, Salvador Minuchin. It is perhaps the most easily understood model as it is based upon changing those features in a family which do not conform to a number of core beliefs or shared family blueprint. In particular these beliefs include a family's need to have appropriate generational boundaries, rules and hierarchies in accordance with its current context. The model's strengths lie in its clarity, relative simplicity and usefulness with a wide range of family problems. However, some therapists may feel unhappy about the degree of directiveness the technique demands, and the influence and power invested in them.

Change is achieved by the therapist using a directive approach to alter family patterns to a 'healthier functioning form'. The family need not gain insight because appropriate change in their interactional patterns should result in a reduction of symptoms. The therapist uses a normative model of healthy family functioning that considers the family in terms of its boundaries, hierarchies and its life cycle stage. Relationships that are regarded as too close and over-involved are described as enmeshed, and those that are too distant as disengaged.

Techniques involved in a structural approach

Engagement (or joining)
This is the process by which the therapist negotiates a contract with the family and establishes a leadership role within the therapy (Minuchin and Fishman, 1981). The therapist will form personal connections with all family members which may be used to promote change.

Using a genogram
Genograms are used with all family therapy approaches and are included here because of their usefulness in laying out family information in a clear graphical form and 'mapping' family processes. Drawing the genogram may

facilitate engagement and subsequent work by the family. It should ideally include three generations of family members, to give information about inter-generational patterns. It may also include other significant people. Figure 14.1 shows a genogram drawn in standard convention and illustrating some significant events and relationships.

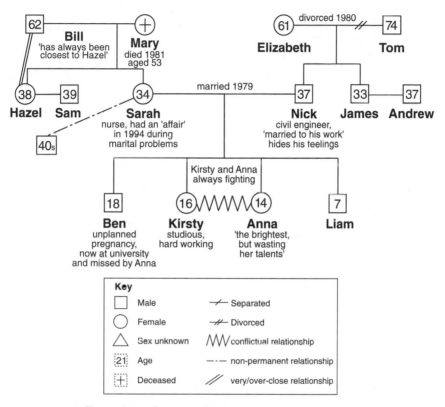

Figure 14.1   Example of a three generational genogram

Mapping the boundaries, sub-systems and relationships
The structural therapist will consider the family structure in terms of sub-systems (see Figure 14.2). These can be core structures of a family, i.e. an individual, a dyad (such as a husband and wife), or a generational grouping (children, grandparents). Sub-systems can also represent a common connection, e.g. family members with the same illness. The family itself can of course also be considered a sub-system of a larger system, such as a cultural or social group.

For example, a parenting sub-system may have a nominal membership of one biological and one step-parent. If the step-parent is helping raise the children of the biological parent but this is not acknowledged within the family then there is confusion over membership of the parenting sub-system. Conversely, if they are never allowed a parenting role this may indicate a too rigid boundary around parenting.

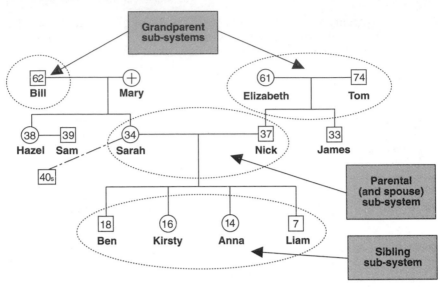

Figure 14.2 Examples of family sub-systems

Once the problems are defined in terms of difficulties within the sub-systems, the therapist will seek to alter them to a more healthy form. In the above example it would be a case of clarifying who was in the parenting role(s) and ensuring this function was consistently carried out.

The properties of each sub-system can be considered in terms of:
- Who participates in it (membership)
- How clear the boundaries are (the degree of consensus on membership)
- How firm the boundaries are (how easily members can move in and out)
- What the functions are (e.g. parenting)

Reframing

In structural therapy a 'reframe' is the process whereby the therapist challenges the existing description of a problem and offers an alternative that fits equally well. The intention is to change existing interactional patterns by the re-description of behaviours. For example, a teenage anorexic's refusal to eat might be reframed from 'illness' to 'challenging behaviour', thereby moving it from the domain of medical treatment to that of parenting problems.

Directive and restructuring interventions

A behavioural way in which the therapist can create change is by intervening directly in family patterns. This may be done by developing an alliance with a particular family member in order to strengthen their position or by interrupting communication between members of the family to break unwanted patterns. Moving individuals within the therapy room, e.g. a child from between two parents, can also help to establish appropriate boundaries.

Strategic family therapy

Strategic therapy works by using interventions that reduce the power which the symptom has over the family thus freeing the system up. Strategic therapy does not use a normative model of functioning but aims to provide a brief intervention that moves the family towards a healthier way of relating. Whilst strategic therapy can change deeply entrenched behaviours, possibly in a short time, some of its techniques may be considered manipulative.

Symptoms are seen as an indication that a family is at a life cycle transitional stage but is having problems re-structuring around it: for example, where a parent develops agoraphobia at a point when their last child is preparing to become more independent, thus necessitating the delay of that independence. Unhelpful repetitive sequences, such as occasional relapses, then occur whenever change is threatened. These will occur in place of more complex adaptive changes, for example adjusting to life without children. Therapy involves getting the family to interrupt these repetitive sequences and move to a new (and more adaptive) range of responses.

Working strategically with behaviour patterns

Reframing
Reframes in strategic therapy are intended to alter interactional patterns. For example, reframing the above agoraphobia as 'the parent giving up their own independence to help their child become independent' would be intended to alter the meaning (and power) attached to the sequence and thereby modify the interactions themselves.

Direct and paradoxical interventions
As previously described, interventions will be intended to interrupt repetitive and unproductive sequences. They may be in the form of messages or tasks having a direct action or, if the family commonly oppose the therapist or change, a paradoxical approach may be called for.

Examples of direct and paradoxical interventions
- Prescribing the symptom: this is a paradoxical intervention that discourages negative behaviours by requiring that they be carried out in an organized and burdensome fashion. (For example, a teenager who never attends Sunday lunch could be told to make announcements at 10 am, 11 am and noon that he is going to miss the meal.)
- Symbolic acts: these attempts to reduce dangerous or destructive behaviours by encouraging them to be acted out in symbolic rather than real fashion. (For example, getting a person to replace visible self-mutilation by drawing or painting injuries to themselves.)
- Prescribing 'pretending to have the symptom' ritualizes the symptomatic behaviour and the gains that follow. (For example, a child who has headaches to receive attention will be asked to pretend to have them and for the parent to continue to provide the attention. In time the headache becomes unnecessary for the child to obtain attention.)

Milan and post-Milan approaches

These methods work through the exploration and clarification of how family ideas, beliefs, relationships and actions relate to the presenting problems. As well as personal beliefs, therapy will explore the influence of family myths and scripts, such as 'we are a family who must always look after each other'. The therapist uses a stance of 'curiosity' to explore and challenge existing links and introduce possible new connections. Post-Milan therapy differs from its predecessor primarily by the greater use of explanations co-constructed by therapist and family rather than by therapist alone.

Working with family belief systems

Neutrality
Neutrality refers to a specific stance originally adopted by the Milan team which has become a core concept of systemic therapy. In its original form, the therapist's aim was to avoid making moral judgements and be seen as a non-allied figure working at a more removed (meta) level (Palazzoli *et al.*, 1980). The concern about this approach is that therapy could endorse a 'moral neutrality' (Jones, 1993), for example where both an abuser and the abused would be afforded equal validation. This is clearly unacceptable, and the concept of neutrality – whilst still of central importance – must be used judiciously and with great care. The post-Milan approach views neutrality more as a recognition and measured use of the therapist's beliefs rather than a suspension of them.

Hypothesizing
A hypothesis is a systemic conjecture of how the presenting problem links with family processes, relationships and beliefs. It will be developed by the therapist and team prior to a session and modified according to subsequent feedback. It is not usually shared explicitly with a family, but used by the therapist to guide their circular questioning. A hypothesis is not necessarily truer than the family's explanation, but it introduces new and potentially more helpful systemic ideas into the system.

Circular questioning
Circular questioning is a process that brings out connections between actions, beliefs and relationships of individuals within a family (Campbell *et al.*, 1991) (see Box on p. 281 for examples). The circularity referred to is the process of using responses to construct further questions that build to form a complex picture of relationships, behaviours and beliefs. Many questions will explore family processes through the eyes of different family members, thus gaining a number of perspectives. Circular questioning will normally involve interweaving the questioning of a number of family members at one time.

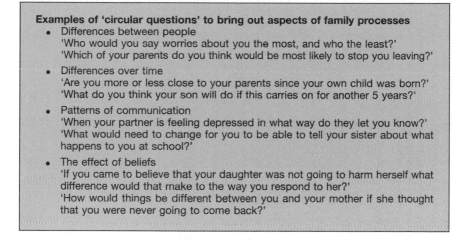

Examples of 'circular questions' to bring out aspects of family processes
- Differences between people
  'Who would you say worries about you the most, and who the least?'
  'Which of your parents do you think would be most likely to stop you leaving?'
- Differences over time
  'Are you more or less close to your parents since your own child was born?'
  'What do you think your son will do if this carries on for another 5 years?'
- Patterns of communication
  'When your partner is feeling depressed in what way do they let you know?'
  'What would need to change for you to be able to tell your sister about what happens to you at school?'
- The effect of beliefs
  'If you came to believe that your daughter was not going to harm herself what difference would that make to the way you respond to her?'
  'How would things be different between you and your mother if she thought that you were never going to come back?'

Reframing

In this context reframing usually offers new meanings to unhelpful beliefs and behaviours. A reframe that explicitly seeks to alter the meaning of a behaviour or belief by putting it in a positive light is described as giving it a positive connotation.

For example, a therapist may wish to use a reframe to help a couple who have become stuck in a pattern of mutual blaming. With a knowledge that each had been raised in a depressed household, the blaming could be reframed as their wish to avoid replicating problems from their own families of origin by energizing the other so that they will not lapse into depression. This would allow the therapy to address their concerns and fears rather than who is at fault.

End of session intervention (message or task)

The purpose of an end of session intervention is not usually disclosed as its effect is through the impact of its content. Interventions may be direct (e.g. giving straight feedback or a task) or paradoxical (where the prescribed message is intended to perturb rather than reinforce). A split message is a technique that allows the therapy team to introduce an awkward or controversial idea without alienating themselves from the family. Two opposing ideas, one of which is the controversial suggestion, are given with the message that both are being offered for the family to consider. This allows the therapist and family to address the merits and disadvantages of each idea.

Working with a team

The Milan Schools use a peer team who observe the therapy specifically to provide the therapist with consultation on the therapy process. The team will assist in the formulation of hypotheses and introduce ideas and comments about the therapist–family system. They are not superior to the therapist but offer a one-removed or 'meta' view of the therapy. A reflecting team

(Anderson, 1987) is where the observing team discuss their thoughts and ideas openly in front of the therapist and family. This enables the family to become observers to a discussion on their own family processes. These processes are discussed more fully in the 'supervision' section.

Other models

There are a number of other models of interest in current family therapy approaches. These include:

- **Brief therapy/solution-focused therapy:** Both these methods seekto achieve expedient resolution of the presenting problems or symptoms. The therapist works with any clients (or 'customers') who are motivated to change by using a range of strategies and techniques that work toward desired change rather than past problems (De Shazer, 1984). Solution-focused therapy is particularly noted for emphasizing clients' coping strategies by concentrating upon the occasions when they have overcome other difficulties.
- **The narrative or 'externalizing the problem' approach:** Aims to help people separate from 'problem saturated' descriptions in their lives (White, 1988). This method entails identifying the dominant problem and co-constructing it as an external force or will that is exerting an unwanted influence. Therapy may help the family or individual resist and then overcome the problem that wishes to 'dominate' their lives.
- **Medical family therapy:** This approach from North America is used to help families and individuals affected with chronic physical conditions that are (or are seen as) having a biological foundation. The family therapist uses a biopsychosocial systems model to address the role which the illness plays in the family dynamics and for the person individually (Doherty et al., 1994). The aim of therapy is to help the patient (and their family) cope with the effects of chronic illness or disability and to reduce conflict around it.
- **Behavioural family therapy:** Following a thorough assessment that may involve individual interviews, interventions are designed to produce specific behavioural change. This model places great emphasis upon using proven techniques, for example, parent training or problem solving. It claims to be particularly useful with conduct disorders and adult mental illness (Falloon, 1991).

Aims of therapy

The aims of therapy will be related to the clinical context and the style of therapy used. Thus family therapy used in a Social Services setting may aim to reunite a child with their family, while in a mental health clinic its aim is to contribute towards recovery from a psychiatric illness. More specifically, each model of therapy will have aims in accordance with its own theory of change. Structural therapy will aim to improve family functioning and reduce symptomatic behaviour through the introduction of appropriate boundaries and structures. In Strategic therapy the aim is to help individuals or a family become 'unstuck' from patterns of behaviour that are problematic and which prevent them from moving on in their life cycle. The aim is not to provide insight but to change behaviour in an expedient and effective fashion. In the Milan systemic therapies the intention is to develop change through systemic understanding that allows individual members to have greater choice and agency.

Which patient and why?

Assessment for family therapy should be regarded as a two-way process. Both the family and the therapist will need to assure themselves that the timing, the setting and the nature of the problem make family therapy the right choice.

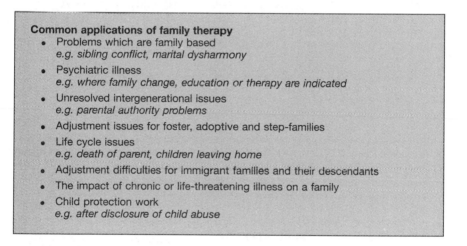

Common applications of family therapy
- Problems which are family based
  e.g. sibling conflict, marital dysharmony
- Psychiatric illness
  e.g. where family change, education or therapy are indicated
- Unresolved intergenerational issues
  e.g. parental authority problems
- Adjustment issues for foster, adoptive and step-families
- Life cycle issues
  e.g. death of parent, children leaving home
- Adjustment difficulties for immigrant families and their descendants
- The impact of chronic or life-threatening illness on a family
- Child protection work
  e.g. after disclosure of child abuse

The referral

Many families find themselves referred for family therapy without sufficient explanation or discussion. It is important to establish the appropriateness of the referral and how well the family have been prepared for therapy. A referral may also indicate how much belief the referrer has in family therapy and whether other treatments are being pursued concurrently.

A good referral will include: a comprehensive description of family composition, ideas of how the problems relate to family dynamics, and a summary of how these issues have been addressed to date. It is also helpful to know what expectations the referrer and family have for outcome. The two principal reasons for rejecting or postponing a referral are either because it is not adequately supported by the referrer or family, or there needs to be a clarification or resolution of other issues, such as court proceedings, first.

Useful information in a referral
- Family members' names, ages and relationship
- History of problem and significant family events
- Referrer's thoughts on the relationship between problems and family function
- Previous and current therapies
- Expectations of therapy (referrer and family)
- Information given to family about what to expect of family therapy

Assessment appointment

The assessment appointment gives the therapist information on who in the family will attend, how motivated they are and what style of therapy is likely to be most helpful. The exploration of these issues also allows the family to judge how they feel about a family approach. As well as information to compile a genogram the assessment appointment needs to explore how the family interact (both currently and in the past) and how this relates to their difficulties. This information will allow the therapist to develop a working hypothesis. It is likely that even after an initial meeting the family will be given feedback and possibly a therapeutic task, both as an intervention and to assess their degree of motivation. If further therapy is agreed, this may be either a fixed number of sessions or a more open contract.

Indications for family therapy

Family therapy is used for individual or interpersonal difficulties that can be addressed through the way they affect and are affected by relationships. This does not necessarily require the presence of the whole family. An individual can be helped to gain a systemic understanding of important processes within their family that can allow them to make changes.

Contraindications for family therapy

Family therapy can be counterproductive where its use inappropriately delays important processes such as child protection, divorce or other legal proceedings. There are also instances where individual therapy needs to precede any family intervention so that an individual is sufficiently prepared to work in a family context. Working with the survivors of sexual abuse commonly falls into this category. Other important contraindications include situations where there is a risk to personal safety within treatment sessions, and where therapy is seen to be maintaining the problem.

Which therapist and why?

The majority of family therapists have primary professional qualifications as psychiatric nurses, psychiatrists, social workers or psychologists, and in the United Kingdom most are employed as such. Many combine family therapy with other responsibilities (e.g. child protection, provision of mental health care) and will use an approach that links therapy, their professional role and the organizational context. Family therapy practised within a specific professional role carries distinct issues. Whilst the theoretical background gives the therapist a broad knowledge base – enabling them to relate the therapy to other organizational and clinical procedures – it can also prejudice therapist neutrality through the conflict of roles. Many family therapists will also integrate systemic practice into their other clinical and managerial work.

Training

Family therapy training is organized into introductory, intermediate and advanced level courses. Most of these courses are part time, and have a strong emphasis on linking training with the students' clinical practice setting. Training takes a minimum of four years with an additional supervised post qualifying practice year. At introductory level, training focuses upon systemic thinking, the different models of therapy, basic family processes and interviewing techniques. Intermediate training involves studying these themes in greater depth and linking them with the students' own clinical work. The advanced training takes an additional two years and has a major element of supervised clinical practice along with a research dissertation and advanced theoretical study. Training at the advanced level will be accredited to MSc standard and teaches students to a level where they can work as independent practitioners. Post-registration courses in supervision, training and research are now becoming increasingly common.

Supervision

There are specific requirements for the supervised practice of trainees and the ongoing professional development of qualified therapists. As discussed previously, many therapists will also use peer supervision as part of their working practice. Although co-working (two therapists working jointly) is common, it does not allow an outside viewpoint and is perhaps the least suitable supervisory arrangement. It is preferable for one therapist to assume a supervisory role in the therapy room and communicate with the therapist rather than participating actively in interviewing the family.

A supervising team will need to communicate freely amongst themselves and will normally work in a separate room. Therapy will be followed either through a one-way screen or via a video link. Communication between team and therapist can occur using a telephone link, an ear bug or by the therapist speaking directly with the team. Additionally, the therapist will take a number of breaks during a session to consult with the supervising team. Some family therapists use the technique of observing team participation (reflecting team or 'Greek chorus'), where the observers come into the room and have a discussion amongst themselves about what is going on in the family.

Therapeutic setting

A purpose designed setting for family therapy will usually include a one-way screen with observation room, a connecting telephone and video equipment. Such a setting will mainly be found in mental health clinics and training agencies, and whilst desirable is not essential. In circumstances where a screen is not available the therapist and supervising team may work within one room, so long as they are accustomed to such an approach and have previously negotiated rules for the session. In these circumstances it is customary for the supervisor(s) to sit outside the circle of therapist and family in order to identify their different function. The therapy room must be big enough not to become oppressive during the 1 to $1\frac{1}{2}$ hours that sessions normally last, particularly where some of the family may be restless or angry. When there are young children involved, toys and drawing materials can prolong their involvement (and therefore that of the adults). Many families will want to leave the therapy room if the team are taking a break of ten minutes or longer, often preferring to wait in the reception or outside. A quiet and private room, comfortable chairs and pleasant surroundings are all obvious contributors to a positive working environment.

Family therapy in the home is only indicated when a family has genuine difficulties attending a clinic or when it is used to engage a family who would otherwise be unlikely to come into therapy (Reimers, 1994). The main arguments against using the family home are firstly the lack of control the therapist has over the setting, for example with interruptions and distractions, and secondly the difficulties in clearly demarcating therapy from everyday activity. While therapy in a home setting is possible, it is only with the full commitment of a family that a reasonably successful outcome could be expected.

Clinical example: a post-Milan approach

Mark Edwards (17), his two brothers, John (19) and James (13), along with their mother, Mary (37), were referred by their general practitioner to the local psychiatric clinic for family therapy. Five years earlier, Mary had separated from her violent husband, Alan, and since then had suffered recurrent bouts of depression. Her GP had treated this with antidepressant medication and tried, unsuccessfully, to get her to accept individual psychotherapy. At her most recent appointment she had sought advice in managing her middle son, Mark, whom she was worried was becoming beyond her control. His behaviour, notably bad tempers and excessive drinking, was upsetting the rest of the family, particularly his younger brother, James. Mary had wanted individual treatment for Mark but after some persuasion by her GP was referred for family therapy.

The hypothesis
Prior to the appointment, the therapist and team constructed an initial hypothesis based upon the referral letter from the GP. Their systemic hypothesis began with the idea that Mary had not resolved her feelings about her ex-husband, Alan, and it was likely the 'family script' would identify him as somebody who

had only been destructive to the family. Given that Mark was now becoming troublesome, it was probable that in some way his behaviour was linked to the story that was being held about his father. From Mark's perspective, he may believe that he had to choose between rejecting his father, or being like him. The hypothesis adopted the idea that Mark was indeed showing loyalty to his father, despite (or because of) the rejection by the rest of his family. In believing that Mark's behaviour could only worsen their mother's depression, his brothers may be trying to scapegoat him to protect her.

The first session
The first session was used by the therapist to engage the family, begin to explore their dynamics and answer their questions about therapy. In the process of engagement the therapist sought to acknowledge the views and situation of each participant. This was partly to shift the focus from Mark but also so that each person felt valued. Guided by the hypothesis, the questioning explored the relationship of the children with their father, each other and the consequences of the current problems. It emerged that Mark had been the only child to regularly see his father and that this was an ongoing source of conflict with his elder brother, John. Since the divorce John had adopted a role of supporting his mother which had developed into a relationship that bound them loyally to each other. John had also come to feel trapped in this relationship, which he saw as now affecting his own life. Both Mark and John were able to recognize how, over time, they had come to take up opposing positions in the family regarding their father. The first session concluded with the family being given positive feedback on their wish for change and that the therapist could see that not only Mark was finding things difficult. An agreement was made for four further sessions, each of one hour.

Following appointments
In the subsequent sessions, therapy looked in greater depth at the difficulties each was facing. Mark and John talked of the mixed feelings each had about their parents and how they were pushed into taking up extreme positions. Mark revealed the jealousy he felt over the closeness of John and his mother, but also came to understand how trapped John felt in this role. Correspondingly, John was able to address his wish to know his father in the way Mark had. Thus the beliefs that had been built up were explored and altered through the conversations. During this process James listened, and seemed to gain from the conversation his brothers were having. John and Mark started meeting together outside of sessions. However, Mary repeatedly said therapy was not working and that the problems at home were continuing (in stark contrast to what her sons were saying). It seemed that she could not easily accept the changes that had been made. The therapist decided not to see the sons for a while but to see Mary alone. The sessions were put to her as a way of helping her as a sole parent. These meetings were able to broaden the discussion from parenting issues to include Mary's own emotional needs. She was praised for having put her own needs second to those of the family, but told she now needed to address them to enable the family to move on. The family was offered occasional supportive sessions and Mary subsequently chose to get counselling for herself in her own right.

Problems in therapy

Becoming 'wedded' to a hypothesis

A hypothesis should be used by the therapist as a way of proposing alternative explanations, and not advocating a 'truth'. If the feedback from the therapy sessions does not fit the hypothesis then the hypothesis should be modified. Becoming wedded to a particular belief and then attributing lack of confirmation to poor therapist skills or family 'denial' will not facilitate positive change.

Symmetrical conflict between therapist and family

This may occur when a therapist or therapists become over-attached or 'wedded' to one idea and fail to address the differences of opinion which are developing between themselves and the family. The more the therapist pushes for one course of action, the stronger the family oppose the push. For example, if a therapist repeatedly sets a task for a father to play with his children, but fails to understand that the father is holding back fearing failure, then the family will oppose the therapist's efforts. If the therapist interprets this opposition as 'resistance' and prescribes further tasks, conflict between therapist and family will escalate.

Attributing blame

It is rarely helpful to attribute blame when understanding the nature or origins of individual or family problems. However, it is essential that individuals (particularly adults) are considered responsible for their own actions, especially when that action is violent or abusive. It is an epistemological error when understanding circular patterns of effect, to deny the effects of inequality of power by believing that each individual has equal influence.

Work against resistance

Most contemporary practitioners would not see resistance as an inherent quality of a family but as a theoretical construction made by the therapist. Neither would they regard resistance purely as the antithesis of cooperation. Perhaps the most helpful stance is to regard the opposition (resistance) a family puts up as an indication that therapy is not providing them with help in a form they can use. Reframing resistance in this way has become a trademark of the brief therapy movement.

Failure to engage with a family

If a therapist is to establish a trusting cooperative relationship with a family it is important that the family feel understood, validated and fairly treated. However, building a therapeutic relationship at the same time as practising new skills can also be difficult. Too much concentration on technique can make the therapist come across as uncaring and mechanical. Similarly, if a therapist does not recognize their own personal biases then this will affect their ability to treat a family with fairness and impartiality.

Loss of neutrality

Similarly, family therapists need to be alert to a danger of marginalizing some members or forming over-strong alliances with others. By acknowledging and addressing the influence of their own family background, gender, race and class a therapist will be more able to adopt a fair and therapeutic position. Emotive issues such as sexual abuse, violence or gender attitudes are all areas that require particularly careful consideration.

Labelling families as dysfunctional or pathological

Labelling families in this way is a process that can both dehumanize them and deny the reality of their experiences. A more helpful approach is to look upon the family's behaviours, however discordant with the therapist's beliefs, as being positively motivated and representing their best attempt to overcome their difficulties. It is more likely an overbearing parent will respond to therapy if the therapist can believe they want the best for their child rather than that they are pathologically controlling.

Evaluation of therapy

Research

There is no doubt that the complexity of family processes coupled with the individuality of therapeutic approaches has favoured the use of clinical description rather than empirical evaluation of family therapy outcomes. However, the increasing demand for evidence based practice has encouraged the development of family rating scales and outcome studies. Many of these studies have been on a small scale and have examined practice in a particular clinical setting or with a certain client group. Consequently, many have been so idiosyncratic that the results can only contribute toward a broad picture of family therapy efficacy. These studies, and the majority of the larger ones, have been in the field of mental health, particularly examining therapy with the families of schizophrenics and adolescents with eating disorders.

Some of the more scientific studies have looked at the effectiveness of family therapy (particularly using a psychoeducational approach) in decreasing expressed emotion (EE) in the families of schizophrenics. High EE (criticism and over-involvement) has thus been shown to increase relapses in schizophrenics (Berkowitz, 1988). There is substantial evidence that adopting such an approach, in addition to medication, can reduce relapse rates from 50% to 9% (Leff et al., 1982).

Dare et al. (1995) have found that the family and personal dynamics of young people with anorexia are too complex to provide a similar generalized measure of the efficacy of family therapy. High parental criticism (EE) of the child was discovered to be an indicator of a high drop-out rate as well as poor therapeutic outcome (Le Grange et al., 1992). As a result of this finding, a model called 'family counselling' has been developed, where family therapy techniques combined with an educative approach are used with the parents and the child in separate sessions. The results of the study concluded that family therapy was more effective than individual psychotherapy when the anorexia had begun in adolescence, and as effective for onset in adulthood. This and other studies also suggest family therapy can play a significant part in the treatment of adolescent bulimia.

Overall, recent research suggests family therapy is most effective for psychiatric disorders when it is applied flexibly, with different treatment approaches being determined by both the clinical condition and family factors. This would include working with different family configurations, the inclusion of psychoeducational methods and the use of family therapy in conjunction with other treatments.

Financial implications

The use of teams in family therapy can lead to it being wrongly considered an inefficient and expensive process. It is only in training contexts that large teams, such as used by the Milan School, are usually found. Many family therapists will work alone, in pairs or as part of small teams. Additionally, whilst family therapy may be used for periods over a year, it will be rare for treatment to extend to more than ten sessions in total. Family therapy has developed as a pragmatic approach, able to address agency as well as family problems, and it is thus an effective and efficient intervention in many therapeutic settings.

Alternatives to family therapy

Family therapy should be a first choice where a presenting problem is seen to be caused or maintained by family factors. It does not necessarily require the whole family to attend, as taking a systemic approach can even enable an individual to consider the impact of different relationships (past, present and future). Some models of family therapy, such as Structural therapy, are less reliant upon complex thinking or language than others, and this may be a consideration in their applicability for certain families or individuals.

Family therapy may be second choice to any short- or medium-term therapy if an individual feels able to address issues in a family or relational context. It may also be used in place of some group therapies and as a substitute for marital or couples therapy. Whilst not providing the degree of personal insight of some individual therapies, family therapy can effect change in individuals, families and professional systems with substantial and lasting effect.

Through the use of a systemic approach family therapy can be compatible with many other treatments, even if their associated beliefs and methods are widely different. Systemic family therapy should not be portrayed to families as the only way to proceed, with other approaches presented as 'wrong' in some way; treatment choices should be made with informed consent. If family therapy is to be used in conjunction with other treatments then the preliminary work with a family would need to include addressing the implications of working concurrently with different treatment modalities. Family therapy is often an important component in the treatment of complex psychological problems, particularly with young people. When used in this way it can be successfully combined with other treatments, including medication and individual psychotherapy.

Further reading

Barker, P. (1981) *Basic Family Therapy*. London: Granada.
Burnham, J. (1988) *Family Therapy*. London: Routledge.
Jones, E. (1993) *Family Systems Therapy*. Chichester: John Wiley.

Bibliography

Anderson, T. (1987) The reflecting team: dialogue and meta-dialogue in clinical work. *Family Process*, **26**, 415–428.
Berkowitz, R. (1988) Family therapy and adult mental illness: schizophrenia and depression. *Journal of Family Therapy*, **10**, 339–356.
Campbell, D., Draper, R. and Crutchley, E. (1991) The Milan systemic approach to family therapy. In: A. Gurman and D. Kniskern (eds), *Handbook of Family Therapy*, Volume II. New York: Brunner/Mazel, pp. 325–362.
Dare, C., Eisler, I., Colahan, M., Crowther, C., Senior, R. and Asen, E. (1995) The Listening Heart and the Chi Square: clinical and empirical perceptions in the family therapy of anorexia nervosa. *Journal of Family Therapy*, **17**, 31–57.
De Shazer, S. (1984) The death of resistance. *Family Process*, **23**, 11–17.
Doherty, W., McDaniel, S. and Hepworth, J. (1994) Medical family therapy: an emerging arena for family therapy. *Journal of Family Therapy*, **16**, 31–46.
Falloon, I. (1991) Behavioural family therapy. In: A. Gurman and D. Kniskern (eds), *Handbook of Family Therapy*, Volume II. New York: Brunner/Mazel, pp. 65–95.
Le Grange, D., Eisler, I., Dare, C. and Hodes, M. (1992) Family criticism and self starvation: a study of expressed emotion. *Journal of Family Therapy*, **14**, 177–192.
Leff, J., Kuipers, L., Berkowitz, R., Eberlein-Vries, R. and Sturgeon, D. (1982) A controlled trial of social intervention in the families of schizophrenic patients. *British Journal of Psychiatry*, **141**, 121–134.
Minuchin, S. and Fishman H. (1981) *Family Therapy Techniques*. Cambridge, MA: Harvard University Press.
Palazzoli, M., Boscolo, L., Cecchin, G. and Prata, G. (1980) Hypothesising-circularity-neutrality: three guidelines for the conductor of the session. *Family Process*, **19**, 3–12.
Reimers, S. (1994) Bringing it back home: putting a user-friendly perspective into practice. In: S. Reimers and A. Treacher (eds), *Introducing User Friendly Family Therapy*. London: Routledge, pp. 220–240.
Von Bertalanffy, L. (1968) *General Systems Theory*. Harmondsworth: Penguin.
White, M. (1989) The externalising of the problem and the re-authoring of lives and relationships. In: *Selected Papers*. Adelaide: Dulwich Centre Publications, pp. 5–28.

15
Therapeutic Communities

Gill McGauley

Introduction

The term 'therapeutic community' is currently applied to a wide range
of institutions which, although united by some common concepts, have
very different histories and have consequently been shaped by different
ideals and therapeutic approaches. The meaning of the term is further
complicated by the fact that it is sometimes applied, without clear
discrimination, to units which have only adopted a few therapeutic
community principles. It is therefore important to differentiate between
those units which have adopted a therapeutic community approach as
compared to those establishments which have maintained the original
therapeutic community ideals and principles. This latter group work much
more actively within the ethos of a therapeutic community, irrespective
of their historical developmental differences, and are best referred to as
therapeutic communities proper.

Historical perspective

The democratic–analytic community

The current therapeutic community approach in Britain derives from two
historical developments which have generated distinct styles of therapeutic
community. The first style developed as a result of the psychiatric and social
problems which were the legacy of the Second World War. There was a need
to treat large numbers of psychiatric casualties, and to focus on problems
such as morale rather than on individual difficulties. Dr Tom Main, in 1946,
first used the term 'therapeutic community' to describe the approach that
developed to deal with these issues at the Northfield Hospital in Birmingham
(Main, 1946). It was a military hospital where several doctors, including
Main, Foulkes and Bion, were posted during the war.

At the same time, Maxwell Jones, a research physiologist by training, was
trying to rehabilitate servicemen suffering from 'effort dyspnoea' – a disorder
in which the symptoms were of doubtful 'organic' origin but equally were
not clearly neurotic. The scarcity of trained staff and the large numbers of

patients resulted in patients' receiving treatment in groups. In this setting, Jones discovered that patients with physiological symptoms of anxiety were best helped by each other in an atmosphere of open communication. Jones therefore set up a structured programme in his unit which de-emphasized medical hierarchy, and stressed the importance of both sociological and psychological concepts.

The work of both Main and Jones revealed two important developments which were to act as the main guiding principles in the development of other therapeutic communities. They demonstrated that patients with psychiatric problems could be better helped when (i) professionals were willing to be less hierarchical and (ii) when the patients themselves were allowed to become involved in understanding the meaning of their symptoms, and in helping one another 'as a community'. Both of these innovators strove to create units where there was a more democratic and open style of relating between staff and patients. The patients were expected to take a more active part in their own care, as well as in the management of fellow patients and in the running of the unit as a whole. However, because of their individual theoretical backgrounds, the units developed by Main and Jones emphasized different components of the treatment approach.

The legacy of the Northfield experiments and T.F. Main
The Northfield Military Hospital in Birmingham was home to a number of psychoanalysts and social psychologists who were posted there between 1943 and 1946. Of this group, Main, Bion and Foulkes are best remembered. W.R. Bion was later to become famous for his experimental groups at the Tavistock Clinic, London and for his contributions to the field of psychoanalysis. Michael Foulkes went on to create a method of therapy called 'group analysis', and later formed the Institute of Group Analysis.

At Northfield, Main aimed to develop and sustain a 'culture of enquiry' where the meaning of people's behaviour could be understood (Main, 1983). He later became Director of the Cassel Hospital at Richmond, Surrey where he placed particular emphasis on traditional analytic techniques within this therapeutic setting. The Cassel Hospital continues to treat young personality disordered patients in a residential setting with a treatment programme that combines elements of the therapeutic community approach with individual psychoanalytic psychotherapy. In addition, the Cassel runs one of the few residential units which treats whole families whose fabric has often been disrupted by physical and sexual abuse.

The legacy of the Mill Hill experiments and Maxwell Jones
Although Main coined the phrase 'therapeutic community', it was Maxwell Jones who came to symbolize the therapeutic community movement. He recognized his indebtedness to the pioneers of group dynamic theories (such as Foulkes and Bion) but added his own particular emphasis which stressed the importance of sociotherapy. His earlier success in rehabilitating prisoners of war prompted the government to open the Industrial Neurosis Unit at Belmont Hospital, South London in 1947 – which is today known as the Henderson Hospital. It is perhaps the best known example of a 'therapeutic community proper', and adheres firmly to the principles laid down by Maxwell Jones. Today Henderson specializes in the treatment of moderate

to severe personality disordered young adults with a treatment programme that incorporates both group psychotherapy and sociotherapy. These young people suffer marked disturbances of emotional, behavioural and social functioning, and have often been seen as 'untreatable' by conventional psychiatric services.

The concept-based community

The second historical influence upon the current therapeutic community approach in Britain came from the importation of the 'concept house' approach which began in California in 1958. Charles Dederich, an alcoholic in recovery and a committed member of Alcoholics Anonymous, became dissatisfied with some of the limitations of this latter organization. He founded an organization called Synanon where ex-alcoholics and ex-drug addicts could live together and help one another to stay drug-free. Whereas the democratic–analytic community in Britain had grown from the psychiatric tradition, Synanon and many of the communities that followed were run by non-professionals who were addicts in recovery. Professionals, such as psychiatrists and psychologists, were often viewed suspiciously and considered to have little to offer. A second difference was that doctors and nurses in British therapeutic communities aimed to dismantle the authoritarian medical hierarchy so that it became 'flattened', whereas organizations such as Synanon developed a graded staff and resident hierarchy. Failure to abide by decisions made at 'the top' resulted in the individual being confronted in the encounter groups held at the end of the day. Synanon and its sister organizations (Day Top Village, Samaritan Village, Gateway Foundation and Phoenix House) took the name of concept-based communities because they adopted clear and simple explanations for the psychological course of addiction, and for the means by which therapeutic communities might help people live without drugs or alcohol. These explanations were known as 'concepts'.

The therapeutic community movement

It would be a mistake to see these two different styles of therapeutic community as polarized. They share the common underlying philosophy that if you are able to understand and communicate to others the reasons for the development of your difficulties, you will become motivated and will feel better able to withstand the necessary effort and pain which characterizes major personal change.

After the end of the Second World War, therapeutic communities were seen as representing a new psychiatric movement. The creation of the National Health Service (NHS) in 1948 brought to public attention the plight of chronic psychotic patients who had been detained in Victorian asylums. Traditional psychiatric care, hampered by the lack of any effective pharmacological treatments, could offer these institutionalized and stigmatized patients very little (Stanton and Schwartz, 1954; Goffman, 1961). The climate was one of social and political change where traditional models of psychiatric care were challenged. The theoretical concepts of therapeutic communities fitted well against this background, and the 1950s and 1960s saw a proliferation of therapeutic communities.

As well as the growth of democratic–analytic and concept-based therapeutic communities, other styles of community evolved. Therapeutic community principles were applied in traditional psychiatric hospital wards, day centres, prisons, educational establishments and in 'group homes', which were ordinary houses in residential neighbourhoods where patients lived together for mutual support.

Another style of community which evolved in the late 1960s grew from the 'anti-psychiatry' movement. In Britain this movement grew from the work of two British psychiatrists, R.D. Laing and David Cooper. It was concerned with the role of the psychiatrist, the nature of mental illness and how society defines normal behaviour. In the view of anti-psychiatry, the psychiatrist's responsibility was only to the patient. They believed that psychiatrists should not act as policemen or jailers, or to persuade patients to behave in a socially acceptable way so that social peace was preserved. Instead they should help the patient as a whole, guiding the patient through their psychic turmoil until they reached health. Some anti-psychiatrists totally rejected the idea of mental illness, although most accepted that people suffered from mad or psychotic states. However, they did not feel that society was justified in either ostracizing these people or 'controlling' their lives by admitting them to psychiatric hospitals and treating them with drugs or electroconvulsive therapy. This movement gave rise to small communities, consisting of six to ten people, such as the Archway Community which later became part of the Philadelphia Association and the Arbours Association founded by Joseph Berke. These communities provided an alternative for those people seeking sanctuary who wished to avoid treatment and hospitalization. The community was seen as 'a place to be', where the emphasis was on 'coming to terms with oneself'.

These different styles of therapeutic communities can be seen as being on a continuum, starting with the highly structured concept-based communities, moving through the democratic analytic type, to those with little structure which had their roots in the anti-psychiatry movement. Although they have their differences, all these styles of therapeutic community can be seen as part of a general movement away from paternalistic authority towards self-help.

In the late 1960s, traditional psychiatric practice was being revolutionized by the success of neuroleptic and anti-depressant drugs which provided effective treatment for the large number of institutionalized patients. By the mid 1970s, many of the communities which had been formed in a wave of enthusiasm had been forced to close. However, the past twenty years have seen a slow but steady recognition that there is a place for therapeutic community treatment within several systems such as health care, education and prisons.

Principles of theory and practice

Although therapeutic communities are united in working towards a common therapeutic aim, there are distinct differences in the theoretical principles which underpin such aims.

Theoretical principles of the democratic–analytic therapeutic community

To successfully achieve Main's 'culture of enquiry', the community concentrates on the *meaning* of an individual's feelings, actions and relationships with others (residents and staff).

The therapeutic principles which underpin the structure of the community are derived from:

- Studies of therapeutic communities
- Psychoanalytic theory
- Theories of group functioning
- Theories of organizational and social systems

Theoretical principles from the study of therapeutic communities

In the 1950s a team of sociologists, led by Robert Rapoport, studied the 'Social Rehabilitation Unit' run by Maxwell Jones (Rapoport, 1960). Rapoport described four themes which emerged as the key values that staff held about treatment, which have subsequently become linked with democratic–analytic style communities.

- **Democratization** is the view that every member of the community should share in making decisions about community affairs, both therapeutic and administrative. As community decisions are often made on the basis of a vote and as residents often outnumber staff, the resident's authority and participation in the therapeutic process is enhanced and the conventional hierarchy flattened. The traditional 'medical model', which puts the patient into a passive role, is minimized. In many communities 'patients' are referred to as 'residents' to denote their active role in their own and others' treatment.
- **Permissiveness** refers to the belief that all members of the unit should tolerate a wide range of behaviours that might be distressing or seem deviant. It allows residents to understand, rather than simply react to, both sides of a social interaction. This does not mean that residents can do whatever they like, whenever they like. There are rules which are made by the community as a whole, and can only be changed by the community as a whole. Often these rules centre around the prohibition of violence to self and others, and illicit drug or alcohol use. They occasion automatic discharge when broken. At Henderson, rule breakers are considered by the community to have discharged themselves but may ask permission to stay on the unit until their behaviour can be discussed at the next community meeting. Greater tolerance of deviance is thus permitted.
- **Communalism**, the sharing of tasks and amenities by staff and residents alike, is well established in the community culture and fosters supportive group acceptance. Everyone's behaviour affects every other person in the community in a powerful way.
- **Reality confrontation** refers to the belief that residents should be repeatedly presented with interpretations of their behaviour as it is seen by others. This is to counteract the use of defensive mechanisms (such as denial, distortion and confusion) that interfere with their capacity

to relate to others in a more mature way. The combination of treatment styles and interventions relating to both the psychological and social world of the residents (i.e. from group psychotherapy to communal cookery) provide multiple forums where residents can examine their own psychological and social interactions and progress.

Therapeutic communities may seem strange places to new members, whether they are residents, staff or visitors such as medical students. Some of this strangeness is the result of being in a community which applies the above therapeutic principles. Democratization means that assuming your decisions will be implemented unquestioned simply because you are the doctor will meet with an early challenge from the community. Communalism fosters staff and residents working alongside each other, and talking to each other without the trappings of status. It allows for a more natural interchange, one that differs from the medical style of talking to patients in which the doctor has to elicit the maximum amount of information in a fixed period of time. New doctors, like new residents, are expected to join in the daily chores such as cleaning. The new staff member is therefore faced not only with an unfamiliar and new physical environment, but also find themselves in a new role. However, the permissiveness of the community allows for an understanding attitude to any mistakes which new staff members may make, while the emphasis on reality confrontation means that residents are able to relay back to each other how they appear to others.

Vignette 1

A new doctor joined the lunchtime cleaning group on her first day in the community. She felt anxious and keen to get along with people but uncertain of her new role. Her anxiety so disorientated her that she entered what she thought was the staff room only to realize she had picked the wrong door and entered a resident's bedroom.

In entering without asking she had transgressed one of the community rules. Both people felt awkward but nothing was said. However, word got around the community and the doctor felt embarrassed when another resident cruelly made fun of her and her error at the next morning's community meeting. The resident whose room she entered spoke up saying that she appreciated that it was a mistake, and that it is difficult being a new community member. She and other residents then pointed out the less forgiving resident's sarcastic attitude, saying they were tired of the way he always put people down and reminding him of how he had been supported by the community when he first arrived.

Theoretical principles derived from psychoanalytic theory

The external setting

In individual out-patient therapy the external setting is attended to by boundaries relating to the time and place of the session. In the therapeutic community the external setting is provided both concretely by the fabric of and metaphorically by the structure of the community. Attention is given to the times of groups, the role of the staff and the rules of the community which act as boundaries helping the resident to feel secure. Within the limits set by the structure, residents are free to participate in whatever way they choose. Their behaviour can then be understood as coming from them as their individual response to the structure of the community.

The internal setting of the residents

One of the advantages of the therapeutic community is that, because residents participate in both the formal and informal psychological and social life of the community, there is an increased opportunity for them to learn about the connections between their feelings and behaviours and the unconscious meanings which may underpin them. In therapeutic communities, as in individual psychodynamic therapy and group analysis, patients and residents bring their habitual ways of relating to others into the community and these can be explored within the transference and countertransference reactions which arise. In a therapeutic community, transference and countertransference reactions may occur in a greater number of configurations as compared with out-patient therapy. The following example illustrates a transference reaction between a resident and the whole community. However, such reactions may occur between a resident and a member of staff, between individuals or between groups of residents.

Vignette 2

As a new resident, Paula was withdrawn and tearful. When she became the focus of attention she would burst into tears or run out of the group meeting. Staff and residents became increasingly frustrated by her behaviour and began to discuss whether she could benefit from the community.

Paula's mother died when she was a young child and her father had remarried. Paula felt her stepmother treated her cruelly and that the arrival of step-siblings resulted in her having a tenuous place in 'her family'. Her behaviour in the face of these traumas was to withdraw.

The meaning of Paula's behaviour in the community was understood as being a replay of a family dynamic. Her withdrawal in the community echoed her earlier withdrawal from her stepmother for fear of being treated cruelly and ejected from the family. Her tendency to retreat was, however, provoking the community to 'get rid of her'. After this dynamic had been understood, Paula no longer hid her tearful face behind her hands, and eventually became a respected member of the community. In this example, Paula behaved as if the whole community was acting against her, like her early experience of her step-mother.

An individual relies, to a greater or lesser extent, on various psychological defence mechanisms to protect themself from unpalatable feelings. In a therapeutic community, defence mechanisms can operate, not only to aid the individual but to help the community avoid pain or conflict.

Vignette 3

Bill entered the community just before Christmas, when it was running on a 'skeleton' staff. Although Bill was late for some groups the residents repeatedly accused him of disrupting their therapy – more forcefully than his occasional lateness warranted. He was 'voted out' of the community as a result of a minor misdemeanour. It seemed that the residents were unable to bear their own feelings of loss connected to the disruption of Christmas holidays. Instead they were projected on to Bill who was attacked and driven out.

This process of projection followed by 'scapegoating' arises from the unconscious idea that Bill's departure would solve this problem. However, the community was no further forward as it still needed to deal with its feelings about the holiday.

In residents who have poor impulse control and who struggle to tolerate even small amounts of frustration, feelings often spill from their internal world into the external structure and get enacted in the community. For example, a resident may be unable to think about her internal explosive state and only express it through action (such as putting her hand through a glass window).

Acting out is enactment outside therapy. Although many therapeutic communities are residential, and therapy is twenty-four hours a day, acting out can still occur: for example, a resident goes on weekend leave feeling angry and, instead of dealing with his feelings in the community, he acts them out by picking a fight.

Therapeutic communities are often able to tolerate much higher levels of enactment and acting out behaviour than can be contained in out-patient settings as a well-functioning community is able to contain the high levels of anxiety which such incidents engender.

The internal setting of the staff

The staff in a therapeutic community must constantly monitor their own countertransference reactions as they may give important clues to the relationship which the patient is unconsciously trying to recreate. Just as with transference phenomena, countertransference phenomena in a therapeutic community may occur in a variety of combinations.

Vignette 4

Ann had been subjected to a prolonged incestuous relationship with her father from an early age. Her mother had turned 'a blind eye' and had frequently left the family home. When both parents had been together, Ann remembers them rowing violently. In the community, she would often seek out female staff but then quickly exclude them. With male staff and residents, she would discuss intimate details of her abuse when there were no females around and hint at current self-harming behaviour which often had a sexualized element to it. The male staff felt invited into a secretive relationship while the female staff felt excluded and impatient with her. This led to a heated staff debate where the male staff felt the female staff were insensitive, and the female staff felt jealous of the secrecy between Ann and the male staff. These countertransference reactions shed light upon how she was unconsciously trying to recreate her parental relationships, only now the arguments were occurring between the staff.

This example illustrates how the unconscious mental mechanism of 'splitting' can occur in a staff team where one group is seen as representing good qualities (i.e. sensitivity) while the other group holds all the bad qualities (i.e. lack of understanding). Such unconscious mechanisms can cause splits between residents and staff, between staff and staff, or between the community and the outside world – all of which hinder the work of the community.

To further open communication and understanding within the community, staff must be aware of both their internal feelings and those of the staff team. This awareness helps staff to resist acting unthinkingly on their countertransference feelings, and can provide residents with new understandings of how they relate to others which can then be put into practice.

Theoretical principles derived from concepts of group functioning

As well as providing a forum where Main developed the democratic–analytic therapeutic community approach, the two Northfield experiments generated ideas which were to lay the foundations for the development of analytic group therapy in Britain through the work of Bion and Foulkes. Although other models of group therapy have evolved, the work of Foulkes in generating a theory of group therapy and applying it in practice, and Bion's work in observing small group processes, are perhaps the most relevant pieces of group-related work which have been applied to democratic–analytic therapeutic communities.

The work of Foulkes and the development of group analysis

As man is a social creature, Foulkes viewed neurotic symptoms as an expression of psychological difficulties which have their origins in relationships. He aimed to treat the individual within the context of the group, where people interact with and behave towards each other based on their assumptions (often unconscious) about themselves and others. As the group develops, all the inter-relationships and patterns of communication contribute to the formation of a group matrix. The significance of any communication can then only be understood fully if it is seen as being within the matrix, inside of which all processes take place. Foulkes regarded the group matrix as providing the common shared ground necessary to determine the meaning of events, as well as all the various levels of communication and interpretation within the group. Such a matrix can develop within therapeutic communities where the therapeutic space, physical space, culture of the community and its relationship within itself and with the outside world all make a contribution. This matrix both generates and provides understanding of the communication of its members.

Within the matrix transference and countertransference relationships are formed. In addition, Foulkes differentiated the following group-specific therapeutic factors which occur over and over again in the many sub-groups that form as well as in the whole therapeutic community as a group.

- **Socialization:** Through the experience of being accepted by and belonging to the group, patients are brought out of their isolation. This experience is vital for patients (like those often referred to therapeutic communities) whose disordered personalities predispose them to problematic interpersonal relationships.
- **Mirror phenomena:** As it is easier to see in others what one cannot recognize in oneself, patients may see aspects of themselves reflected in the image, behaviour and problems of other group members. This enables the residents to gradually reorganize and take responsibility for traits in their own personalities.
- **Chain and condenser phenomena:** When the group pools its associations, a loosening of group resistances can occur resulting in a sudden discharge of unconscious material.

Bion's observations on group dynamics

Bion (1961) recognized that recurrent emotional patterns occurred in groups. He described well-functioning groups where both the individuals comprising the group and the group itself developed an understanding of how they related to each other. If, in addition, spontaneous communication existed at many levels, Bion described this as a 'work group'. In contrast, 'basic assumption states' in groups may arise when the group culture is defensive and is aimed at opposing therapeutic work.

Bion described three styles of group interactions which could lead to the development of basic assumption groups.

- In the dependent group, the group behaves as if someone will magically satisfy the group's needs and longings. In a therapeutic community, this style of group initially expects all the answers and solutions from the staff group. When these are not instantly proffered, staff are often attacked and the group searches for an alternative leader.
- In the fight–flight group, the group avoids working by means of conflict or absence. Members of the therapeutic community, when in this state of mind, may critically attack others or erode the therapeutic work by missing groups or other community activities.
- In the pairing group, two or more members of the therapeutic community (staff or residents) may join forces to exclude other group members and avoid discussing their own problems.

Theoretical principles derived from studies of organizations and social systems

Historically, democratic–analytic communities developed as an attempt to move away from the harmful aspects of traditionally run psychiatric hospitals. Their aim was to avoid the damaging effects of institutionalization and stigmatization, replacing these by fostering residents' individuality and autonomy. This concept, derived from organizational studies, developed into a therapeutic community principle.

Another principle is that staff behaviour and expectations can impact powerfully on the residents' level of functioning. For example, if covert disagreements exist between the staff, the team may notice an increased collective level of disturbance amongst the residents. In this way, repeated lateness and non-attendance at groups by the residents in the community may increase when a high proportion of staff are 'off sick' or coming in late as a result of low morale stemming from unresolved conflicts within the staff team. Such obvious connections can be easily passed over as they create anxious and uncomfortable feelings.

In addition to observable staff behaviour, the unconscious group dynamics within the staff team can have a powerful effect upon individual members and on the whole community. For example, a staff team which over-protects new staff because of an anxiety that they will find the work too stressful limits the opportunity for these staff to become meaningfully involved in community life. New staff members may then feel disillusioned and leave.

Theoretical principles of the concept-based communities

These communities aim to provide their residents with a set of simple, direct concepts or clear explanations of the psychological causes of their addictions and how the community will help them live without their particular addictive substances. If residents can grasp these principles or 'concepts', they can gain a sense of mastery over their previous situation. The concept-based communities see drug addicts or alcoholics as people with impulsive personalities which drive their actions. They stress that the residents must be responsible for their own situation and choice to change.

The concepts are grouped into three sorts. Those which:

- explain the nature of the addicts' problems;
- explain how therapy might be effective; and
- give guidance on community conduct – the resident is expected to behave in a calm, tolerant manner.

Aims of therapy

The democratic–analytic and concept-based therapeutic communities share some common therapeutic aims.

- Both styles of community aim to enable the individual to learn more about their problems and difficulties, and how these effect relationships with other people within the society in which they live. Both types of community encourage the individual to take personal responsibility for their situation and role in maintaining or perpetuating this.
- Therapeutic communities aim to increase a person's knowledge of themselves so that they are in an optimum position to face the difficult and painful process that is involved in personal change.
- The final goal of therapy is that the individual is able to live successfully in society without the need to fall back on their previous maladaptive behavioural strategies, especially when presented with stressful or conflictual situations.

How do therapeutic communities differ from other therapies?

Whether communities adopt a democratic–analytic or concept-based style, they differ from other therapeutic modalities by the fact that there is a community which provides a method for bringing about psychological change. De Leon (1994) distinguished therapeutic communities from other treatment approaches by their 'purposive use of peer community to facilitate social and psychological change in individuals'. Thus, all activities in a therapeutic community are designed to provide a forum for therapeutic and educational change, and all residents are mediators of these changes.

Which patients and why?

Therapeutic communities proper often function as specialist resources and, as such, are referred patients who are often labelled as 'difficult to treat'. Within psychiatric services, the group of patients who commonly attract this label are those with personality disorders. Consequently, patients with this diagnosis form the majority of residents who are referred to and accepted by such therapeutic communities as the Henderson and Cassel Hospitals in London.

Therapeutic community residents are not easily categorized within the international mental health classifications (ICD-10/DSM-IV) as the community culture emphasizes understanding of behaviour rather than concentrating on diagnostic and symptomatic presentation. However, failure to communicate effectively with the outside world and other mental health professionals, who may think within this diagnostic framework, can lead to the isolation and marginalization of communities.

Most therapeutic community patients would probably be diagnosed as having several severe personality disorders according to the DSM-IV classificatory system. Those most often represented are the borderline, antisocial and narcissistic types. In addition, many patients have histories of receiving psychiatric treatment, being in care, alcohol or drug abuse, physical and sexual abuse, previous self-harming and suicide attempts.

Vignette 5

James was referred to the therapeutic community by a consultant psychiatrist because of his persistent self-harming behaviour which included overdosing, inflicting deep lacerations to his wrists and bouts of uncontrolled drinking. His mother died when he was eleven and he had never known his father. After his mother's death, he lived with his step-father but this relationship broke down because of the repeated beatings he inflicted on James who was then taken into care.

James left school with no qualifications and worked occasionally, such as labouring on building sites. During his adolescence he began to drink and would sometimes steal cars while intoxicated. By the time he applied for admission, he had been fined several times and spent a few months in a Youth

Custody Centre. He had not attended any of his psychiatric out-patient appointments and was currently an in-patient in his local psychiatric hospital after a recent overdose.

His referrer described him isolating himself on the ward, maintaining that he had no problems, and greeting any approaches by staff with an outburst of verbal abuse. At interview, he was initially sullen and suspicious wanting to know who were staff and who were residents. He was able to give a reasonably good account of himself and, when questioned by residents, he was able to confide in them his worries about his escalating drinking and his increasing feelings of loneliness.

In general, the patients who are referred to therapeutic communities lead chaotic lives which are a reflection of their internal disorganization. Traditional psychiatric care, including out-patient psychotherapy, cannot provide the degree of therapeutic structure required to help them. The highly structured 'therapeutic community day' provides this external support and functions to contain the anxieties that can drive acting out behaviour.

There are few absolute indications or contraindications for admission to a therapeutic community. An important factor is whether the person's problems are seen as appropriate by the community. However people who can verbalize their feelings and difficulties, and who function in a group setting, are often preferentially selected. In general, residents have to satisfy the individual rules and conditions of entry of a particular community. For example, a patient on a probation order which specifies that they must reside in the community would not be accepted by a community where residents must be free to leave unconditionally.

Similar principles apply to indicate or contraindicate acceptance to a particular community as apply to selection for a small group. Having one resident who could be isolated from the community group because of their age, ethnicity, physical disability or radically different mental state is a relative contraindication.

Therapeutic communities for specific populations

Some therapeutic communities have developed to help specific populations, such as:

- Concept-based communities which treat and rehabilitate people with drug and alcohol problems
- Therapeutic communities of both styles which have developed in the prison system
- Communities which have developed in maximum secure hospitals
- The therapeutic community prison for men, HMP Grendon Underwood in Buckinghamshire, England
- Communities which treat adolescents in secure or open settings

These communities aim to select residents who they feel will benefit from their programme. Although residents may be united by a form of behaviour, i.e. addiction or offending, they may vary in the degree and nature of their underlying psychological problems.

Assessment

Unlike acceptance into individual psychotherapy, acceptance into a therapeutic community not only depends on the characteristics of the individual, but on the interplay of these with the characteristics of the community. Each therapeutic community operates a different style of assessment procedure. The following description outlines some common elements. Staff often screen out patients who are obviously unsuitable for the community in a pre-referral process. For example, a person who is actively psychotic would not be offered an assessment to enter a community whose members had neurotic or personality problems. The potential resident is often invited to spend some time in the community and explain the reasons why they want to join the community to a multi-disciplinary admission panel. In some communities, current residents are involved in this selection process.

At assessment, candidates are invited to talk about their current and past difficulties, aspects of their childhood and adolescence, and asked about the problems they would like to address if selected. The group is particularly concerned with the individual's motivation to change, their psychological-mindedness and the ability to accept responsibility for their problems. In addition, the group will want to assess the individual's capacity to live alongside them as part of the community. They will be interested to know how the potential resident feels about joining different groups, having to abide by the community rules and taking on various jobs that ensure the smooth running of the community.

Unconscious dynamic interactions are present in any assessment process, but they may be particularly pronounced where residents are involved. The selection process is also an important part of residents' treatment as they are exposed to new candidates who echo their own difficulties and they may realize (consciously and unconsciously) how they appear or have appeared to others. Aspects of themselves which they find difficult to accept may be displaced and projected into the selection candidate.

> Vignette 6
>
> *Months after Anna joined the community, another resident, Jane, now her friend, told her that she had voted against her admission. Jane recalled that listening to Anna's description of her sexual abuse had reminded Jane of many more details of her own sexual abuse. She later realized that by voting against Anna she was unconsciously trying to distance herself from her distress.*

Which therapist and why?

There is no standard template which qualifies a person to work in a therapeutic community; however there are certain qualities and abilities which are advantageous. Of crucial importance is the ability to maintain therapeutic integrity and boundaries while being a part of the community as, in contrast to out-patient psychotherapy, staff spend considerable informal time with residents, including evenings and weekends. In the community, staff work in a variety of different groups. They may be involved in individual and group psychodynamic work, art therapy, psychodrama and more task-oriented groups, such as cooking or gardening. The capacity to be flexible while maintaining an individual therapeutic stance is an advantageous combination. It is harder to 'hide behind' psychotherapy clichés when outside the traditional setting of the psychotherapy session.

New staff often feel deskilled and, in an attempt to recover their position, can often resort to the 'stock phrases' of therapy, such as 'why don't you talk about it in the group?' or 'you seem to feel angry'. Such phrases miss the emotional point when the staff member is faced by a suspicious and distressed resident who has just cut themselves. In these difficult situations, it is often better to trust the structure of the community by alerting the senior residents who can mobilize the community resources. The practical aspects can then be attended to. The crisis meeting, which will inevitably follow such an incident, is the time to try to understand the resident's behaviour.

Staff must be willing to move out of traditional hierarchical roles as this is of therapeutic benefit to residents who are only too willing to relate to staff in a fixed way, involving hostility towards and suspicion of authority. This style of relating to staff, which is often the legacy of earlier harsh, neglectful or erratic parenting, is harder to maintain in the face of a community structure which flattens hierarchical roles.

The role of the staff team in a therapeutic community is complex and requires the staff to continually monitor and reflect on the dynamics within the resident group, the staff group and the interactions between them. Using this information, the staff team must then evaluate their performance. A staff member should be prepared to tell the staff team about their work and actively participate in staff business meetings, sensitivity or support groups, as well as supervision groups to try to understand the conscious and unconscious processes alive within the community.

Training in concept-based communities, for both ex-addicts and professional staff, is primarily the experience of going through the community as a resident. These communities often have their own career structure. The democratic–analytic communities usually expect their staff to have a recognized professional qualification; for example, in nursing, psychology, social work, psychiatry or the creative therapies. They often expect staff to continue their training. This can be accomplished in a number of ways: either by an organized in-house programme or by external psychotherapy or psychoanalytical training, group or individual, which involves personal therapy.

Therapeutic setting

Although therapeutic communities developed from different roots, and offer treatment to a spectrum of very different people with psychological difficulties, they share some similarities in their therapeutic setting.

The community day is highly structured, with group meetings occupying a central place in the programme. The form of these groups will vary immensely between communities but will include a regular meeting where the whole community joins to discuss and organize community business. Throughout the rest of the day residents participate in groups of various sizes and orientations.

Types of groups offered within therapeutic communities
- Small psychodynamic groups
- Art, music or drama therapy groups
- Psychodrama groups
- Task-oriented work groups (e.g. gardening, cookery)
- Communal sports groups
- Cleaning groups

The therapeutic day is lengthy and there is often an evening 'wind-down' group to resolve any left-over problems. The therapeutic structure also provides space for emergency meetings, and groups to review progress and allocate community jobs to residents.

In concept-based therapeutic communities encounter groups, held two or three times a week, are the main therapy sessions. They are highly confrontational, aimed at challenging the residents' defences. In psychoanalytic psychotherapy residents are expected to contain their emotional reactions between groups, while in concept-based communities individual counselling programmes supplement group sessions. Concept-based communities often offer several educational seminars each week as well as extended groups or 'marathons', lasting between twenty-four and forty-eight hours, which many regard as providing profound and lasting insights.

Staff in a democratic–analytic community participate in a wide range of groups, as well as meeting regularly as a staff group to attend to community business, discuss the dynamics of the day's groups and examine the functioning of the staff team. Failure in this area may lead to unacknowledged difficulties interfering with the therapeutic work.

In concept-based communities a charismatic leader heads the hierarchy. As former addicts, these leaders are important role models. The concept of a credible role model who has demonstrated the efficacy of treatment, by their own personal achievement, is a major component of the programme. All staff and residents are in a chain of command. As residents demonstrate increased competency and emotional growth, they increase their status and privileges.

Time spent in therapy varies between communities but an average range is between eight and sixteen months. Concept-based community principles have been modified for use within a prison setting, and many of these programmes have an associated community limb where the resident can choose to continue treatment after release.

Problems in therapy

The powerful dynamic forces which operate within and between groups in therapeutic communities, if unaddressed, can give rise to destructive processes. These processes, which can lead to problems for the community, can arise from:

- Dynamics within the resident group
- Dynamics within the staff group
- A 'messianic' group dynamic
- Dynamics between the community and the outside world

Problems within the resident group

Personality disordered residents frequently test the strength of the treatment alliance. The nature of their difficulties, such as their impulsive behaviour and limited capacity to tolerate frustration, means that there will inevitably be acts of aggression in every community. Attacks may be aimed primarily at themselves – self-harming behaviour, damaging the culture of the community by attacking the fabric of the building, and flaunting the rules (for example, by bringing drugs on to the unit).

The type of response 'chosen' by a community is crucial to determining whether the treatment alliance is repaired or further damaged. If the community reacts by displaying a narrow repertoire of relatively inflexible responses, such as immediately isolating or expelling the resident, the motives leading to the behaviour and the unconscious meaning underlying the behaviour do not get examined or understood (Norton and Dolan, 1995). Residents often invite staff to relate to them in such punitive and exploitative ways as they unconsciously desire a relationship based on the community exerting power and control over them. This allows perpetuation of a victim/perpetrator style of relating which is familiar ground to many residents. If such an invitation is taken up, then destructive processes (such as scapegoating and the unconscious encouragement of unhealthy dependency in residents) gain the ascendant position.

De-emphasizing 'vertical' authoritarian relationships and strengthening horizontal peer group relationships can minimize these processes, encouraging residents to ask for support from other community members.

Problems within the staff group

In general, the role of the staff in a therapeutic community is to maintain its ethos and culture and to facilitate its health. To achieve this, the staff group must be alert to maintaining the community's internal boundaries as well as seeing and modifying the destructive processes at work within the resident and staff groups, in order to preserve the 'culture of enquiry'.

Vignette 7

The climate of a democratic–analytic community changed when a third of the residents admitted had served custodial prison sentences. A 'them and us' (staff versus residents) mentality was foremost. Talking in groups with and about others was regarded as 'grassing' (sneaking). References that being in the community was like being 'on trial' abounded and, if a resident was on a vote for contravening the rules, staff were accused of 'block voting' (i.e. voting en masse against a resident). Staff were required to tolerate these projections, and not take up the resident's invitation to behave punitively towards them, while trying to unlock the dynamic mechanisms which resulted in this therapeutic stalemate.

Staff can often remain blind to such projections from the resident group, especially when they resonate with rivalrous dynamics within the staff team. Main's paper 'The Ailment' (1957) describes the splits and resulting rivalry which can occur in a staff team when a resident or group of residents become special. Some staff see only the 'good' aspects of these patients, 'denying' their bad aspects. The envious competition generated can lead to failures of communication in the team, resulting in confusion. This is often felt most acutely by the resident group, who may resort to destructive acting out.

The 'Messianic Community'

Unconscious mechanisms may occur in groups with destructive results, including the unconscious splitting of the staff team and the 'messianic fantasy' as described by Bion. In this fantasy, the community elevate a 'charismatic' leader to an idealized status while another non-community group perceives the leader as a danger. In an idealized split, the leader and his or her colleagues collude in their view of the idealized (or 'good') unit which then engages in a battle with the externalized 'badness' located in other aspects of the psychiatric or social establishment. The community ceases to be a work group as it is worshipping the charismatic leader. Other variations of the fantasy involve staff and residents looking for past or future messiahs, and preoccupying themselves with grieving or hoping as opposed to working. This messianic fantasy has been especially linked to destructive processes in therapeutic communities (for example Hobson's (1979) paper on 'The Messianic Community').

Problems between the community and the outside world

The principles and culture that therapeutic communities strive to maintain (for example, the increased levels of permissiveness and democratization present in democratic–analytic communities) can often differ from the values held by the wider community comprising other professionals, the NHS, residents' families, the media and the general public.

Such differences can lead to misunderstandings and breakdown in communications between the therapeutic and external community. However, the therapeutic community exists and functions within this wider system and is dependent upon it. Failures of communication, especially when communities feel criticized and misunderstood, can lead them to withdraw from contact with external systems. Such an isolated position renders them vulnerable to the wider community further misunderstanding and criticizing their work. It is often the task of the leaders in the therapeutic community to maintain a system of open communication with the outside world.

Evaluation of therapy

Because of the range and number of therapeutic communities, there is a considerable body of research literature concerning therapeutic outcome. However, many studies are flawed by methodological problems. Communities, both democratic–analytic and concept-based, which treat personality disordered patients have been particularly productive in generating outcome data.

Democratic–analytic therapeutic community outcome research

Dolan and Coid (1993) comprehensively review outcome and other research data from democratic–analytic NHS and prison communities, non-British therapeutic communities and concept-based communities. This work is recommended for a detailed analysis of outcome studies.

They highlight the common research pitfalls, which include the lack of rigorous diagnostic criteria for subjects, the lack of control samples and the paucity of objective outcome measures. Uncontrolled studies of change during therapeutic community treatment have generally demonstrated improvement on psychological testing (Norris, 1985). However, research as to whether these changes are maintained after discharge are limited by a lack of control groups and a short follow-up period, although some research has shown a significant improvement in residents' psychological distress which is maintained for up to three years (Vaglum et al., 1990).

Studies which have looked at long-term progress have mainly concentrated on offender populations, and have used recidivism as an outcome measure. Some studies show no difference between a treated group of male offenders versus the untreated group (Robertson and Gunn, 1987). However, the five-year follow-up study from the Henderson Hospital (Copas et al., 1984) found a significantly lower 'relapse' rate in the treated group. The same study showed that the length of stay in the therapeutic community was positively correlated with improved outcome, a finding echoed by studies from prison therapeutic communities.

Concept-based therapeutic community outcome research

Wexler et al. (1990) evaluated a voluntary concept-based therapeutic community in a New York prison. The study compared all clients completing the therapeutic community programme with inmates who had volunteered and been placed on the waiting list. The study confirmed the view that therapeutic treatment within prison settings can reduce recidivism in drug addicts more effectively than other treatments. Wexler warns of the risk of generalizing these results to other populations who may present with personality disorders as well as addictive problems.

There is also a significant body of literature which documents the effectiveness of the therapeutic community approach in rehabilitating drug abusers in non-custodial settings. These studies show significant improvements on the outcome variables of drug use, criminality and employment. There is a consistent positive relationship between time in residential treatment and post-treatment outcome status, although some work suggests that there is a plateau beyond which additional therapy may no longer improve outcome.

The drug abusers in the outcome studies were mainly opiate addicts. Since the 1980s, the drug usage profile of most admissions to residential therapeutic communities has been one of poly-drug abuse. Therefore, new studies are needed to evaluate the effectiveness of the therapeutic community in treating this more recent generation of abusers.

The efficacy of the therapeutic community approach

The efficacy of therapeutic community treatment may be considered in terms of whether the private and public costs are reduced as a result of treatment. Private costs are the personal cost to the individual (in terms of their productivity and health) that are compromised by their addictive or personality problems as addressed in the discussion on outcome research. Public costs refer to the social costs of these disorders – the expenditure borne by the public as a result of the medical, social and legal support these people require plus the costs inflicted on society by their antisocial and criminal activities. These latter costs are more difficult to assess. However, findings from cost-of-treatment studies regarding concept-based communities support a general conclusion that these treatment methods reduce public costs. Hubbard and colleagues' (1989) work suggests that residential therapeutic communities yield favourable cost-benefit value, particularly in respect of savings in crime and positive gains in employment.

Research undertaken by Menzies et al. (1993), conducted in a democratic-analytic therapeutic community, suggests that personality disordered patients who are not treated are likely to remain high service users at a considerable cost to the nation. Although treatment in a residential therapeutic community may, at first sight, appear expensive, the cost of admission can be recouped when the therapeutic gains reduce future service use.

Further reading

Hinshelwood, R.D. and Manning, N. (eds) (1979) *Therapeutic Communities: Reflections and Progress*. London: Routledge and Kegan Paul.
Kennard, D. (1983) *Introduction to Therapeutic Communities*. London: Routledge and Kegan Paul.
Kennard, D. (1988) The therapeutic community. In: M. Aveline and W. Dryden (eds), *Group Therapy in Britain*. Milton Keynes: Open University Press, pp. 153–184.

Bibliography

Bion, W.R. (1961) *Experiences in Groups*. London: Tavistock Social Sciences Paperbacks.
Copas, J.B., O'Brien, M., Roberts, J. and Whiteley, J.S. (1984) Treatment outcome in personality disorder: the effect of social, psychological and behavioural variables. *Personality and Individual Differences*, **5**, 565–573.

De Leon, G. (1994) Therapeutic communities. In: M. Galanter and H.D. Kleber (eds), *Textbook of Substance Abuse Treatment*. Chicago: American Psychiatric Press, pp. 391–414.

Dolan, B. and Coid, J. (1993) Therapeutic community approaches. In: B. Dolan and J. Coid (eds), *Psychopathic and Antisocial Personality Disorders: Treatment and Research Issues*. London: Gaskell, pp. 146–180.

Goffman, E. (1961) *Asylums*. New York: Doubleday. Republished Harmondsworth: Penguin, 1968.

Hobson, R.F. (1979) The Messianic community. In: R.D. Hinshelwood and N. Manning (eds), *Therapeutic Communities: Reflections and Progress*. London: Routledge and Kegan Paul, pp. 231–244.

Hubbard, R.L., Marsden, M.E., Valley, R.J., Harwood, H.J., Cavanaugh, E.R. and Ginzburg, H.M. (1989) *Drug Abuse Treatment: A National Study of Effectiveness*. Chapel Hill: University of North Carolina Press.

Main, T.F. (1946) The hospital as a therapeutic institution. *Bulletin of the Menninger Clinic*, **10**, 66–70.

Main, T.F. (1957) The Ailment. *British Journal of Medical Psychology*, **30**, 129–145.

Main, T.F. (1983) The concept of the therapeutic community: variations and vicissitudes. In: M. Pines (ed.), *The Evolution of Group Analysis*. London: Routledge and Kegan Paul, pp. 197–217.

Menzies, D., Dolan, B.M. and Norton, K.R.W. (1993) Are short term savings worth long term costs? Funding treatment for personality disorders. *Psychiatric Bulletin*, **17**, 517–519.

Norris, M. (1985) Changes in patients during treatment at Henderson Hospital Therapeutic Community during 1977–1981. *British Journal of Medical Psychology*, **56**, 135–143.

Norton, K.R.W. and Dolan, B. (1995) Acting out and the institutional response. *Journal of Forensic Psychiatry*, **6**, 317–332.

Rapoport, R.N. (1960) *Community as Doctor*. London: Tavistock.

Robertson, G. and Gunn, J. (1987) A ten year follow-up of men discharged from Grendon Prison. *British Journal of Psychiatry*, **151**, 674–678.

Stanton, A. and Schwartz, M. (1954) *The Mental Hospital*. New York: Basic Books.

Vaglum, P., Friis, S., Irion, T. et al. (1990) Treatment response of severe and non-severe personality disorders in a therapeutic community day unit. *Journal of Personality Disorders*, **2**, 161–172.

Wexler, H.K., Falkin, G.P. and Lipton, D.S. (1990) Outcome evaluation of a prison therapeutic community for substance abuse treatment. *Criminal Justice and Behaviour*, **17**, 71–92.

16

Humanistic Therapies

Fiona Blyth

Introduction

An important feature of the humanistic therapies is that there is no single theory or method identified with one person. The term applies to a group of therapies with diverse theoretical perspectives and treatment methods that evolved alongside psychoanalysis and behaviourism in the early part of the twentieth century. The unifying factor is a shared existential philosophy relating to personal responsibility, and a fundamental trust in the innate human capacity for growth and 'self-actualization'. One of the main exponents of existentialism, Soren Kierkegaard, believed that attempts by philosophers such as Hegel to define human existence imposed false perceptions that facilitated avoidance of free choice and personal responsibility. He challenged the authority of religious dogma and asserted that human beings were essentially alone and responsible for themselves.

In order to summarize an extensive field, the examples of transactional analysis, Gestalt, psychodrama and person-centred therapy have been used to illustrate humanistic therapy practice. There are many other humanistic approaches, some of which are indicated in the bibliography.

Historical perspective

The humanistic therapies evolved out of the political, social and cultural upheaval in Europe during the early part of the twentieth century. However, the movement flourished mainly in America where charismatic individuals such as Moreno, Perls, Rogers and Berne were practising in circumstances distinctly different from those of their colleagues in wartime and post-war Europe. It is perhaps not surprising that this group was focused on human possibilities for growth and development while their colleagues in Europe concerned themselves with darker, self-destructive drives.

The primary training of these individuals undoubtedly influenced the conceptualization of their models, although they rejected what they perceived as the determinism of psychoanalysis and behaviourism. Following the lead of Moreno, the founder of psychodrama, the humanists recognized patients as having a central role in realizing their own potential for health and growth, thus placing the authority to effect change in the patient rather than in the therapist. This was a major shift away from the passive role traditionally expected of patients.

In 1908 *Jacob Moreno*, a Romanian psychiatrist practising in Austria, was pioneering group psychotherapy with children. From his observations of children at play he came to recognize the therapeutic possibilities in their spontaneity and use of 'make believe'. He brought together a group of actors and interested colleagues to form the Theatre of Spontaneity, where he used dramatic improvisation to facilitate this spontaneity in children and adults. By 1921, *psychodrama* was recognizable as a distinct therapeutic approach and one of the first humanistic therapies.

In 1925, because of the changing political climate in Europe, Moreno emigrated to America and established an institute in New York where he lectured and taught psychodrama. He was a major influence on the development of humanistic therapy, family therapy and group psychotherapy – a term he coined along with 'encounter' and 'here and now'. Moreno's approach attracted considerable interest from professional colleagues who participated in open group sessions. In 1942 he founded the American Society for Group Psychotherapy and Psychodrama, the first professional group psychotherapy organization. Despite this significant contribution, he is often given little credit in the psychotherapy literature.

In neighbouring Germany during the 1920s, a dynamic young couple, *Fritz and Laura Perls*, were working at the Goldstein Institute in Frankfurt. They were exposed to a range of theoretical and philosophical ideas, including Kurt Goldstein's view that human beings were, in his terms, 'self-actualizing' and 'organismically regulating'. Fritz and Laura Perls became interested in existential philosophy and the human potential movement. In an increasingly oppressive political climate, their beliefs in people being personally responsible, innately healthy and capable of growing beyond their knowledge and experience were regarded as inflammatory and the Perls were blacklisted as radical activists by the Nazi regime. In 1933 they fled, via Holland, to South Africa where they met the philosopher Smuts. He introduced them to Eastern philosophy and the concept of Holism.

Fritz Perls was an analysand of Karen Horney, and later of Wilhelm Reich. Initially, he and his wife practised as classical analysts but they became dissatisfied with the limitations of the approach and began to develop their own methods. This may have been influenced by a deep sense of disillusionment which Fritz Perls experienced on meeting Freud at a conference in Czechoslovakia in 1938. By 1946 the Perls had emigrated to New York where they established a practice and attracted the attention of political activists and the literary set. They combined their considerable clinical experience, creative flair and existential philosophy to form *Gestalt* psychotherapy, and proposed that this was a radical new alternative to psychoanalysis. The first Gestalt institute was established in New York in 1952, where Laura Perls remained active until her death in 1992. Fritz Perls never stayed in one place for long and travelled extensively, setting up training groups. In the 1960s, at the age of seventy, he was appointed Consultant Psychiatrist at the Esalen Center in Big Sur, California. By this time Gestalt had become widely recognized, and many attempts were made to emulate Perls' unconventional and charismatic style.

During the 1930s, *Carl Rogers*, a psychologist who studied theology and trained as a teacher before practising psychotherapy, was experiencing doubts about the classical analytic approach. He had trained as an analyst in the hope that it would enhance his clinical effectiveness and was disappointed when he discovered that this was not the case. In December 1940 Rogers presented a modestly titled paper, 'Some Newer Concepts in Psychotherapy' at the University of Minnesota. This was the launch of his approach based on clinical experience and years of careful research. He dispensed with opacity, transference and interpretation, believing that these methods encouraged the client to be dependent on the therapist and hindered their natural capacity for self-healing and actualization. He proposed that a trust-based, authentic, empathic relationship created the optimum conditions for the client to express and resolve psychological disturbance. The seminar was well received and prompted him to publish *Counselling and Psychotherapy* (1942), which provided a detailed account of his theory and practice.

During the 1950s Rogers became internationally renowned for the psychotherapy outcome research he carried out and inspired, and he is widely credited with gaining widespread acceptance of psychotherapy as a valid psychological treatment. Several studies conducted by Rogers and other therapists supported the hypothesis that an authentic, accepting, empathic relationship could effect positive change in people across a broad diagnostic range. In the last two decades of his life, Rogers established the Centre for the Study of the Person in California and turned his attention to world politics. He firmly believed that the humanistic approach had wider application, and travelled extensively to meet with political and religious leaders in South Africa, Eastern Europe and Northern Ireland. Rogers proposed that the way forward for humankind was by means of what he called 'the quiet revolution'. *Person-centred therapy* is now practised extensively and forms the foundation of many counselling and psychotherapy courses.

In the meantime, during the 1940s and 1950s, a group of like-minded psychologists and psychiatrists in Europe developed a philosophical approach which focused on the 'givens' of existence: death, freedom, isolation and meaninglessness. *Rollo May, Ernst Angel, Henri Ellenberger* and Irvin Yalom were influential exponents of this approach in America, and it was Rollo May who formulated what was to become recognized as *existential psychotherapy*. The psychiatrist *R.D. Laing* was a leading exponent of existentialism in the United Kingdom. Existential ideas were an important influence on the development of humanistic therapy, although the existentialists are often critical of its optimistic stance. As the existential approach is philosophical and does not define psychopathology in theoretical constructs or establish training institutes, there are relatively few practitioners. This is compounded by the value placed on accepted scientific paradigms by many medically based practitioners.

In 1957, *Eric Berne* (1910–71), a Canadian-born psychiatrist practising in the United States, published a series of papers on intuition. This heralded the emergence of *transactional analysis*, which was a model of psychotherapy and theory of personality that integrated psychodynamic concepts and humanistic principles. Berne trained at the New York Institute for Psychoanalysis and was an analysand of Paul Federn. Other important influences were ego psychologists Heinz Hartman and Ernst Kris and the neurosurgeon Wilder Penfield. Berne's first application for full membership of the New York Institute for Psychoanalysis was refused, and although Berne reputedly denies any rift between himself and the analysts, it is widely held that this rejection was the catalyst that spurred him on to develop transactional analysis.

Berne was an early exponent of 'open communication', and is reputedly one of the first psychiatrists to include patients in ward rounds and case conferences which, at the time, was revolutionary. Berne's original published works were intended for professional colleagues with an understanding of psychoanalytic concepts. Unexpectedly *Games People Play* (1968), with its immediately recognizable repetition-compulsions expressed in colloquial terms, gripped the imagination of the public and became an international best seller. The success of *Games People Play* and Thomas Harris' *I'm OK – You're OK* launched transactional analysis into a ten year period of popularity. This achieved Berne's aim of making psychoanalytic concepts accessible, but did little to endear him to his colleagues in the psychoanalytic establishment, who responded by effectively relegating transactional analysis to the realms of popular psychology.

Eric Berne was a serious and dedicated clinician who was committed to discovering the most effective way to treat psychological trauma. He made a significant contribution to psychotherapy and his concepts such as 'psychological games', 'scripts', and 'the child in the adult' have been incorporated into mainstream psychodynamic language and theory. He is rarely acknowledged in psychotherapy texts and this may reflect a long-held resentment of his apparent rejection of analytic theory. In the past thirty years transactional analysis has developed to a point where it is widely respected as an effective treatment model with broad clinical application. Transactional analysis has also developed as a specialist training with organizational and educational applications.

Humanistic therapies are now recognized and practised throughout the world. In the United Kingdom, they are mainly available in the private sector, with humanistic and integrative psychotherapists representing 25% of the United Kingdom Council for Psychotherapy register of qualified members.

Principles of theory and practice

Humanistic therapies view psychological disturbance as an interruption of the natural tendency for healthy growth. The focus of the humanistic therapist is therefore less on *why* people limit themselves and more on *how*. Insight is recognized as important, but not necessarily as the main focus of the therapeutic work. Material from the past is regarded as useful in that it can inform the therapist and client, but the main thrust of treatment is to increase awareness and enable clients to access their innate human instinct to thrive. Eric Berne called this life force *physis* and Carl Rogers identified it as the *formative tendency*. Maslow's 'hierarchy of human needs' with its *growing tip* is a well-known description.

Transactional analysis

Transactional analysis (TA) is a model of psychotherapy and theory of personality which integrates psychoanalytic concepts with humanistic philosophy. There are three distinct yet inter-related schools of theory and practice which have developed from Eric Berne's original teaching. The basic philosophical assumptions are:

- People are 'born OK'; psychological disturbance is acquired.
- People are capable of thinking independently (unless severely brain damaged).
- People are responsible for the decisions they make, and their consequences.

A distinguishing feature of TA is the use of formal treatment contracts. Client and therapist negotiate a treatment contract with a clearly defined observable outcome. This makes explicit the joint responsibility of client and therapist in the relationship, and acknowledges their equal worth.

An important principle of TA practice is the sharing of information. Clients have access to records, plan their treatment and are encouraged to learn the theory so that they can work with the therapist as they map the nature of their problems. To facilitate understanding of the basic theoretical principles, TA uses clear diagrams and colloquial language. This reduces the mystique of therapy and the therapist, and it acknowledges the client's capacity to think independently. The four cornerstones of TA theory which underpin the three TA schools are *ego states*, *transactions*, *games* and *scripts*.

Ego states

Ego states are dynamic aspects of personality originally called exteropsyche, neopsyche and archeopsyche, which Berne later renamed *Parent, Adult* and *Child* ego states (Figure 16.1). In the Parent ego state 'introjected' parent figures from the past are evoked in the present. They are the beliefs, mannerisms and emotional responses of an actual person from the past. The Adult ego state is the congruent, aware person attuned to themselves and their environment, who responds congruently without the contamination

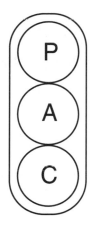

Figure 16.1   Structural ego state model (Berne, 1968)

of parental prejudice or childhood fantasy. The Child ego state is the archive of a person's total life experience to date, moments of which may be evoked and re-experienced in the present. It is therefore the Child ego state that holds the early decisions that may impede potential for psychological health and growth. These early decisions are often framed in catastrophic terms for example 'If I get angry I might kill you, so I will never show my feelings'.

In *structural analysis* the content of the ego states is explored, and the individual is encouraged to become aware of the internal dialogues between their ego states. As the client 'tunes in' to their internal conversations they become aware of the origins of the dialogue – 'Oh that was my mother's voice, telling me to keep quiet or I'll embarrass her in front of her friends'. The mother's voice is 'heard' in the Child ego state and the client cringes as they re-experience the original shame in the present (Figure 16.2).

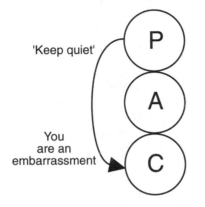

Figure 16.2   Structural analysis

Functional analysis focuses on the manifestation of five functional aspects. 'Nurturing Parent', 'Controlling Parent', 'Free Child', 'Adapted Child' and 'Adult' (Figure 16.3). For instance, a person in their Controlling Parent ego state may be rather rigid in thought and lacking in creative responses, especially when faced with the prospect of change. In Nurturing Parent they

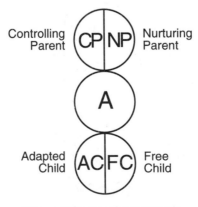

Figure 16.3   Functional analysis

may notice a friend is looking tired and express concern. When in Adapted Child they may agree to do something they do not want to do in order to avoid a confrontation. Their Free Child is often characterized by a spontaneous quality and expansive gestures. Healthy people move fluidly between their ego states.

A restricted flow of energy between ego states is evidence of psychological disturbance, which is shown as *contamination* of the Adult ego state with Parental beliefs and Child fantasies. When ego states are undifferentiated, the capacity for reality testing and self-awareness is compromised: for example, when the Parent ego state impinges on or contaminates the Adult ego state, prejudices ensue. When the Child ego state contaminates the Adult ego state a range of psychological disturbance such as 'magical thinking', phobias and delusions become apparent. The resulting 'script beliefs' are based on Parental influence and Child assumption. When there is a double contamination script beliefs based on Parental influence and Child assumption significantly impair the capacity for reality testing and rational Adult functioning (Figures 16.4–16.6). The therapist will use a range of interventions, including confrontation of 'discounts' (distortions of reality), to enable the client to de-contaminate and strengthen their Adult ego state.

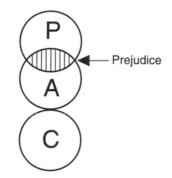

Figure 16.4 Parent contamination of Adult

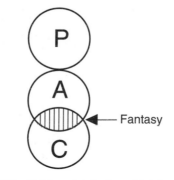

Figure 16.5 Child contamination of Adult

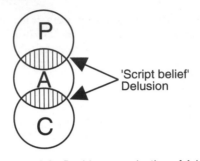

Figure 16.6   Double contamination of Adult

Transactions

These are basic units of human communication: a stimulus plus a response. In transactional analysis proper diagrams are used to identify transactional patterns between the ego states of the people involved (Figures 16.7–16.9). There are two basic levels of transacting: the overt *social level*, which is

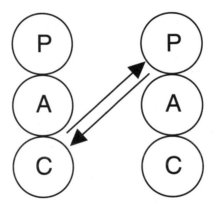

Figure 16.7   Complementary transaction

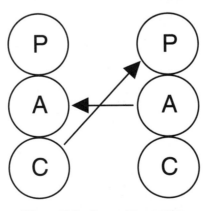

Figure 16.8   Crossed transaction

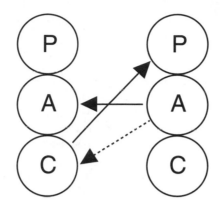

Figure 16.9 Duplex transaction showing ulterior transaction

observable, and the covert *psychological level*, which is sensed. A basic 'rule' of communication is that when transactions are made at both levels, the outcome of the communication will be determined at the ulterior, psychological level.

Games
Games are a series of transactions with a familiar pattern and predictable outcome. Those who are involved start out in one of three classical game roles – Persecutor, Rescuer or Victim. A game is characterized by the sudden switching of roles and the collection of a payoff. For example, the Victim may suddenly round on the Rescuer who ends up bewildered and thinking, 'I was only trying to help'. These games are played outside awareness as a means of generating familiar, often negative, units of recognition or 'strokes' in TA terms. In infancy, strokes are essential for survival and come mainly from close physical contact with a primary parent figure. Later, strokes are symbolized by words and gestures. Human beings will therefore settle for, and even actively seek, negative strokes rather than risk having none at all. As individuals become more autonomous the need to manipulate strokes through game playing diminishes. Relationships generally improve but, as not all complementary players are willing to change, some relationships are abandoned.

Script
This is the life plan which is constructed in infancy in response to parental influence. This script passes from consciousness but it is often faithfully acted out, with the author 'casting' for complementary players and 'setting up' the final scene. Infants, dependent on parental figures for survival, reach conclusions about themselves and others on the basis of perceived 'messages' or *injunctions* from parent figures and adapt accordingly. These parental 'messages' cannot make a person develop in a certain way but they do exert a significant influence on the formation of life scripts (Figure 16.10). Berne identified four basic life positions: I'm OK, You're OK, I'm not OK, You're not OK. Robert and Mary Goulding (1979) identified twelve messages or injunctions that are recurring themes in the formation of life scripts. The

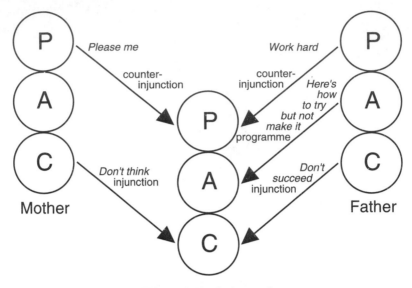

Figure 16.10   Script matrix

script decisions in response to these messages reflect a fundamental belief about the self in relation to others. The aim of therapy is to access the original messages, and the decisions made in response to them. The client can then update these decisions in the present.

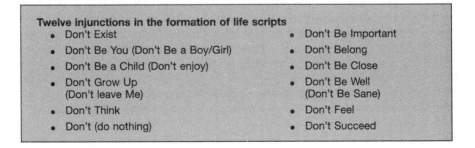

Twelve injunctions in the formation of life scripts
- Don't Exist
- Don't Be You (Don't Be a Boy/Girl)
- Don't Be a Child (Don't enjoy)
- Don't Grow Up
  (Don't leave Me)
- Don't Think
- Don't (do nothing)

- Don't Be Important
- Don't Belong
- Don't Be Close
- Don't Be Well
  (Don't Be Sane)
- Don't Feel
- Don't Succeed

Therapeutic relationship
Transactional analysis is not limited to a single type of relationship. The therapist will initially be concerned with establishing a working alliance with the client, which forms the basis of any therapeutic work. The presenting issues of the client, the therapeutic context (for example short- or long-term therapy) and the experience and preferred style of the therapist will determine the nature of the therapeutic relationship that develops. Therapists who practise the classical model may, if appropriate, work with a transference/countertransference relationship, or favour the redecision model which actively discourages the development of transference. Clarkson (1995) gives

a good account of the multiplicity of therapeutic relationships, and how the therapeutic relationship can change through the course of treatment. In common with all humanistic psychotherapies, the therapist aims to demonstrate healthy functioning and emotional literacy.

Stages of treatment
1 Establishing a working alliance with the client, mapping the nature of problems and negotiating a preliminary contract.
2 Decontamination of the client's Adult ego state. The therapist helps the client to identify the parental prejudices and childhood fantasies that they have used to distort reality and reinforce their life script. This increases self-awareness, awareness of others and the capacity for self-support.
3 De-confusing the Child ego state and developing an internal nurturing parent. This involves relinquishing fundamental strategies and beliefs that have been held as essential for survival from the Child ego state. It is important to establish that they have decided to keep themselves safe, act safely with others and stay in touch with reality: the therapeutic relationship and the potency of the therapist provides the necessary containment.
4 The final stage of therapy is the integration of new decisions and bringing to a close the therapeutic relationship. This stage often involves the client reviewing other relationships, discovering disowned aspects of their authentic self and experimenting with new ways of being.

Person-centred therapy

A fundamental *trust* in the human capacity for health and self-actualization underpins the theoretical concepts of person-centred therapy. Rogers' focus was the innate instinct to thrive present in all living organisms, even in the most challenging circumstances. His model is based on the assumption that, given the conditions conducive to healthy growth, the *formative tendency* towards actualization and fulfilment of potential is activated (Rogers, 1980). Rogers identified three essential qualities or *core conditions* that the therapist must develop: *congruence*, *empathy* and *unconditional positive regard*.

Self concept
The *self concept* represents a 'false' image of the self, constructed in response to the attitudes of significant others. This internalized perception is often characterized by a sense of worthlessness and confusion. For some people raised in a climate of criticism this negative self-view is pervasive and impedes or obscures the real, potentially actualizing *organismic* self.

Conditions of worth
Infants instinctively know what they feel and want. However, being totally dependent on others to meet their survival needs, they soon learn to adapt their feelings and expressions to the demands of primary carers. If mother recoils at an expression of rage, the infant learns to suppress that feeling and substitute an alternative response perceived to be acceptable. From the perceived message 'If you express rage, I will leave you' the infant deduces

'If I am quiet and make no demands, I'll be loved'. In adulthood, securing the approval of others involves manipulating thoughts, feelings and actions into an acceptable form. For some people the terror of abandonment, symbolized by disapproval, is so great that any authentic expression of feelings is perceived as potentially catastrophic. The individual's focus on the conditions for approval from others suppresses the authentic, organismic self and adapts to satisfy the perceived conditions of worth.

The organismic self
The organismic self is essentially the real self: aware, experiencing and highly attuned to themselves and others. This instinctive self can be trusted to seek out what is required for healthy growth. In psychological disturbance, this natural instinct for survival becomes distorted by the conditions of worth which influence the development of the 'false self' or self concept. Some people who are highly dependent on approval learn to mistrust their own instincts and, when the growing edge of the organismic self opposes the individual's belief systems, the self concept is threatened and the person experiences intrapsychic conflict. When the organismic self is accessed and expressed, the capacity for psychological health and self-actualization is activated.

Locus of evaluation
The locus of evaluation is said to be *external* when the individual is heavily invested in gaining approval from others. The organismic self is suppressed to such an extent that the individual identifies almost exclusively with their self concept. Power and wisdom is located in others and, prohibited from knowing what they really think or feel, the individual is plagued by self-doubt. When the locus of evaluation is *external*, psychological health depends on securing approval from others. This precarious conditional existence is characterized by psychological disturbance, often expressed as worthlessness and confusion.

Psychologically healthy or *fully functioning* people (Rogers, 1963) are, by contrast, secure in their sense of self-worth and trust their instincts. Attuned to themselves and others, they respond to experiences openly and creatively, making decisions on the basis of their own judgement. These people have a highly developed sense of self worth and an *internal* locus of evaluation.

The primary focus of person-centred therapy is the 'real' relationship between therapist and client. The importance of this principle cannot be overstated because it is the therapist's capacity for authenticity, acceptance and empathy in the relationship with the individual which provides the optimum conditions for self-healing and fulfilment of potential. To be effective in this encounter with the client, the therapists must be willing to attend to their own psychological health and capacity for self-actualization. This will involve personal therapy and a commitment to ongoing personal development and supervision. The emphasis on the psychological health and development of the therapist is essential because the therapist will be entering into a 'real' relationship with the client. The therapist does not have a set of techniques or theories to apply, therapist and client 'encounter' each other and, as trust develops, the conditions are created for the client to access and express their authentic, organismic self.

Congruence

In the context of person-centred therapy, congruence is the therapist's capacity for self-awareness and authentic expression of thoughts and feelings towards others. Communicating honestly and sensitively is a crucial factor in the development of trust in the relationship. The therapist actively seeks to identify and set aside thoughts and feelings which may not be relevant in the relationship with the client, and does not burden the client with their own issues. If, however, the therapist experiences a *persistent* response, perhaps over several sessions, then disclosure is viewed as relevant. To withhold or shelter clients from the therapist's authentic response, however uncomfortable it may be, undermines the development of trust and can do more harm than good.

Unconditional positive regard

Rogers considered the cultivation of a climate of acceptance as essential in the creation of the conditions required for change and growth. This affirming or *prizing* of the client confronts their negative self view. Developing this attitude presents the therapist with a considerable challenge as they learn to suspend their own value systems and seek a non-judgemental position. To be effective the therapist embraces the philosophy that living organisms, including human beings, are intrinsically worthwhile. The client is therefore not required to adapt to conditions imposed by the therapist. It is widely accepted amongst person-centred therapists that total unconditional acceptance is not possible, and that the therapist must continuously monitor their value systems in relation to the client and consider this in supervision.

Empathy

The main focus of the therapist in the relationship is to intuit and understand the meaning of the client's moment-by-moment experience, and to communicate this understanding sensitively. The therapist seeks to experience the client's inner world, to feel as the client is feeling yet with the awareness that these are the client's feelings. A common misconception about empathy is that it involves simply reflecting back the client's words, as for example, 'you are feeling sad about that'. While this response indicates that the therapist has registered what the client said, it does not demonstrate the therapist's understanding of the client's experience of sadness. One of the measures used in research studies was an empathy scale that rated the therapist's responses. The results of several studies, notably Truax (1970), show that clients of therapists who were rated as accurately empathic showed improvement while clients of therapists with low empathy scores showed some increase in psychological disturbance.

In person-centred therapy the therapeutic relationship creates a safe environment for the client to risk knowing and expressing previously denied aspects of their 'real' self. As the need to 'please' the therapist and adapt to their imagined demands is relinquished, dependency on approval diminishes. The client attunes to their own needs, and develops a sense of trust in their capacity to get these needs met.

Psychodrama

Psychodrama is primarily concerned with action, and less emphasis is placed on theory than in other models. The theoretical concepts that inform the therapist therefore focus on human qualities, and how people experience themselves in the moment rather than explaining psychopathology in depth. This is in keeping with the existentialist view that what matters is the 'here and now' process.

Role theory

As the term implies, there is a difference between the roles adopted in response to the expectations of others and the performer. In psychodrama, the therapist or director focuses on an individual or protagonist in the group and facilitates enactments of roles that the performer has assumed. The aim is for the individual or protagonist to access the authentic, uninhibited and expressive aspect of self which Otto Rank (1945) called the 'will'.

Exploring *roles* in this way offers the individual a useful structure to understand interpersonal relationships. As the group members re-enact past roles, observe other roles and experiment with different ways of being, they develop their role repertoire and their capacity for *role distance*. This is the ability to evaluate self, others and situations without the constraints imposed by the expectation of being in *role*. Moreno believed that people should constantly evaluate the roles they have assumed and be willing to experiment and change, lest they become inflexible and lacking in creativity. This may be why he always remained on the periphery of 'the establishment'.

Spontaneity

This was the quality Moreno observed in children at play and which he believed was essential for creative and effective responses to the challenges posed by daily living. Spontaneity, in Moreno's view, is not an impulsive superficial quality; it is the instinctive life force that characterizes the human capacity for actualization and fulfilment of potential. The aim of the therapist is to create the conditions for protagonists to access their spontaneity. This quality is modelled for the group by the therapist, who will be actively setting the scene and creatively using available props to facilitate the enactment.

Physical activity

It is generally accepted that the mind influences the body. In psychodrama the opposite is also accepted; the body influences the mind, and physical activity counters the feelings of passivity and helplessness so often manifested by people with psychological disturbance. In re-enactments, physically moving between one role and another makes explicit the boundaries between the self and others that may have become blurred.

Concretization

Inviting the protagonist to demonstrate rather than talk about their situation bypasses defences that are often characterized by vague intellectualizations, and uncovers inadequate or obsolete coping strategies. The director might intervene with 'don't talk about it, show us'.

Sublimation

The vital, exciting and playful nature of the psychodrama approach provides the group member with a safe and containing space to express their natural imagination and experiment with ways of accessing and channelling creative energy. This healthy, motivating experience sometimes comes as a surprise to those who associate psychotherapy with suffering and gloom.

Catharsis

The cathartic release of creative energy is a fundamental element of psychodrama and an important factor in psychological healing. Following cathartic release, individuals often report a sense of engaging with their 'real' self that they have previously denied or disowned.

The therapeutic process

The essential elements of a psychodrama group
- The **director**: the therapist who conducts the group
- The **protagonist**: the group member who is the focus of an enactment
- The **auxiliary**: another group member who plays a supporting role, such as a sibling or parent of the protagonist in the enactment
- The **stage**: the area where enactments take place. This may be a special stage or a space set aside for the work
- The **audience**: other group members who play the important role of supporting and encouraging the *protagonist*. Members of the audience may be invited to supplement the *auxiliaries*

The director or therapist does not have a pre-specified set of procedures to support the therapeutic work; each protagonist's enactment is unique. The director will be formulating strategies as the drama unfolds, assessing the material that the protagonist is presenting and improvising with whatever is available in the environment to bring to life the protagonist's 'primordial drama'. This requires sound clinical judgement and considerable creativity on the part of the therapist.

A psychodrama group session typically has three identifiable stages. The preliminary warm-up slot where the director uses an exercise or series of exercises designed to 'drum up' energy and create the group cohesion necessary for safe containment of the main body of the work. The warm-up also gives the director an opportunity to monitor group process and detect group members who might be ready to work. The second stage will be the psychodramatic enactment or enactments. This is followed by the third stage of the process, feedback, which is described in the clinical example (see pp. 333–4).

Gestalt psychotherapy

Gestalt is a model of psychotherapy derived from a synthesis of existential thought, Eastern philosophy, psychoanalytic theory and phenomenology. Together, these elements form an approach that uses active methods to facilitate *awareness* which is essential for the individual to achieve *self-regulation* and *self-actualization*. People are understood as complex bio-socio-physio-logical organisms existing in relationship with the environment and concerned with achieving and maintaining a state of balance or 'wholeness'.

Each person has an instinctive capacity to sense what is needed from the environment for healthy growth. For instance, a person may be attentively listening to a lecture when they become aware of tension in their legs. The stiffness becomes the focus of attention and the speaker's words recede; when the listener adjusts position, the stiffness eases and the speaker becomes the focus of attention again. The healthy individual adjusts fluidly between what is, at any given moment, *figure* or *ground*. Left to their own devices, the individual will sense and *aggress* or actively seek what they need to maintain their equilibrium. This ongoing process of sensing, seeking satisfaction and returning to balance forms the natural *organismic flow*, an ongoing process of Gestalt formation and destruction (Figure 16.11).

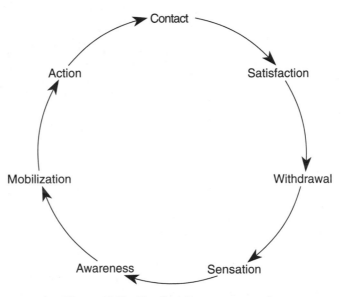

Figure 16.11 The Gestalt awareness cycle

Stages of the 'Gestalt' or 'awareness' cycle
The individual experiences a sensation and becomes aware that the cause is stiffness in their limbs. This is followed by an urge to relieve the tension and the identified action is to shift position. As the individual stretches, the tension is released and a state of physical comfort returns.

Disturbance of the Gestalt cycle
The Gestalt approach strongly resists categorizing or conceptualizing people in terms of psychopathology, and individuals are regarded as basically healthy with a natural tendency to thrive. People are not born with flawed

personalities but rather psychological symptoms are the consequence of impediments (which are often self-imposed) of the natural growth process, which is a uniquely human characteristic.

The fully functioning individual is characterized by awareness, flexibility and creative self-regulation in response to internal and external stimuli. Dysfunction manifests as a disruption of the natural organismic flow, which produces anxiety, rigidity and resistance to change. Unresolved situations or *fixed Gestalts* block the natural capacity for healthy growth. An experience in the past, which has not been resolved, will result in *unfinished business*. For example, a young man who had been repeatedly humiliated about his appearance at college withdrew to his room and created a fantasy world where he was an omnipotent superhero. He lived with his elderly grandmother and, when she died, he finally sought therapy and began to express the rage and helplessness he had denied for many years.

Contact

All living organisms exist in relationship with their environment. That which is 'me' and that which is 'not-me' differentiates the ego boundary between an individual and their environment. The individual 'lives' at the point of contact between the ego boundary and the environment, moving in and out of contact. Contact at the ego boundary can be experienced as a moment of oneness or completeness; following cathartic expression of a long held resentment an individual may experience a deep sense of connectedness. When the ego boundary becomes either undifferentiated or rigid the quality of contact is compromised and neurotic symptoms arise.

Introjection/deflection

Information is either 'swallowed whole' or 'spat out' without question. For example, an individual may accept a statement from a significant person in their life that they are insensitive without testing the reality of this belief. The contact boundary in this case is too permeable. Alternatively, when the contact boundary is rigid and impermeable, they may reject this feedback without considering that it might be useful. The healthy individual will 'chew it over' before deciding whether to accept it or not.

Retroflection

A person who does not allow themselves to express their thoughts and feelings may turn them inwards. For instance, a person who is holding back sadness may hold their breath, while a person retroflecting anger may make a fist or bite their fingers. Similarly if an individual needs reassurance, and is afraid that their demand will be denied, they may retroflect their need and sit huddled up, rocking back and forth.

Projection

Sometimes a person projects unacceptable aspects of self into the environment. For instance, a person who is suppressing angry feelings may attribute them to someone else and say, 'you're obviously angry with me'. In these cases, the projected aspects of self are not necessarily negative: for example, a student may project her creativity onto an admired tutor rather than accept that she has matured and no longer needs the relationship.

Confluence
This occurs when the ego boundary is not differentiated and the individual does not have a clear sense of what is 'me' and what is 'not-me'. The confluent individual often becomes involved with others very quickly and then feels overwhelmed and retaliates or withdraws. When a person makes contact without awareness, perhaps agreeing to something they do not feel comfortable with, they are said to be *confluent*.

These mechanisms all have positive aspects. For example, projection is closely allied to empathy and it is prudent not to hit someone in anger but to hold on and find a safe way to express the feeling. Reassuring oneself can also be a healthy way of coping. The important factor is the individual's capacity for awareness and flexible contact at the boundary.

Gestalt in practice
The primary aim of the Gestalt therapist is to facilitate the individual's capacity for awareness, to identify and resolve interrupted Gestalts or unfinished business, and to promote healthy functioning. The therapist encounters the patient in a real relationship, actively confronting the development of transference. Instead, the individual is invited to tune in to their authentic thoughts, feelings and expressions.

Gestalt is traditionally practised in groups, where the therapist works with an individual who takes the 'hot seat' whilst the other group members witness the work. This draws on the experience of the working members to facilitate a form of self-therapy. The group ends with people sharing and processing the impact of the therapeutic work. Gestalt therapy is now increasingly used as an individual therapy with a broad range of application, including the treatment of people with severe psychological disturbance.

Gestalt therapists create experiments to facilitate awareness and authentic expression. These include techniques such as empty chair work, role reversal and enactments. They also use careful tracking of the individual's moment-by-moment responses, such as a shift in the pattern of breathing which may indicate a retroflection. Some of these experiments may involve 'heightening' the internal conflict between the individual's authentic need and the self-imposed prohibition, which can result in the cathartic release of suppressed feelings. The therapist will assess the individual's capacity to withstand this depth of work and their capacity for self-support. As in other humanistic models where the therapist encounters the patient in a real relationship, they must develop a high level of self-awareness and personal effectiveness. This facilitates trust in the therapeutic relationship and models healthy functioning for the client.

Which patient and why?

Everyone can, potentially, benefit from humanistic therapy: from the individual seeking to enhance their potential for self-awareness and personal growth, to the severely psychologically disturbed individual requiring intensive longer-term treatment. Humanistic therapy actively promotes independence, the capacity to think effectively and taking personal responsibility for actions. People with psychological disturbance are not regarded as being 'ill'.

Some models, such as Gestalt and transactional analysis, are effective with people who have disorders of personality, particularly in the context of therapeutic communities where a high level of continuing support and the normalizing effect of the milieu creates the optimum conditions for intensive therapeutic regression, such as re-parenting and cathartic experiments. Transactional analysis is applied successfully with client groups who are often excluded by other psychotherapy approaches, such as people with learning disabilities and addictions. It is based on a treatment model of assessment, diagnosis, treatment planning and reassessment and therefore integrates well with medically based services such as acute psychiatry. Rogers demonstrated in his research that the person-centred approach is effective with people from broad diagnostic categories, including psychosis, and is also applicable in educational and organizational settings.

It is the competence of the therapist in relation to the individual's level of psychological disturbance and the therapeutic context that is the determining factor in selection. Therefore it is the responsibility of the therapist to assess a client carefully, to decide if the therapeutic environment is adequate, to establish if client and therapist can work together safely and whether they are competent to practise with a particular client.

Considerations at assessment for humanistic psychotherapy

- What is the nature of the client's difficulty?

- What is the therapist's experience, and is the therapeutic setting viable?

- What is the client's current capacity for reality testing and self-support?

- What is the client's motivation for therapy? Do they want to have therapy or are they under pressure from someone else? Are they willing to change?

- What is missing? What have they not emphasized? A person may seem very disturbed but on the other hand is competent at work; equally they may seem very composed and be concealing an intention to self-harm.

- What is the client's agenda? What does the client expect from the therapy? Is the therapist willing to facilitate this? For instance a client may imagine that the therapist will 'make them better'; highlighting unrealistic expectations is important.

Transference is usually discouraged because it can create long-term dependence on the therapist, unnecessarily prolonging treatment. Many people do not have the time, inclination or financial resources to commit themselves to therapy several times a week for a number of years. This is also an important consideration for services with finite resources where it is in the best interests of the client and the organization to support the client's capacity to function independently.

There are no specific contraindications for humanistic therapy, although there are cautionary notes. Humanistic therapists are mindful of the potency of their approach and will carefully match the 'dose' of therapeutic intervention to the client's level of tolerance.

Which therapist and why?

Training in humanistic therapy is an advanced training. The majority of humanistic therapists are graduates of medicine, psychology, social work, psychiatric nursing or an equivalent profession. They also have additional relevant training and experience, such as counselling or other psychotherapy qualifications.

Training is by accumulation of specified learning activities, supervision and personal therapy hours. Trainees are usually 'sponsored' by a named supervisor who monitors the professional and personal development of the trainee throughout training, and who will endorse any application for final examination. Many trainees choose to affiliate to a particular training establishment, and there are a growing number of institutes affiliated to universities. It is also possible to accumulate accredited training hours and supervision hours at other centres and this practice is often encouraged as it broadens the trainees' range of experience.

The personal development of the trainee is crucial in any humanistic training. Training is therefore as much about self-development and actualization as it is about building a sound theoretical base and effective clinical practice. Trainees may at any time during the training be advised to take 'time out' to work with their own issues and will not be supported to take their final assessment if there are any doubts about their fitness to practise.

Final examination and endorsement to practise usually involves three stages:

- A written dissertation or series of papers that must demonstrate the candidate's grasp of the theoretical concepts relating to their particular model as well as a working knowledge of psychodynamic principles and psychiatric diagnosis. Candidates who do not have a mental health qualification are required to undertake a psychiatric placement.
- A clinical case study, which shows their integration of theory and practices, and which is usually supported by audio-tapes of sessions.
- When the written stage has been passed the candidate can apply for a final assessment that will involve live supervision of practice, sometimes over several days, by external examiners and peers.

The whole training process usually takes from three to five years to complete. As the course requirements are personally demanding, often inviting significant change in the trainee, it is not unusual for some to take longer to reach the stage of final assessment.

No humanistic training is ever fully complete. Implicit in all humanistic therapies is the expectation that practitioners will continue to develop, and that as part of their actualization process will test, question and experiment. Postgraduate supervision and professional development is therefore recommended, and is a requirement for continuing endorsement to practise by most bodies of humanistic therapy. There is no better way to discover the nature of such an active approach than by personal experience.

Therapeutic setting

Flexibility is one of the most significant advantages of humanistic therapy. Moreno took his troupe and set up the Theatre of Spontaneity at venues all over Vienna. This capacity to adapt to a wide range of client groups and therapeutic settings is useful. The therapist is not tied to the same room at the same hour on the same days, although this level of consistency is possible if it is appropriate in the context of the therapeutic contract. This capacity for flexibility means that humanistic models of therapy can be integrated with other treatment programmes and models such as psychodrama, Gestalt and transactional analysis are particularly effective in the context of intensive treatment settings such as therapeutic communities.

There is little provision of humanistic therapy in the National Health Service (NHS) and limited opportunities to gain experience of these methods in NHS services. A gradual process of rapprochement is emerging in the form of innovative NHS services which recognize the value of diversity and which provide a range of therapeutic expertise, including humanistic therapy (Knowles, 1997).

Currently, humanistic therapy is mainly practised in the private sector, individually and in groups. These may be mixed or gender-specific and will range from weekly slow-open groups to a series of weekend marathons. Because humanistic therapists are not restricted to a particular method of practice and type of setting the creative possibilities are endless. The therapeutic setting will largely depend on the professional background of the therapist and the context of the therapeutic work. Humanistic therapists are usually creative people with wide interests and this is often reflected in the spaces they create to work in. Seating is comfortable and there are usually plenty of cushions and other materials for use in active work. However, this is not a requirement and, in stark contrast, the psychodramatist may set up a stage in a disused ward in an old psychiatric hospital with just a few large cushions. Some therapists, such as those who work with creative arts and drama, will require art materials, musical instruments and sand trays, and any of the therapists using active methods will need sufficient space for the client or group to move around.

Clinical example

A psychodrama group starts with a warm-up theme of 'waltzing around the group', which is centred on families and relationships. After a few minutes of this, Anna is clearly warmed up to an issue involving her mother, and she anxiously recalls an argument they had the previous night.

As this is a psychodrama group, we soon stop talking about it and move into action with Anna as our protagonist. Although psychodrama is a group method, the main part of the drama is usually focused on one protagonist with other group members participating in various ways. We start building the scene and increasingly seeing it, hearing it and experiencing it, as the level of exploration and understanding deepens. Often the extra dimension of stimuli that the re-enactment offers triggers this intensity. Various group members are 'roled in' to represent Anna's family members, and the scene is reconstructed and examined. Role reversal is the main tool in psychodrama, and it extends emotional and intellectual awareness.

All participants in the scene re-enactment become truly involved and engaged, highlighting and opening up unresolved and unconscious issues for Anna to work with. Classical psychodrama 'follows the emotional smoke' (as Moreno used to say) and will try to work from the periphery to the core. In Anna's case, last night's row re-enactment triggers off a memory of a previous time when she felt similar which is then re-enacted. This pathway through past scenes is followed until the original trauma is reached and the emotional intensity of the experience is understood in the core situation. Often this core experience is traced back to childhood. The experienced helplessness, as in Anna's case is, of course, very real: when growing up, the core experience of realistic helplessness becomes a neurotic habitual response to certain triggers.

Once the core experience is explored and understood and suppressed emotions (often anger) expressed, the protagonist may need to experience the event differently from the original experience. The psychodrama director may encourage the protagonist to act in 'surplus reality', in order for them to experience something new. In Anna's case this was expressing her anger towards her mother as a little girl, and acting out a fantasy of gagging her at will and being in control. Having now internalized the experience of expressing emotion and taking control in a situation, the psychodrama returns to the 'here and now' and Anna is encouraged to handle the argument differently.

Going from the periphery to the core and back to the here and now has meant moving through exploration, catharsis, increased understanding, reparation and finally a rehearsal for living. In Anna's case, the action part of the drama concludes with an enactment of a future confrontation with her mother, and the group coaches Anna in a range of behavioural options. The extensive role reversal, the relief of unexpressed emotion and the 'surplus reality' experience has unblocked and strengthened Anna, giving her the resources, and the tools to deal with the situation differently next time.

The session ends with a 'group sharing'. Group members are encouraged to share their emotions and experiences with the protagonist, Anna, which helps her to feel less exposed. It also serves as a time for group members to ask for support, if needed. Processing the work, intellectualizing, or any kind of 'talking about' the session, is discouraged in the sharing.

Problems in therapy

Myths about humanistic psychotherapies abound and are generally fuelled by mistrust and fear. Some of the more commonly held myths are:
- 'There is no sound theory.'
- 'It is only applicable for people with mild psychological disturbance.'
- 'Humanistic therapists stir up people's feelings, which is dangerous.'
- 'They are unprofessional and not "proper" psychotherapists.'

Touch
There is also considerable misunderstanding about the use of touch, with a failure to recognize its value when used with careful clinical judgement and supervision. Clarkson (1995) gives an excellent account of the use of touch, and also self-disclosure in a clinical context.

Creativity in the face of distress
Another widely held belief is that any treatment which actively encourages behavioural change and creative expression cannot be as valid as treatment

which focuses on painful and distressing feelings. Humanistic therapy does encourage independence and self-actualization, and to achieve this painful and difficult feelings and beliefs are often explored. For many clients this is familiar territory, and the challenge is to access creative, healthy responses and thus promote autonomy.

Cultural context
The humanistic approach is characterized by a high level of emotional literacy. This capacity for authentic expression is not as highly prized in Western culture as intellectualization and this may account for some of the misunderstandings that occur. The philosophical approach is also very different from a medical or scientific paradigm, and may be difficult for the more scientifically orientated individual to accept.

Effectiveness and risk
Humanistic therapy is a highly effective method of treatment. This is sometimes underestimated and people attempt to use powerful treatment techniques without an understanding of the theoretical principles. Humanistic therapy is concerned with the release of suppressed emotion but is also, in competent hands, a safe and containing way of working with difficult client groups, particularly those with personality disorders. Active methods are not always employed.

Past or present focus
Working 'in the moment' with a borderline client can be far more effective than working with material from the past which a client can use to fuel disturbance. Any technique that invites separating out aspects of personality, such as empty chair work, is to be avoided in the early stages of treatment as the client uses this splitting as a defence. Instead, the therapist invites the client to stay with their current sensations, which has a grounding and containing effect.

Insufficient training
A therapist untrained in the humanistic approach may not have sufficient training to make these clinical decisions and adjust the focus of treatment, the result of which may be an uncontained outburst or deterioration and the end of therapy. This can perpetuate the myth that active methods are dangerous. But any psychotherapy is potentially ineffective, or harmful, when practised by untrained or incompetent therapists. Humanistic therapists who are properly trained can work safely with suppressed feelings in clients with high levels of disturbance and facilitate healthy expression of these emotions.

Evaluation of therapy

Humanistic psychotherapy evolved out of dissatisfaction with traditional methods of working. As part of the rejection of established scientific practice, outcome research has not played a significant role. Rogers was one of the few humanistic therapists committed to research, which he pursued throughout his academic career.

In 1957, he was appointed Professor of Psychiatry and Psychology at Wisconsin University and launched a major project researching the effectiveness of the person-centred approach in the treatment of people diagnosed with schizophrenia. One of the notable conclusions of this study was significant improvement in subjects who reported the therapist as accurately empathic. Several studies carried out by Rogers and others support the hypothesis that an authentic, accepting, empathic relationship effects positive change in people across a broad diagnostic range.

Despite Rogers' efforts and Abraham Maslow's recommendation that research would secure the future of the humanistic therapies, there has been relatively little published. This situation is changing as the national associations and training establishments have become aware of the importance of rigorous evidence-based research, and are now investing in research programmes. There is also a significant rise in the number of training establishments affiliated to universities and offering higher degrees. Most would see this as a positive development for the humanistic movement and look forward to the publication of humanistic-related psychotherapy research.

However, there is some disquiet amongst those practitioners who view these efforts to capture and define aspects of people as antithetical to the ethos of humanism. It remains to be seen if practitioners accept the call for research, and whether papers relating to humanistic therapies are submitted to and accepted for publication in mainstream psychotherapy journals.

Alternatives to therapy

Person-centred therapy is applicable in a wide range of settings, including education and large organizations. The core conditions of congruence, empathy and positive regard form the foundation of most psychotherapy and counselling practice, and can be widely used as part of other mental health treatments.

Transactional analysis is arguably one of the most adaptable humanistic models. It has a broad theoretical base and a range of treatment options. As it is based on a model of assessment, diagnosis, treatment planning and reassessment it integrates well with medically based services such as acute psychiatry. Psychodrama has been integrated with a number of other approaches, including family therapy. Gestalt experiments have been adopted by therapists of many orientations and practised in a variety of settings.

Contrary to popular belief, it is also possible for humanistic and analytic approaches to integrate well. When there is a willingness to work collaboratively with a genuine mutual interest in the knowledge and experience of the other, analysts and humanistic therapists can have useful dialogue, enhance their effectiveness and both learn more about their own approach by comparison with another.

Acknowledgements
I would like to thank Ineke Powell for contributing the clinical example to this chapter.

Further reading

Berne, E. (1961) *Transactional Analysis in Psychotherapy.* London: Souvenir Press.
Boy, A. and Pine, G. (1982) *Client Centred Counselling: A Renewal.* Boston: Allyn and Bacon.
Clarkson, P. (1989) *Gestalt Counselling in Action.* London: Sage.
Clarkson, P. (1992) *Transactional Analysis Psychotherapy: An Integrated Approach.* London: Routledge.
Clarkson, P. (1995) *The Therapeutic Relationship.* UK: Whurr Publications.
Global, F. (1970) *The Third Force.* New York: Grossman.
Greenberg, I.E. (1975) *Psychodrama: Theory and Therapy.* London: Souvenir Press.
Hatcher, C. and Himelstein, P. (1995) *The Handbook of Gestalt Therapy.* New York: Jason Aronson.
Johnson, F. (1985) *Characterological Transformation.* New York: Naughton.
Kurtz, R. (1990) *Body-Centred Psychotherapy.* California: Life Rhythm.
Perls, F.S. (1969) *Ego, Hunger and Aggression.* New York: Random House.
Polster, E. (1987) *Every Person's Life is Worth a Novel.* London: Norton.
Rogers, C.R. (1951) *Client-Centred Therapy.* London: Constable.
Rogers, C.R. (1980) *A Way of Being.* Boston, MA: Houghton, Mifflin.
Stewart, I. (1989) *TA Counselling in Action.* London: Sage.
Stewart, I. and Joines, V. (1987) *TA Today: A New Introduction to Transactional Analysis.* Nottingham: Life Space Publishing.
Tillich, P. (1960) *The Courage To Be.* London: Fontana/Collins.
Van Duerzen Smith, E. (1988) *Existential Counselling in Practice.* London: Sage.
Wilbur, K. (1979) *No Boundary: Eastern and Western Approaches to Personal Growth.* Boston, MA: Shambhala.

Bibliography

Barnes, G. (1977) *Transactional Analysis After Eric Berne: Teachings and Practices of Three TA Schools.* New York: Harper and Row.
Berne, E. (1957) Ego states in psychotherapy. *American Journal of Psychotherapy,* **11**, 239–309.
Berne, E. (1966) *Principles of Group Treatment.* New York: Grove.
Berne, E. (1968) *Games People Play.* Harmondsworth: Penguin.
Berne, E. (1973) *What Do You Say After You Say Hello?* New York: Bantam.
Clarkson, P. (1995) *The Therapeutic Relationship.* UK: Whurr Publications.
Clarkson, P. and Pokorny, M. (1994) *The Handbook of Psychotherapy.* London: Routledge.
Corsini, R. and Wedding, D. (1984) *Current Psychotherapies.* USA: F.C. Peacock.
Dryden, W. (1984) *Individual Therapy in Britain.* Milton Keynes: Open University Press.
Frick, W.B. (1971) *Humanistic Psychology: Interviews with Marlow, Murphy and Rogers.* Columbus, OH: Charles E. Merrill.
Goulding, M.M. and Goulding, R.L. (1979) *Changing Lives Through Reduction Therapy.* New York: Brunner/Mazel.
Harris, T.A. (1973) *I'm OK – You're OK.* London: Pan Books.
Knowles, J. (1997) The Reading Model: an integrated psychotherapy service. *Psychiatric Bulletin,* **21**, 84–87.
Mace, C. (1995) *The Art and Science of Assessment in Psychotherapy.* London: Routledge.

Maslow, A. (1968) *Toward a Psychology of Being*, 2nd edn. New York: Van Nostrand Reinhold.

Maslow, A. (1987) *Motivation and Personality*, 2nd edn. New York: Harper and Row.

McNeel, J. (1976) The parent interview. *Transactional Analysis Journal*, **6**, 61–68.

Mellor, K. and Andrewartha, G. (1980) Reparenting the parent in support of redecisions. *Transactional Analysis Journal*, **10**, 197–203.

Moiso, C. (1985) Ego states and transference. *Transactional Analysis Journal*, **15**, 194–201.

Moreno, J. (1965) Therapeutic vehicles and the concept of surplus reality. *Group Psychotherapy*, **18**, 211–16.

Perls, F.S. (1969) *Gestalt Therapy Verbatim*. Utah: Real People Press.

Rank, O. (1945) *Truth and Reality*. New York: Knopf.

Rogers, C.R. (1942) *Counselling and Psychotherapy*. Boston: Houghton, Mifflin.

Rogers, C.R. (1961) *On Becoming a Person*. Boston, MA: Houghton, Mifflin.

Rogers, C.R. (1963) The concept of the fully functioning person. *Psychotherapy: Theory, Research and Practice,* **1**, 17–26.

Rogers, C.R. (1980) *A Way of Being.* Boston, MA: Houghton, Mifflin.

Steiner, C. (1974) *Scripts People Live*. New York: Grove.

Truax, C.B. (1970) Length of therapist's intervention, accurate empathy and patient improvement. *Journal of Clinical Psychology*, **26**, 539–541.

Woollams, S. and Brown, M. (1978) *Transactional Analysis*. Dexter, MI: Huron Valley Institute.

17

Forensic Psychotherapy

Samuel M. Stein and Gwen Adshead

There is a better way of dealing with criminals than putting them in prison.
Edward Glover (1888–1972)

Introduction

What is forensic psychotherapy: is it a separate discipline in itself, a special branch of forensic psychiatry or a variant of psychotherapy? Over the past decade, there has been an explosion of interest in this field which reflects a number of different factors (Adshead, 1991). First, looking back over the past one hundred years, the problem of interpersonal violence has never seemed more pressing. Secondly, there is growing evidence that retributive actions and increasingly punitive measures by society do not reduce violence, and may even increase it. Thirdly, research developments in cognitive neuropsychology and developmental psychopathology are starting to confirm our common intuition that most human behaviour has meaning. This holds true even for violence in the context of mental illness, where 'rationality-within-irrationality' can be found (Link and Stueve, 1994).

However, some types of criminality and violence leave us with a sense of psychological bereavement and bafflement which requires thought. Forensic psychotherapy looks to address this process by attempting to understand both the conscious and the unconscious motivations in the criminal mind which underlie the offence. Forensic psychotherapy does not seek to condone the crime or excuse the criminal, but rather to consider the individual offender within the context of the family, the group, the institution and, more broadly, within society (Welldon, 1993; Cordess and Cox, 1996).

Historical perspective

For centuries, the psychological causes of crime and violence have intrigued those interested in human nature, including psychologists, criminologists, sociologists, anthropologists, physiologists and psychoanalysts. In this sense, forensic psychotherapy is not a new discipline (Evans *et al.*, 1996).

Freud himself made a major contribution to the development of this field as his theories relating to criminality, delinquency and violence paved the way for an understanding of anti-social behaviour, and for understanding crime as a sequel to unconscious criminal intention (Winnicott, 1965). Freud (1916) suggested that acts of criminality stem from an unconscious sense of guilt – the criminal unconsciously sets himself up to be punished for unacceptable unconscious fantasies. As described by Cordess (1992), criminal acts are therefore committed as a consequence of the individual's sense of unconscious guilt and not because of the absence of a capacity for guilt. Reik added to Freud's work in his 1925 paper entitled 'Compulsion to Confessing and Need for Punishment'. Freud also made an active contribution to understanding perversion and perverse behaviour. He initially believed that perversion was simply a carrying into adult life of a fixated piece of infantile sexuality, but went on to postulate that 'neuroses are, so to say, the negative of perversion'. In other words, perversion seeks to increase sexual pleasure whereas neurosis seeks to reduce the conflict caused by the possibility of sexual pleasure (Freud, 1905; Stoller, 1986).

Klein's contributions have also been important in the development of forensic psychotherapy. She acknowledged the role of innate aggression and the death instinct, and suggested that all children utilize unconscious primitive mechanisms in order to manage their hatred and aggression toward loved objects. Such mechanisms may persist into adult unconscious life and be replicated in conscious relationships with others. The development of object relations theory enhanced the evolution of forensic psychotherapy as most violence takes place within the context of a relationship. For example, the victim may unconsciously symbolize an important figure from the offender's past.

Psychoanalysts such as Bion, Fairbairn, Bowlby and Winnicott all contributed to the understanding of criminal behaviour. Fairbairn suggested the existence of an 'internal saboteur' which might account for disordered relationships in adulthood (Guntrip, 1982). Bion (1970) elaborated a model of containment whereby the baby's intolerable thoughts are projected into the mother, digested and then returned to the child in a more manageable form. This constitutes the origin of the capacity for thought, which will make an immediate resort to action in times of stress less likely later in life. Both Bowlby (1969, 1973) and Winnicott (1984) believed that the failure to provide adequate care in childhood led to insecure attachment and impaired self-identity, which directly contributed to delinquency and violence. Bowlby's 'Forty-four Juvenile Thieves' (1944) also helped to bring these issues to public attention.

Cordess (1992), describing the fragile legacy of psychoanalysis and crime, details the more recent history of the forensic psychotherapy movement in the United Kingdom. Several important psychoanalytic papers on criminality were published in the 1920s, and led to the foundation of the Institute for the Study and Treatment of Delinquency (ISTD) in London in 1931. Edward Glover was a co-founder of the ISTD and, by 1933, the vice-presidents included Adler, Havelock Ellis, Freud, Jung and Otto Rank. Therapeutic work at the ISTD led to adaptation of classical psychoanalytic techniques, and the 'Psychopathic Clinic' was opened at the West End Hospital in 1933. Staff included Wilfred Bion, Melitta Schmideberg and John Bowlby, all of whom worked without payment. With the advent of the National Health

Service (NHS) in 1948, this institution became known as the Portman Clinic, which continues to play a leading role in the development of forensic psychotherapy today, including the provision of an established Diploma Course in Forensic Psychotherapy. An International Association for Forensic Psychotherapy has also been established, and held its eighth annual meeting in 1998.

Principles of theory and practice

Principles of theory

According to Cordess and Williams (1996), the criminal act is multi-determined. As such, sexuality and aggression are neither inherently good nor bad, and both have a positive and adaptive role to play in human behaviour. However these behaviours can be distorted by internal and external experiences, leading to delinquency, criminality, addiction, violence and perversion. According to McDougall (1990), these serious acting-out behaviours may all have similar mental mechanisms and may simply represent different methods of solving the same basic unconscious conflict (which is the approach followed in this chapter to explain the general principles of the many different forms of deviant behaviour). This 'solution' may take the form of a neurotic symptom, a perversion, a psychosis, a criminal career or even a work of art. As described by Welldon (1994), the forensic psychotherapist therefore needs to investigate the crimes in detail, especially the sequence of events leading up to the action as well as the offender's reaction to it. This can give clues to early traumatic experiences, and to the unconscious way through which an individual tries to resolve conflicts resulting from these experiences. The more we can understand about the criminal mind, the more we can take positive preventative action and implement better management and treatment.

The meaning of the criminal act

The criminal act may be calculated and associated with professional careerist criminality; however, many criminal acts are a consequence of unconscious processes and fantasies which tell us something about the internal world of the perpetrator (Welldon, 1994; Cordess and Williams, 1996). The deviant acts may have a specific unconscious meaning and function, or may represent the offender's desperate attempt to give some meaning to his life. The significant themes and images which underlie the offence can be used by the perpetrator to render otherwise incomprehensible aims and object choices meaningful (McDougall, 1990). It is therefore important to define the deviant act according to the intrapsychic meaning which it has for the offender, based on his feelings, thoughts and the psychological necessity of criminal behaviour rather than simply defining deviant behaviour according to societal expectations (Stoller, 1986). The same deviant act may thus have a significantly different meaning and function for different people according to their level of personality development (McDougall, 1990).

The influence of appropriate parenting

Deviant behaviour is often the result of disturbed family dynamics, and many offenders have experienced a past history of childhood abuse, deprivation and neglect (Stoller, 1986; Welldon, 1994). Winnicott (1965) viewed crime as a symptom of failure in childcare, with deviant behaviour being deeply rooted in the mother–child experience and associated with very primitive anxieties. In these situations, the mother seems unable to enter into a state of reverie or to provide 'good-enough' parenting by containing and modifying the infant's intolerable anxieties. Instead, the mother treats the child as an extension of herself and uses the relationship to meet her own psychological needs.

The mother presents to the child as 'contradiction itself', being both seductive and forbidding, gratifying and frustrating, welcoming and rejecting (McDougall, 1990). As a result, the child is subjected to excessive stimulation with which it cannot cope and develops an enormous sense of helplessness, vulnerability, fear and defencelessness (Welldon, 1994). This situation is compounded by a failure in paternal function as it is the task of the father to protect the child from the relationship with the mother, and to help his children become independent of her. This failure makes it difficult for the child to identify with a worthwhile father, or to develop an internal image of a parental couple that may be complementary to one another. The resulting interpersonal dynamics interfere with the child's process of separation and individuation. Overwhelming feelings of dependency, loneliness, emptiness and object-loss occur, which the child attempts to master by developing psychological defences (McDougall, 1990). These separation anxieties can easily produce dangerous acting out in later life, especially when experiences of separation and loss are evoked (Welldon, 1994). However, childhood difficulties cannot provide the whole explanation since not all children who receive inadequate parenting become criminal or violent.

Aggression and hostility

The child, as a result of anxiety, fear, bewilderment and frustration, develops enraged and aggressive feelings towards its mother and father. This anger serves a discharge function which alleviates anxiety and tension (Glasser, 1979). However, any aggression towards the parents on whom he depends may threaten the child's self-preservation and endanger his psychic health (Anna Freud, 1936). The problem then is how to master hatred of the parents and achieve control over murderous rage. Aggression and hostility therefore need to be deflected, transformed into more acceptable social functions or repressed. The child who is healthy is able to master these emotions (Winnicott, 1958; McDougall, 1990).

Excitement is one of the ways in which aggressive anxieties can be defended against, when overwhelmed by feelings of fear, rage and violence. Aggression is thus important in the aetiology of criminality and perversion. The deviant scenario serves as a container for rage, mortification and violently destructive impulses, and aggressive wishes are held in check by compulsive behaviour (Rosen, 1979; McDougall, 1990). At the core of the perverse act, according to Stoller (1986), is the desire to harm others and deviant behaviour is therefore more of a study of hostility than of libido. Unfortunately, aggressive impulses do not provide any satisfaction unless there is opposition to the resultant behaviour, and the environment must be tested and re-tested in its capacity to stand the aggression (Winnicott, 1958). This is to demonstrate to the perpetrator that he has not destroyed his loved objects or been destroyed by them himself. In the exchange, the mother's idealized image remains non-conflictual, the mother is constantly repaired and assurance is provided that no one is destroyed (McDougall, 1990). The aim of the deviant behaviour is therefore to protect the people on whom one is dependent, whilst still satisfying one's need to destroy and attack.

Failure of symbolic thinking

Segal (1957) described the child's capacity to deal with unresolved conflicts by symbolizing them. An inner fantasy world is created to deal with intolerable aspects of reality and to render them understandable. Loss is made tolerable by introjection of lost objects which become internalized and eventually a part of the self. This development of internal representations or symbols permits the child to free himself from helpless dependence on the environment and important external objects.

In contrast, the perpetrator of deviant acts demonstrates a clear failure of symbolization, with a cutting of associative links and a limited capacity to develop an internal world. Instead, they function at a pre-symbolic level in which the image is seen only as it presents in concrete reality rather than as a psychic representation. The offender therefore has to use external objects to fill the gap created by symbolic failure. In other words, they substitute objects in the external world to do duty for absent internal symbolic objects. This leads to concrete thinking and the use of violent projective mechanisms rather than symbol formation in mediating internal conflict – for example, hitting a total stranger who reminds one of one's mother rather than dealing with the hostility towards her within one's own mind. The lack of symbolic internal objects means an endless repetition and addictive attachment to the outer world and external objects (McDougall, 1990).

The perpetrator is compulsively driven to repeat the action endlessly as the traumatic childhood experience is memorialized in the offence rather than symbolized (McDougall, 1990). This piece of infantile history is re-enacted ritualistically as a means of gaining ego mastery of the event. The offence is restricted and unvarying, with the plot being the same in every instance. The perpetrators lack imagination, and there is poverty of both fantasy and invention. With minor variations the scene always involves the punishment of an innocent victim, such as a child being chastised by its mother. These rituals serve the function of undoing separation, and are resorted to when the offender feels threatened (Stoller, 1986; McDougall, 1990).

The 'core complex'

According to Winnicott (1965), the infant is either in a permanent state of being merged with the mother or else staging a total rejection of the mother. Glasser (1979) described a similar 'core complex' evident in deviant patients which comes into play very early on and, based on a love–hate relationship, develops into a vicious circle. A deep-seated longing for an intense and intimate closeness to another person arises, amounting to a state of merging, oneness or 'blissful union'. This longed-for state implies complete gratification with absolute security and containment of any destructive feelings towards the object in question. However, with this merging comes a loss of self and a sense of annihilation by the object. This results in flight from the object to an emotionally safe distance and a premium is placed on independence and self-sufficiency. Unfortunately, the distance and isolation again bring separation anxieties and a desire to be merged with the object, and relief is sought through renewed contact with the object. The deviant individual is thus caught in a cycle whereby intimacy is annihilatory and yet separation is isolating, prompting a tendency to repeat the experience again and again. It is simultaneously a search for, and fear of, fusion with the other.

The anti-social tendency

In 1958, Winnicott described what he called the anti-social tendency. He said that it arose as a reaction to deprivation, usually based on good-enough early experiences that had since failed or been lost. The anti-social tendency was an attempt at self-cure, aimed at repairing a break in the continuity of environmental provision, and thus implied an expression of hope. The anti-social tendency is in essence object-seeking, and the anti-social child who steals an object is not looking for the object stolen but seeks a mother or father on whom he can make a claim because he feels deprived of their love. Greediness as a result of deprivation is the precursor of stealing, and can be seen as an attempt to recover one's lost internal objects by laying claim to substitute objects in the external world. By stealing, the anti-social child is compelling someone to re-establish environmental stability. The compulsion to go out and buy something (instead of stealing it) is a common manifestation of the anti-social tendency in non-deviant individuals. The anti-social tendency therefore represents hopefulness in a deprived child who is otherwise hopeless, hapless and harmless. This understanding that the anti-social act is an expression of hope is vital in the treatment of those who manifest with anti-social tendencies.

Childhood trauma to adult triumph

Freud (1920) described how changing from a passive to an active role may serve as a means for assimilating unpleasant or traumatic experiences. For example, the infant playing with a cotton reel to master its sense of helplessness at the mother's unwanted absence. The aim is to actively reverse roles, especially if they involved humiliation and deception, converting childhood trauma into adult triumph and allowing the victim to become the victor. Thus revenge is hidden in almost all deviant actions, as is the desire for mastery, control, humiliation of others and defiance. This relates mainly to the internalized parents and is acted out in the external world. As a result, each time a deviant act is committed, a triumph is celebrated. The essential purpose of deviant behaviour is therefore to be superior to, harmful to, triumphant over and in control of another (Stoller, 1986). However, the triumph is only celebrated if the offender has a sense of having overcome the same risks as existed during the childhood episodes. The risk is not that of being caught or sent to gaol, but of suffering the repeated humiliation of a childhood trauma. Running these risks introduces an element of excitement, leading to an elevated sense of self-esteem and courage. It is important to recognize that the offender will want to gain a sense of having overcome terrible odds, but the sense of risk must only be an impression as if the risk is too high, anxiety will escalate instead of being dissipated (McDougall, 1990).

Identification with the aggressor

Identification with the aggressor is the core of Anna Freud's contribution to the study of defence mechanisms. It is a powerful device for combating objective, external anxiety situations by denial of vulnerability and help-lessness. The victim tries to master his anxiety by involuntarily imitating the aggressor, identifying with the dreaded external object. Using mechanisms of both projection and identification, roles are reversed between the attacker and the attacked. By impersonating the aggressor, assuming his attributes or imitating his aggression, the child transforms himself from the person threatened into the person who makes the threat (Anna Freud, 1936). It is important to note that the victim identifies not with the person of the aggressor but with his aggression. As described by Dyer (1983), the individual introjects the characteristics of the forces in the outside world which are perceived as threatening. The sense of being threatened is transformed into a sense of being threatening within the individual by impersonation and identification. These threatening and aggressive aspects are then projected back on to the outside world. Thus victims who become perpetrators experience a conscious or unconscious desire to take revenge for the pain inflicted on them, and act out the nature of their abuse on someone who reminds them of their own powerlessness. In this way, they find someone else to take over their own traumatized self-representation, someone who will experience the unwanted feelings instead of themselves. Unfortunately, this leads to three-generational processes and cycles of abuse.

The nature of perversion

Freud (1905), in his 'Three Essays on the Theory of Sexuality', clarified the features common to all perversions. Wakeling has since defined sexual deviation as the persistent and compulsive substitution of some other act for heterosexual genital intercourse. However not all aberrant sexual acts are perversions, and there is no succinct generally accepted theory of the perversions (Rosen, 1979).

Conditions that determine the development of sexually deviant behaviour are laid down in early childhood, and a relationship has been demonstrated between the severity of an adult perversion and the severity of the traumatic experience in childhood. In this sense, perverse behaviour derives from infantile sexuality and has a grain of historical reality, as historical events are represented in the details of the manifest sexual act (Rosen, 1979; Stoller, 1986).

Deviant behaviour is dictated more by non-sexual than by erotic needs, and serious offences such as rape and incest are committed virtually unaccompanied by pleasure (Rosen, 1979). What is important is the partner's response, and his lack of control or reduction to childlike helplessness. The partner may also be reduced to the level of a part-object and dehumanized to serve as an inanimate container for destructive wishes (McDougall, 1990). Perversion is thus the product of anxiety and always contains the element of conflict. Anxiety and pain are transformed into pleasure in what amounts to the libidinization or eroticization of anxiety, hatred and aggression (Stoller, 1986).

The perverse act often alternates between being ego-syntonic before the event but ego-dystonic afterwards. The consequent sense of shame and guilt which follows the feelings of excitement and pleasure then results in a re-creation of the initial sense of anxiety that initiated the episode in the first place. Relief is again sought by engaging in pleasurable and ego-syntonic deviant behaviour, and an ever-narrowing cycle of deviant behaviour is set in motion. The more ego-syntonic the individual's deviance, the less likely he is to change (Rosen, 1979).

Aims of therapy

Norwood East, a founding father of forensic psychiatry, wrote in 1949 that 'treatment must be directed towards the long and difficult task of amending the character of the offender rather than the speedy dissipation of a collection of acquired symptoms' (Cordess, 1992). Similarly Winnicott (1965) wrote that we must supply the criminal with an environment that corresponds to that which is normally needed by the immature infant and which is able to take up all the strains resulting from ruthlessness and impulsiveness.

Forensic psychotherapists are in an unusual position with regard to the aims of therapy because they may have more than one role. It is rare for the patient to self-refer, or to have actively sought out psychotherapeutic treatment; so psychotherapy is often being offered to someone at a third

---

Aims of forensic psychotherapy
- The development of a psychodynamic understanding of the offender and the consequent treatment regardless of the seriousness of the offence
- An ability to act as an attachment figure and container who can help the patient to learn to think and to experience affects safely
- A capacity to help impose conscious thought between the offender's impulses and actions
- A willingness to assist the patient to speak and develop an emotional language, especially about their offences
- Establishment of realistic goals which are geared towards the patient's needs and abilities
- Encouragement of the individual to take greater responsibility for their actions

party's request. The patient may ask 'Are you here for me?' Similarly, the court or institutional framework of the therapy may ask 'Are you here for us?' The answers to these questions may be in conflict, and can lead to ethical dilemmas.

How does forensic psychotherapy differ from other therapies?

Forensic psychotherapy is not a separate school, with a complete set of theories and practice to accompany it. It involves work with a particular patient group; those who act rather than think, and who alternate between a victim and a perpetrator identity. The patients are disabled and damaged individuals who do not fit the customary criteria for psychotherapy; indeed they may be people specifically thought unsuitable for such treatment.

Forensic psychotherapy is different from other forms of therapy because society is directly involved. It is a triangular situation between patient, therapist and society which goes beyond the special relationship between the patient and the therapist (Welldon, 1994). Instead, forensic psychotherapy is the handling of three interacting positions – the psychotherapist's, the patient's and that of society's criminal justice system.

Forensic psychotherapy differs in a number of other ways. The vast majority of patients will be young males, and many will have histories of at least transient psychosis. It is also unusual for a forensic psychotherapist to work outside an institution or team. Although some forensic psychotherapy does take place in out-patient settings, such as the Portman Clinic in London, these are the exception. Forensic psychotherapy is most often the psychotherapy of in-patients and institutions, and implies a collaborative endeavour between a range of different agencies (Cordess and Cox, 1996).

Finally, forensic psychotherapy differs by virtue of its attention to security. Although the emphasis will be on internal security (states of mind, affect and dreams), the psychotherapist has to be aware of the external security context as well. This includes not only the question of risk to others, but also the question of the therapists' own safety and the need to make the therapeutic space secure.

Principles of practice

The term 'forensic' derives from the Latin *forum*, where the Roman equivalent of a court was held. Thus forensic mental health services, including psychotherapy, offer care to offenders with mental health needs. The patient population is highly heterogeneous and the forensic psychotherapist works with very different groups of patients.

Group psychotherapy for offender patients

Welldon (1993, 1994, 1996) has described in detail the role of forensic group therapy and the considerable potential which this treatment option offers.

A group setting may provide containment and enlightenment to both victims and perpetrators of abuse, and successfully mix patients with sexual deviancy, social deviancy and criminal behaviour. Group therapy aims to facilitate a move towards acting less and suffering more.

Some patients are more suitable for group therapy than others, and therapists should err on the side of caution when setting up a therapy group. The attrition rate can be reduced by careful preparation of patients prior to entering the group. Patients who have been subjected to an intense, suffocating relationship with one parent often do best in group therapy. In contrast, patients who have never experienced satisfactory relationships in early life are more likely to benefit from individual therapy. Those with large and chaotic families are likely to find groups threatening and frightening. The only significant contraindication to group therapy is voyeurism.

According to Welldon, a slow-open group may be offered which is run by a single therapist (as a couple may trigger destructive and envious attacks). Within the group setting, individuals have the opportunity to deal with the externalized representations of many of their internal objects. However, the multiple transferences that arise within the group provide the patient with more than one target for their aggression, which they find very reassuring. In this sense, the group structure makes it more difficult for transference/countertransference processes to take place. A firm and rigorous style is advocated which allows confrontation, although all interpretations are linked to here and now dynamics.

Group analytic therapy breaks through the patterns of self-deception, fraud, secrecy and collusion present in deviant behaviour. Secrecy is especially prevalent in cases of childhood sexual abuse, and extreme secretiveness is one of the contraindications for working within a group setting. The group also provides sources of identification and role modelling, and allows perpetrators to become aware of the extensive consequences of their actions when confronted by other members of the group. The group acts as an auxiliary ego and superego, with a greater capacity than individual therapy to deal with violent behaviour. However, the therapist must remain vigilant for any attempt by individuals to pervert the group process, or attempts to encourage either peers or the therapist to collude with perverse behaviour.

Application of psychodynamic theories to forensic institutions

The forensic psychotherapist tries to understand the effects of managing forensic psychiatric patients on the treating institution as the nature of the clinical material affects not only staff–patient relationships, but also staff–staff relationships and the relationships of clinicians with managers.

Most forensic settings also have a custodial aspect, so that security matters add an additional source of concern, and sometimes conflict, with the therapy. Concerns about 'security' at an institutional level (e.g. walls, keys, uniforms) are often manifestations of staff members' inner insecurity, and will escalate as staff feel less internally secure. Lack of internal security may reflect the personal histories of staff but may also be a manifestation of a change in the institutional dynamics on the staff. A different patient mix, the admission of a notorious killer or the departure of the much valued cleaner may all affect the dynamics of life on a ward.

Winnicott (1955) suggested that the therapist's role in treating some regressed and damaged individuals was simply to survive. The forensic psychotherapist needs to survive, and to represent thinking as a reasonable strategy in the face of anxiety. Given that most offending takes place when thought gives way to action, there will be enormous pressures on staff to act first and think afterwards. The forensic psychotherapist 'stands for' thinking, and can act as a type of psychic brake on runaway action in an institution.

Contributing to risk assessment

There is increasing concern about violent acts carried out by mentally ill patients. Several recent psychotherapy publications (Cordess and Cox, 1996; McGauley, 1997) have addressed the contribution of forensic psychotherapy to the assessment of risk.

Forensic psychotherapists can offer a way of understanding the meaning of violent thoughts, feelings and acts for the individual patient. The relevance of a psychoanalytically oriented risk assessment is demonstrated by the relationships between victims and offenders. Seventy per cent of homicide victims are related to their killers; 80% of children killed each year are killed by their parents. Sixty per cent of rapists know their victims, and a similar percentage holds for child abuse perpetrators. As most crimes of interpersonal violence (sexual or non-sexual) occur between people who have been emotionally attached at one time, a psychodynamic approach to risk assessment, which focuses on psychological development and symbolic representations of caregivers, can be useful.

The forensic psychotherapist may be in a position to consider any risks which the patient presents for staff. Replication of internal world relationships is just as likely to occur with psychiatric staff as with other adults; in fact, it may be more common because of the staff's conscious identity as caregivers. The power of the repetition compulsion in violent patients with childhood histories of trauma should not be underestimated, and can lead to dangerous therapeutic situations in both in-patient and out-patient settings. The psychotherapist can also provide information on any changes, internal or external, which the patient has made while in therapy.

Supervision and support of staff working with offender patients

Supervision is possibly the forensic psychotherapist's most important task because working with forensic patients is difficult, especially living in the shadow of violence without becoming violent oneself. Nursing staff may be in twenty-four hour contact with offender patients, and all forensic professionals have to survive listening to dreadful accounts of violence and cruelty. The task of the forensic psychotherapist is to try to help colleagues to survive in constructive rather than destructive ways.

One difficulty for staff in forensic settings lies in constructing therapeutic alliances with patients who may be profoundly suspicious of any care offered. The internal world of many offender patients is a frightening one, where carers cannot be trusted. Any disappointment by carers is experienced as excruciatingly painful, and stimulates powerful feelings of rage and grief.

Attack being the best form of defence, offender patients may be likely to attack the carer whom they perceive as such a threat to internal homeostasis.

> Vignette 1
>
> *On the ward, Jane was repeatedly verbally abusive to staff, using obscene language and demeaning staff by calling them 'screws'. She also made derogatory remarks about or veiled threats towards their children and families. Jane was repeatedly physically restrained, and often placed in seclusion. In this way, Jane re-enacted with staff her previous experiences of failed care or abuse. She projected on to staff her negative internalized object relationships from the past. Jane was also able to keep her own identity as a perpetrator of violence hidden by locating such behaviour only in the staff. She may well have done the same thing to her victims.*

Staff have to contain violent projections from patients which may resonate with their own capacity for violence, or with feelings of rage and humiliation, and cause a sense of loss of control. Loss of psychological control induces fears of loss of physical control, which then raises conscious and unconscious anxiety. Such anxiety can result in unduly punitive measures against patients. This results in patients' feeling victimized and seeing the staff as aggressors (perhaps very similar to their previous abusers), and the whole cycle begins again.

It is important not to underestimate the degree of real physical risk that there may be to staff in both out-patient and in-patient settings. In secure settings, staff have a contractual responsibility for external safety. Staffing levels are usually precarious, and the patients have committed frightening offences in the past. Given this situation, it is understandable why staff anxieties can sometimes overwhelm their abilities to think appropriately.

Staff support is notoriously difficult to provide in mental health or criminal justice settings. Staff may fear they will become 'a patient' and may also resist coming to terms with their own fantasies of violence. Despite these difficulties, it is vital to provide a 'psychological space' for staff to use in this way. Thinking through clinical controversies may help to separate the patient's pathology from the staff or institutional pathology, especially by paying attention to uncomfortable conscious as well as unconscious feelings. Even if staff can only talk about their work with patients, rather than about themselves, the forensic psychotherapist has a role in helping staff to survive, and to think, which in turn contributes to the maintenance of hope.

Damage limitation: long-term management of very ill patients

For some patients, the psychological damage done in childhood and intensified in adulthood will be too great. Just as there is a need for palliative care in general medicine, so there may be those for whom only psychological palliative care, or damage limitation, can be offered. However, such patients may make significant demands on clinical teams and individual therapists.

As Cox (1976) said, 'If no-one ever left Broadmoor [Special Hospital], you would need more psychotherapists, not less.'

In out-patient settings, such patients often need indefinite psycho-therapeutic support with occasional in-patient admissions. In secure settings, such patients may never appear safe enough to be released. There are also those individuals whose past offences are so notorious that they have been completely rejected by society and can never be released because society would not tolerate it. Such patients need long-term supportive psychotherapy, which is a task in its own right, including supported grieving for all that has been lost (Holmes, 1993).

Staff working with this level of damage and disability need particular support. Patients who are not going to 'get better' challenge professional identity and achievement, and arouse feelings of grief, anger and anxiety. Unless thought about and understood, these feelings may result in unconscious aggression towards patients. This may be acted out by staff as abuse, neglect, dismissal of patients as 'untreatable' or excessive use of medication.

Which patient and why?

By and large, patients who are suitable for other forms of dynamic psychotherapy would benefit from forensic psychotherapy. Referrals come primarily from prisons, the probation service and consultant forensic psychiatrists. As with all referrals for psychotherapy, the question of 'Why has this patient been referred, why now and why by this person?' is well worth asking. It may also prove helpful to discuss with the referrer their expectations of the team, and any previous experience of therapy which the patient has undergone. Although most psychotherapy patients have experienced loss or abuse in childhood, forensic psychotherapy patients have often suffered extremes of trauma or deprivation which make them quantitatively as well as qualitatively different.

There has been surprisingly little written about assessment in forensic psychotherapy, and one should not be too dogmatic about indications and contraindications for therapy. Given that the index offence must be discussed at some point in the therapy, experience suggests that complete denial of the offence means that the patient is probably not yet ready for psychotherapy. However, reassessment or consideration of other forms of therapy should always be considered.

Intermittent psychotic episodes are not a bar to therapy provided there is adequate containment, either physical or pharmacological (Cox, 1990). Any history of a positive attachment which has lasted several years is a hopeful sign, as is a history of getting into and staying in education. A history of current addiction may render therapy unworkable since the patient will be literally 'out of their mind' in the sessions.

Some types of offending may necessarily suggest a particular therapeutic strategy. Sex offenders and patients with psychopathic personalities may do better in groups (Cox, 1973, 1976), or therapeutic communities (Dolan, 1994). Many forensic patients may find groups daunting because they lack communication skills, and short periods of individual therapy may be indicated prior to joining a group. Some patients may benefit from more structured forms of therapy before they begin analytic therapy.

Despite common psychiatric folk lore, there is no evidence to support the assumption that personality disorders are untreatable (Dolan and Coid, 1993). Research evidence increasingly suggests that different forms of personality disorder may respond positively to different types of psychotherapeutic approach (Fonagy *et al.*, 1996). However, patients may get worse before they get better, and the possibility of deterioration may influence the considerations about the venue of therapy. Patients may not be able to begin psychotherapy unless they are in a secure environment.

In an out-patient setting, the therapist may find referral prompted by a pending court case in which the defence wishes to suggest to the court that the offender is motivated to change. Such referrals can create interesting dilemmas as a positive assessment may influence the judge to make a non-custodial disposal, enabling the offender to have treatment. However, the offender patient's motivation may dwindle once freed of the threat of prison, and the therapist may feel 'conned'.

Which therapist and why?

There are many types of forensic psychotherapists, including nurses, psychologists, creative therapists, social workers and medically qualified psychotherapists. The range of professional groups reflects the range of roles a forensic psychotherapist can play; however some therapists may concentrate more on one activity than another.

Forensic psychotherapists may come from various background professions. Whatever the therapist's initial training, it is essential that they have extensive clinical experience as both psychotherapists and as forensic professionals. They need to be fully conversant with the range of forensic settings and psychopathology. Ideally, they will have spent some time working as forensic health care professionals. Guidelines are currently under consideration by the Royal College of Psychiatrists in regard to developing an integrated four or five year training for forensic psychotherapists.

Professional career choices often reflect unconscious processes. Those who choose to work with patients with histories of perversion and violence will need to carefully explore their choice of forensic psychotherapy in their own analysis. It is not possible to practise as a forensic psychotherapist without having undergone such a therapy and ongoing supervision is important, no matter how experienced the therapist.

As a theoretical school, forensic psychotherapy is unlikely to avoid the splits traditionally associated with psychoanalysis and related movements. Indeed, the clinical material itself promotes such splitting as affects of envy, rage and grief may rapidly become too much to bear. Forensic psychotherapy therefore needs to retain a capacity for eclecticism, and maintain an open mind in every sense, because there is still so much to learn and understand.

Therapeutic setting

Secure settings

In purely custodial settings, such as prisons, the forensic psychotherapist is likely to work principally with extremely disturbed young men. They are often from deprived ethnic groups, with histories of severe mental illness, and may have committed serious interpersonal violence. Therapists may also be asked to work with sex offenders, or those with a history of addiction. Very few prisons have access to a psychotherapist but, where such a service is available, the psychotherapist also has a role in supervising and supporting staff.

In the setting of medium or maximum security hospitals, the forensic psychotherapist will see similar patients and some even more disturbed or dangerous individuals. The psychotherapist may see more female offenders, and also women who repeatedly self-harm. Many patients will have committed homicide, and many may have attacked health care professionals. Patients in such settings may be notorious, and the therapist's association with them may be viewed by others with horror, anger or anxiety.

Out-patient or non-secure settings

In an out-patient setting, the forensic psychotherapist is likely to see patients who are less behaviourally volatile than those in in-patient or custodial settings. However, such patients may be no less complex or potentially dangerous. Their psychological disturbance may be more encapsulated and patients may be gainfully employed, may be in long-term relationships and may even be quite socially successful. Non-fatal child abusers and patients with sexually deviant behaviour may commonly be seen as out-patients. It is not unusual for patients to self-refer to out-patient settings.

The Portman Clinic in London offers an NHS psychotherapy service to many such patients, and to patients who may have been discharged from more secure settings. Therapeutic communities like the Henderson Hospital, and to a lesser extent the Cassel Hospital, offer therapy for a subset of personality-disordered forensic patients who are motivated to accept help, and who can tolerate the boundaries set by the community.

Problems in therapy

Boundary maintenance

Every criminal or violent act involves the breaching of a boundary. Given the power of the patients unconsciously to repeat previous relationships, and the destructive quality of those relationships, the forensic psychotherapist needs to be vigilant about boundary maintenance. Boundary violations in therapy most often represent an enactment of previous abuse, or the index offence.

Attacks on the therapeutic boundary can come in many forms: reluctance to come to the sessions, late arrivals, attempts to obtain extra time or special information from the therapist, and (rarely) personal attacks. Attempts may also be made to split the therapist off from others who are involved with the patient's care; this is especially true in the out-patient setting where the therapist may be dependent on the patient for information about their situation.

Physical and psychological boundary violations easily occur between staff and patients. Patients may unconsciously attempt to split staff teams by forming unboundaried relationships with one member of staff. If the staff member responds in an unthinking way, then they too can breach boundaries. Occasionally, these can develop into sexual relationships which may be repetitions of previous abusive relationships.

Vignette 2

Sue described having violent thoughts towards her children, and was admitted to a local psychiatric hospital. There she disclosed a long history of sexual abuse by her father, and began treatment with a psychotherapist. Both parties agreed that no information about the sessions would be disclosed to anyone. The sessions became more frequent, often taking place in the evening. Sue was discharged from the hospital but the sessions continued in the psychotherapist's home. Sue and her therapist also began to meet socially. Then the psychotherapist abruptly withdrew, expressing concerns about boundaries, leaving Sue distressed and angry. She made threats to harm someone, and was found to have a large knife in her possession. Anxieties about her risk to others caused her to be admitted to a maximum security hospital.

Another common way in which boundaries may be tested or broken lies in the tension between victim and perpetrator identity. Most patients have both identities, and so may members of staff. Tensions arise when some staff see the patient as a victim, whilst others see the patient as a perpetrator.

Vignette 3

Jim presented with a long history of armed robbery and mental illness. The clinical team believed that his most recent offence was caused by a lack of medication. Jim said that he did not take his medication because his father told him not to. The clinical team perceived the father to be a difficult man, who undermined their efforts. One clinician said, 'Jim is a nice man really, his offence was his father's fault.' Although Jim's father may indeed have been a bully, who subverted the therapeutic process, Jim's own perpetrator identity was hidden by the clinical team. They (and Jim) focused on his identity as a victim of his father, whereas Jim's own capacity for violence needed to be addressed and could not be as long as it was blamed on his father. Unconsciously, the therapeutic work of the team had been undermined.

The maintenance of boundaries is also about the provision of safety. In forensic psychotherapeutic practice, safety and security need to be maintained both internally and externally. Only by strict attention to therapeutic boundaries and, more especially, to any violation of those boundaries, can the space be made safe enough for the exploration of pain and violence. In the words of Robert Frost, 'Good fences make good neighbours'.

Countertransference

The work of the forensic psychotherapist is profoundly affected by counter-transference feelings. When working with very traumatized individuals, where the damage has taken place at a pre-verbal stage or traumatic events have caused a lack of voice, then countertransference may be the best indicator of what is happening in the room at that moment.

> Vignette 4
>
> *In an early session with a man convicted of sexual violence, the therapist felt an inability to breathe. The windows were wide open, the therapist was quite well, the sensation came on quite suddenly and began several minutes after she entered the room. The therapist felt really quite desperate, and the patient said very little. As she struggled for breath, the therapist recalled that the patient had nearly killed a man by strangulation and that this assault had never been reported to the police. The feeling left as suddenly as it came, without any further intervention. Subsequently it was possible for the patient to tell the therapist how difficult he found it to express feelings of rage and violence in the sessions.*

The forensic psychotherapist needs to pay close attention to feelings, especially those feelings which are strongly positive or negative. In the absence of language, somatic feelings (like those described above) may be indicators of literally 'unspeakable' feelings which patients have to project in order to maintain their sense of self. These projected emotions may resonate with the therapist's own internal world, especially with their own experiences of violence, rage and grief.

All professional staff may act out countertransferentially, from the cleaner to the general manager. Staff and patients' ambivalence about thinking may manifest itself as institutional resistance to psychotherapy, a curious absence of rooms available for psychotherapeutic sessions or the mysterious removal of the patient without any warning. Such behaviour may also represent an unconscious hatred of the patients and their offences, or destructive envy that the patients can have anything as 'nice' as therapy. The task for the forensic psychotherapist is to tolerate and understand both their own countertransference and that of others (Carpy, 1989).

Ethical dilemmas

Ethical dilemmas arise because psychotherapy with offender patients has a moral valence that other types of therapy lack. Classical psychoanalytic theory, as well as other forms of psychodynamic therapy, are essentially non-judgemental. But in custodial institutions it may be necessary (and inevitable) that the therapist does make judgements about the patient's actions as boundary violations may arise, leading to collusion between staff and patients. It is arguably not possible (and possibly not lawful) for the therapist to fail to disclose a patient's threats to escape or harm someone.

Evaluation of therapy

At present, only limited research exists. Very little is known about the mechanisms of change in forensic psychotherapy and there is a paucity of process research. Outcome research is based largely on recidivism, which is notoriously unreliable, and forensic psychotherapy is not yet at a stage where formal meta-analysis is possible (Evans *et al.*, 1996). Epidemiological studies are also needed to provide established baselines for subsequent psychotherapy research (Levinson, 1997).

Early research into deviancy included Bowlby's (1944) study of juvenile delinquents which demonstrated a link between deprivation, trauma and offending. Similarly, Winnicott (1958) found a link between deprivation and an antisocial tendency. These findings have been confirmed in subsequent studies which demonstrated a higher incidence of childhood maltreatment, specifically physical abuse and neglect, in prison populations (Levinson, 1997). Also there is a positive correlation between negative childhood experiences and adult psychopathology (Evans *et al.*, 1996), and a link between sexual abuse and later substance misuse, delinquency and criminal behaviour (Burgess *et al.*, 1987).

Unfortunately, forensic psychotherapy research is fraught with difficulties. The prison culture may interfere with psychotherapy practice, the attrition rate tends to be high, the population is mobile, confidentiality is limited and the reliability of the information provided by offenders needs to be treated with caution (Evans *et al.*, 1996; Levinson, 1997). Ethical issues are legion, and written consent and ethical approval should be obtained for all research projects.

Research must be aligned with the clinical aims of treatment, and caution must be exercised as statistical significance does not always reflect clinical significance. In the early stages of forensic psychotherapy research, single case studies and small sample studies may contribute enormously to our understanding of offenders, their actions and possible treatment options (Levinson, 1997). Unfortunately, these findings cannot automatically be generalized to other clinical populations.

There is also a need for forensic psychotherapy research in order to justify ongoing funding of clinical services. This is especially important in the face of criticisms regarding the psychoanalytically oriented treatment of offenders in the past. Audit projects may therefore play an important part in future evaluation as forensic patients are heavy users of health services (Evans *et al.*, 1996).

Alternatives to therapy

At present, most mentally-ill offenders are treated with medication, although this is often combined with psychotherapeutic approaches. In contrast to general psychotherapy settings, where multiple therapeutic approaches are discouraged, forensic patients may be engaged with a number of different forms of therapy simultaneously. In an in-patient setting, patients may have access to a variety of therapeutic opportunities, whereas in out-patient settings there may unfortunately be little on offer. There is certainly scope for more joint working between psychotherapy and other forensic services.

Offender patients may be offered cognitive or behavioural therapy, and specific behavioural treatments have been developed to enhance socially appropriate behaviour. Cognitive behavioural therapy has also been developed for the treatment of sex offenders (Marshall *et al.*, 1990) and for borderline personality disorder (Linehan, 1993). Evaluation of these approaches has shown a degree of efficacy which persists over time. The main limitation is that any repetition of dysfunctional relationships with the therapist is not explored in any depth. This can result in acting out behaviour on the part of the therapist being missed. The symbolic significance of the act for the patient may also be missed, with the risk that the patient feels misunderstood. However, such therapies may be indicated for those who become too aroused by the affects that accompany dependence in inter-personal relationships, and who may need to feel cognitively contained.

Bentovim (in Cordess and Cox, 1996) describes the nature of trauma-organized systems and the role of systemic thinking in the treatment of offenders. Offending behaviour is a problem that needs to be understood in context as the nature and degree of the offence is often socially constructed. The offender needs to be considered in relation to his family and the wider network as the deviant symptom may play a part in stabilizing the family and maintaining the system's coherence.

Other psychotherapeutic approaches are commonly used in forensic settings, and patients may later progress to more intensive psychodynamic work. The creative therapies (music, art, dance and drama therapy) have developed strongly in forensic settings. These approaches recognize the educational limitations of some forensic patients and also recognize that, for many patients, childhood trauma may have occurred at a pre-verbal stage. Helping the patient to find a voice and language can be the first step in providing forensic psychotherapy.

Further reading

Cordess, C. and Cox, M. (1996) *Forensic Psychotherapy: Crime, Psychodynamics and the Offender Patient.* London: Jessica Kingsley.

McDougall, J. (1990) *Plea for a Measure of Abnormality.* London: Free Association Books.

Rosen, I. (1979) *Sexual Deviation*, 2nd edn. Oxford: Oxford University Press.

Stoller, R. (1986) *Perversion: the Erotic Form of Hatred.* London: Karnac Books.

Welldon, E. and van Velsen, C. (1997) *A Practical Guide to Forensic Psychotherapy.* London: Jessica Kingsley.

Bibliography

Adshead, G. (1991) The forensic psychotherapist: dying breed or evolving species? *Psychiatric Bulletin*, **15**, 410–412.

Bion, W. (1970) Container and contained. In: *Attention and Interpretation*. London: Maresfield Reprints.

Bowlby, J. (1944) Forty-four juvenile thieves: their character and home life. *International Journal of Psychoanalysis*, **25**, 207–228.

Bowlby, J. (1969) *Attachment and Loss. Volume I: Attachment*. London: Hogarth Press.

Bowlby, J. (1973) *Attachment and Loss. Volume II: Separation*. London: Hogarth Press.

Burgess, A.W., Hartman, C.R. and McCormack, A. (1987) Abuser to abused: antecedents of socially deviant behaviours. *American Journal of Psychiatry*, **144**, 1431–1436.

Carpy, D. (1989) Tolerating the countertransference: a mutative process. *International Journal of Psychoanalysis*, **70**, 287–294.

Cordess, C. (1992) Pioneers in forensic psychiatry. Edward Glover (1888–1972): psychoanalysis and crime – a fragile legacy. *Journal of Forensic Psychiatry*, **3**, 509–530.

Cordess, C. and Cox, M. (1996) *Forensic Psychotherapy: Crime, Psychodynamics and the Offender Patient*. London: Jessica Kingsley.

Cordess, C. and Williams, A.H. (1996) The criminal act and acting out. In: C. Cordess and M. Cox (eds), *Forensic Psychotherapy: Crime, Psychodynamics and the Offender Patient*. London: Jessica Kingsley, pp. 13–21.

Cox, M. (1973) Group psychotherapy as a redefining process. *International Journal of Group Psychotherapy*, **23**, 465–473.

Cox, M. (1976) Group psychotherapy in a secure setting. *Proceedings of the Royal Society of Medicine*, **69**, 215–220.

Cox, M. (1990) Psychopathology and treatment of psychotic aggression. In: P. Bowden and R. Bluglass (eds), *Principles and Practice of Forensic Psychiatry*. Edinburgh: Churchill Livingstone, pp. 631–639.

Dolan, B. (ed.) (1994) Therapeutic communities for offenders. *Therapeutic Communities*, **15**, 227–329 (the entire volume is dedicated to the role of therapeutic communities in the treatment of offenders).

Dolan, B. and Coid, J. (1993) *Psychopathic and Antisocial Personality Disorders: Treatment and Research Issues*. London: Royal College of Psychiatrists, Gaskell.

Dyer, R. (1983) *Her Father's Daughter: the Work of Anna Freud*. London: Jason Aronson.

Evans, C., Carlyle, J. and Dolan, B. (1996) Research: an overview. In: C. Cordess and M. Cox (eds), *Forensic Psychotherapy: Crime, Psychodynamics and the Offender Patient*. London: Jessica Kingsley, pp. 509–542.

Fonagy, P., Steele, M., Steele, H. *et al.* (1996) The relation of attachment status, psychiatric classification and response to psychotherapy. *Journal of Consulting and Clinical Psychology*, **64**, 22–23.

Freud, A. (1936) *The Ego and Mechanisms of Defence*. London: Hogarth Press.

Freud. S. (1905) Three essays on the theory of sexuality. In: *The Standard Edition of the Complete Psychological Works of Sigmund Freud*, vol. 7. London: Hogarth Press.

Freud, S. (1916) Criminals from a sense of guilt. In: *The Standard Edition of the Complete Psychological Works of Sigmund Freud*, vol. 14. London: Hogarth Press.

Freud, S. (1920) Beyond the pleasure principle. In: *The Standard Edition of the Complete Psychological Works of Sigmund Freud*, vol. 18. London: Hogarth Press.

Glasser, M. (1979) Some aspects of the role of aggression in perversions. In: I. Rosen (ed.), *Sexual Deviation*, 2nd edn. Oxford: Oxford University Press, pp. 278–305.

Guntrip, H. (1982) *Personality Structure and Human Interaction*. London: Hogarth Press.

Holmes, J. (1993) Supportive analytic therapy. In: *Between Art and Science: Essays in Psychotherapy and Psychiatry*. London: Routledge.

Levinson, A. (1997) Research. In: E. Welldon and C. van Velsen (eds), *A Practical Guide to Forensic Psychotherapy*. London: Jessica Kingsley, pp. 261–269.

Linehan, M. (1993) *Cognitive-Behavioural Treatment of Borderline Personality Disorder.* New York: Guilford Press.

Link, B. and Stueve, A. (1994) Psychotic symptoms and the violent/illegal behaviour of mental patients compared to community controls. In J. Monahan and H. Steadman (eds), *Violence and Mental Disorder: Developments in Risk Assessment.* Chicago: Chicago University Press.

Marshall, W.L., Laws, R. and Barbaree, H.E. (1990) *Handbook of Sexual Assault.* New York: Plenum Press.

McDougall, J. (1990) *Plea for a Measure of Abnormality.* London: Free Association Books.

McGauley, G. (1997) The actor, the act and the environment: forensic psychotherapy and risk. *International Review of Psychiatry,* **9**, 257–264.

Reik, T. (1925) Geständniszwang und strafbedürfnis; Probleme der Psychoanalyse und der Kriminologie. Reprinted as 'The compulsion to confess: on the psychoanalysis of crime and punishment', *From the Works of Theodor Reik.* New York: Farrar, Straus and Cudahy, 1959.

Rosen, I. (1979) *Sexual Deviation,* 2nd edn. Oxford: Oxford University Press.

Segal, H. (1957) Notes on symbol formation. *International Journal of Psychoanalysis,* **38**, 391–397.

Stoller, R. (1986) *Perversion: the Erotic Form of Hatred.* London: Karnac Books.

Welldon, E. (1993) Forensic psychotherapy and group analysis. *Group Analysis,* **26**, 487–502.

Welldon, E. (1994) Forensic psychotherapy. In: P. Clarkson and M. Pokorny (eds), *The Handbook of Psychotherapy.* London: Routledge, pp. 470–493.

Welldon, E. (1996) Contrasts in male and female sexual perversions. In: C. Cordess and M. Cox (eds), *Forensic Psychotherapy: Crime, Psychodynamics and the Offender Patient.* London: Jessica Kingsley, pp. 273–289.

Winnicott, D.W. (1955) Metapsychological and clinical aspects of regression within the psychoanalytical set-up. *International Journal of Psychoanalysis,* **36**, 16–26.

Winnicott, D.W. (1958) *Collected Papers: Through Paediatrics to Psycho-analysis.* London: Tavistock.

Winnicott, D.W. (1965) *The Maturational Process and the Facilitating Environment.* London: Hogarth Press.

Winnicott, D.W. (1984) *Deprivation and Delinquency.* London: Tavistock.

18

Psychotherapy and General Practice

James Herdman

Historical perspective

He who asks questions will get answers – but hardly anything else.
Michael Balint, 1957

This paradoxical statement by one of the most influential thinkers on general practice encapsulates the dilemma faced when working in this area, particularly as a general practitioner trying to take a good clinical history while paying heed to any number of underlying agendas.

The demands of this situation have always been different from those of psychotherapy within a hospital or clinic. Textbooks, dogma and theory have less place than wide experience of life, common sense, intuition, empathy and lateral thinking. For a patient, the general practitioner (GP) has many roles: physician, surgeon, gynaecologist, servant of the state, confidante, social acquaintance, community figure and sometimes psychotherapist too. Somehow all these roles must be consolidated without jeopardizing the validity of any one of them. It is not an easy act to balance and becomes more complicated when the GP engages a patient in some form of psychotherapy.

In contrast to the more compartmentalized role of the specialist, the role of a GP is much broader. This can make their work more difficult and yet potentially more rewarding. One GP may see the work as a series of often minor complaints requiring liberal use of the prescription pad, whereas another may see beyond the confines of the presenting symptom deep into the patient's life – the mere tip of an iceberg which he may be given permission to explore further.

To understand the need for psychiatric and psychotherapeutic help in a general practice setting, it helps to appreciate the high levels of psychiatric morbidity in the community. Cheyne, in 1733, wrote of 'those nervous disorders being computed to make almost one-third of the complaints of the people of condition in England'. The Second World War and its attendant psychological morbidity generated a new interest in this area, especially since neurotic disorders accounted for a large proportion of absenteeism from work, quite apart from the impact of the war itself. A later study by Pemberton (1949) reported a prevalence for mental illness of 6.5%.

In 1966, Michael Shepherd published his important and detailed study of *Psychiatric Illness in General Practice* (second edition, 1981). He looked at the degree and nature of psychiatric morbidity in the community and the work of the GP in identifying and treating such problems. A preponderance of neurotic disorders was found, and GPs agreed that the treatment of these conditions was an integral part of their work. Psychological disorders were the second most common reason for consultation in women and the seventh in men. However, few general practitioners felt equipped to treat them. Not surprisingly, then as today, drug treatments were predominant, along with advice and reassurance. This picture was confirmed in a later general practice study in which 90% of depressed patients were treated with drugs, and only 2% received counselling. Huxley *et al.* (1979) demonstrated that a person's social and financial circumstances were a better predictor of outcome than clinical factors.

There has been a marked change in the pattern of family medicine over the course of this century, from an earlier emphasis on severe acute illnesses, especially infections, to a more recent concern with chronic illness, developmental disorders, behavioural problems and plain unhappiness. Demographic changes have resulted in an increased elderly population, and in people living alone. Social changes have manifested in frequent breakdown of families, more single parents, chronic unemployment and an increasing polarization of the poor and the wealthy. Alongside all this, late twentieth century life carries its own particular stresses, including the immediate broadcasting of traumatic news from all over the world, ever-increasing traffic and urbanization, and considerable concern with the environment and the fate of our planet. The GP is often the first port of call for people suffering from the consequences to health of all these developments. Simultaneously, the pressures on GPs and other health professionals have multiplied, and there is a perceived lack of time and energy to attend to psychological problems at a time when help is needed most.

Principles of theory and practice

In a primary care setting, the term psychotherapy is used to describe any specifically psychological treatment that a GP is able to employ, either as the prime therapist or by referral to an appropriate specialist. It includes brief focal psychotherapy, cognitive therapy, anxiety management, behaviour therapy, family therapy, counselling and occasionally formal psychodynamic psychotherapy.

Balint, psychotherapy and general practice

Any account of psychotherapy in general practice, or of the processes of consultation itself, must start with the seminal contribution of Michael Balint, a Hungarian-born psychoanalyst. His 1957 book *The Doctor, His Patient and the Illness* had a profound influence on the whole style of general practice consultation. At times controversial, his work is now regarded by some as peripheral or not easily applicable to the needs of current general practice. However, just as it remains important for analysts of all schools to know about Freud, so it is essential for GPs to know about Balint. This book set out to describe the most frequently used drug in general practice, what he called *the drug 'Doctor'*. He lamented the paucity of information about the nature of this drug, its dosage and frequency and its side-effects. In order to prescribe himself effectively, the doctor needed to make an accurate diagnosis which took into account all aspects of the problem.

Balint's model of illness behaviour described the use of an *'overall diagnosis'* in which the GP was 'not content with comprehending all the physical signs and symptoms, but tries to evaluate the pertinence of so-called neurotic symptoms'. This can be considered as an attempt to arrive at a holistic understanding of the patient's condition, taking into account physical, psychological and psychosocial factors alongside the doctor's intuitive understanding of the presentation. Before *'organizing'* an illness, a patient may *'offer'* or *'propose'* various illnesses to the GP. The patient will continue to present with new symptoms until some agreement is reached between doctor and patient, based on some mutual understanding about the fundamental nature of the illness. The doctor's response to these offers has an important effect on the final organization of the illness.

In making the overall diagnosis, the doctor is using a different technique from that of a standard psychiatric interview. As Balint said: 'He who asks questions will get answers – though hardly anything else.' Instead, the emphasis is on listening and observing, selective attention and selective neglect. This may assist in distinguishing a *'focal area'* of difficulty where readjustment may help, not only in this area, but in the patient's whole life situation. The ability to listen 'necessitates a considerable though limited change in the doctor's personality'.

Clinical vignette

Mrs B, a 43-year-old manager, presented with recurrent sore throats. She was prescribed several courses of antibiotics, some of which resulted in symptomatic improvement but never for long. Her throat was usually unremarkable on examination and her GP thought that she was becoming neurotic. After a chance discussion with a more psychologically minded colleague he decided to take a fresh look at things and enquired more generally into her life. It then emerged that she had never really grieved for the loss of her mother 5 years previously. She often felt like crying but had been unable to let go. She also felt awkward about the whole situation, and believed that she should simply have been able to cope. In retrospect, her GP realized that he had consistently overlooked her sombre attire and rather false smiles. He had been about to refer her to a throat specialist, but he instead gave Mrs B several brief sessions of bereavement counselling until she joined a group run by the local bereavement service. She began to work through her feelings and experienced no further problems with her throat.

Many patients in general practice present with physical symptoms as an expression of a neurotic complaint. Yet, influenced by medico-legal considerations and a training biased towards mechanistic explanations, GPs fear missing some physical illness when concentrating on psychological issues. In fact, the reverse happens far more commonly and the example above is not unusual. Balint describes the need for elimination by appropriate physical examination.

However, finding 'nothing wrong' is no answer to a patient's legitimate desire and need to find a name for their illness. Work in general practice is frequently with patients who present collections of symptoms that do not add up to any known illness. It may be necessary to seek a specialist's advice, investigation or treatment, although it may be difficult to decide which specialist is most appropriate. The referral may result in a true diagnosis, a false diagnosis or a further statement that nothing is wrong. Only at this point it may become apparent that psychological factors are important, and perhaps even causative. All too often a blind eye is turned to this, each professional involved assuming that someone else is dealing with the situation. This is the *'collusion of anonymity'* described by Balint, where vital decisions are taken, or not taken, without any one person being responsible overall. This results in a general undermining of the patient's confidence in the doctor.

Balint went on to describe the *'apostolic function'* of the doctor. This is a manifestation of the doctor's individual personality or charisma, and gives rise to the following roles:

- The GP may *convert* patients to his point of view, and sometimes organize their illness for them. This occurs when the doctor holds a firm view of his patient's condition to which the patient is expected to conform. This might include naming an illness, and consequently seeing all the symptoms in the light of this illness. Problems occur if the doctor is wrong, too rigid or introduces moral judgement.
- In the *pastoral* role, the GP visits and comforts the sick. This role is never taught formally, yet it is integral to the role of the GP. It relies upon the personality, kindness and natural empathy of the doctor.
- As *father-confessor*; many doctors, particularly those working in psychological medicine, carry out much secular work traditionally done by priests.
- *Reassurance* may be offered to relieve the doctor's anxiety as much as the patients. Some prescriptions are written for the sole reason of giving the patient something concrete, a 'good object' which makes use of the *placebo* effect.

Unfortunately, this apostolic function may contribute to a paternalistic and powerful relationship in which the patient is unduly dependent on the doctor. It is therefore important for the doctor to use these apostolic skills with caution and awareness, forming a *'mutual investment company'* in which both GP and patient have an equal stake.

Balint viewed illness as being related to a *'basic fault'* in the psycho-biological structure of a person, involving both mind and body. His use of the term *fault* is deliberately derived from its geological sense to emphasize the structural nature of a certain pattern laid down in formative years by a discrepancy between needs and care. This could lead to irreversible consequences. It is therefore the GP's task to help patients acknowledge and integrate the pain they are suffering as much as it is to diagnose and 'organize' an illness, which might be partially treatable but which would leave the underlying problem untouched.

Subsequently, as an alternative to long interviews which used the '*technique of the great detective*', Balint and his co-workers developed the '*flash technique*', as described in his book *Six Minutes For the Patient* (1973). It is a short, psychologically oriented interview tailored to the time constraints of general practice and designed to 'tune in' to the patient's wavelength so that it can result in generating a 'flash' of understanding. There is an emphasis upon observation of the patient's whole presentation and manner, as well as the content of his complaint. In this way, it is not dissimilar to the process underlying a mental state examination. Responses and inter-pretations are offered, guided by the doctor's continual internal understanding of his observations, with the hope of arriving at a focus of mutual understanding – the '*flash*'. There are risks in such an intuitive, subjective technique, including collusion and projective identification. Balint considered that the best prevention for problems of this sort was in the doctor having successfully concluded his own personal analysis.

Principles of the flash technique
- The doctor is not driven by dogma or theory.
- An attitude of attentive observation is pursued.
- There is respect for the patient's defences, his privacy and right to hide.

The effects of the 'flash' may result in an intense, intimate contact without cultivating dependency or leading to strong transference, both potential features of formal psychotherapy. The 'flash' involves a tacit or overt revelation of a core issue which the patient may later explore alone or in conjunction with the doctor. Above all, nothing is forced and a position of mutual respect is maintained such that the patient retains a feeling of being in control.

Balint and his co-workers took pains to quantify the results of this technique by looking at changes in the doctor/patient relationship, the patient's symptoms and the emotional tensions in the patient's relationships with those close to him. Whilst few GPs work consistently with this model, the face of general practice as a whole was profoundly and lastingly changed by Balint's contribution. As his wife, Enid Balint, said (1974):

> Balint's work stands or falls by whether each GP can realize what his function is, to know in his heart how he wants to spend his life as a doctor. Thus patients will know where they stand, what to expect and what not to. If what they need is ignored or misunderstood, then the hope for help will waver and the patient will be left alone. The world of medicine will have let him down.

Critics of Balint see his approach as irrelevant to many general practice complaints, or unworkable because of the time and energy it requires of the doctor. According to them, it is simply not possible to see twenty patients in a surgery and to give each one the same attentive concentration. They also feel that the techniques can be used inappropriately to the point of being invasive – this has been called '*Balinting*' or '*mind rape*'.

Selection of patients relies very much on the intuition of the doctor and his reading of messages, spoken or unspoken, given by the patient. Burach and Carpenter (1983) demonstrated that, in new consultations, 76% of somatic complaints but only 6% of psychosocial problems were identified. Balint also recognized cases where the child is the presenting symptom for a problem in another family member. There is continual need for vigilance and reassessment, and awareness of the difficulties in selecting patients who are in need of something more than physical management alone.

The GP and psychotherapy

The basis of a GP's interaction with a patient is the consultation: Balint's work underlined the importance of what happens, on various levels, during this interaction. Whilst he also describes a form of psychotherapy that can take place within the parameters of the consultation, the techniques for this remain rather elusive. It is heavily based on intuition and personality, so only a proportion of GPs can practise it effectively. This led to several other techniques being explored.

Simple *counselling* is the most obvious alternative available to GPs. Essentially this consists of a three-fold process, as described by Egan (1986), beginning with an identification, description and exploration of the problem. It then progresses to a proposal of potential solutions and finishes with some sort of resolution. The qualities required of the GP include empathy, acceptance, reflection, challenging of ideas and cooperative planning.

A recent major development is the very fast growth in provision of specifically designated counsellors in primary health care teams, as described by Salinsky and Curtis-Jenkins (1994). For numerous reasons, including public demand, increased management responsibilities and the time-consuming nature of psychological work for GPs in a busy surgery setting, counselling provision has rapidly increased. There are some concerns that the growth has happened in an unregulated way with little check on professional standards or effectiveness. There are moves to define standards and training, provide coordination and encourage appropriate research.

Problem-solving treatment is helpful, especially for a more pragmatic GP. Mynors-Wallis and colleagues (1995) describe the success of this approach as an alternative to drug treatment. They conducted a randomized controlled trial comparing problem-solving with anti-depressant medication and placebo for major depression in primary care and found that problem-solving treatment was 'effective, feasible and acceptable to patients'. Six sessions were given by a GP and lasted an average total of three and a half hours. Problem-solving was as effective as amitriptyline and more so than placebo. Encouragingly, two of the GPs in the study had no previous specialized psychiatric experience.

Cognitive behavioural therapy has become increasingly popular for conditions such as depression, eating disorders and now even schizophrenia. Although simple in concept, it undoubtedly helps to have further training in this technique and most GPs would refer on to a specialist. Being focused, structured and time-limited as well as equipping patients with a new self-sustaining skill, it is very suitable for primary care.

Teasdale and colleagues studied the effects of cognitive therapy in major depressive disorder (1984). They showed that its addition to existing treatment, mostly anti-depressants, allowed significantly faster recovery. Although at three months the advantage was no longer apparent, speed of recovery is important in itself. The longer the delay, the more likely that potentially irreversible consequences will have occurred, such as the loss of a job or breakdown of a marriage.

Brief dynamic psychotherapy necessitates working in a focused way for an agreed number of sessions. A focus is important for therapy to be brief. A presenting problem is identified, and then explored within the context of any unresolved previous experiences with the whole therapeutic relationship available for transferential interpretation. Selection of patients may be more difficult than with other therapies, although it is well established that there are some patients with very longstanding problems who do well. Predictors of good outcome include high motivation, a history of mature adjustment at some point and a 'deep involvement' between therapist and patient. Few GPs would undertake this sort of work without a particular interest and further training.

There are many other areas in which the psychological skills of a GP may be in demand. *Marital therapy* is one, although couples may often choose to attend a specific relationship service such as Relate. Sexual problems present commonly to GPs and many can be helped by relatively simple *sex therapy* techniques with or without relationship counselling. Formal *family therapy* may not often be practised but variations of family counselling are a part of a GP's job, as is the treatment of behavioural problems in children. Familiarity with *bereavement counselling* is also important. *Group therapy* has a role in areas such as stress management, weight loss and giving up smoking.

Which patient and why?

Estimates of total psychological morbidity in the community vary between 5% and 65%. About 1 in 10 people per year are detected by their GPs as having conspicuous psychological morbidity. This represents about 200 cases on an average GP's list of under 2000 patients, and may be only half the actual morbidity. Of these, 5% are likely to suffer from a psychotic condition (25% in psychiatric hospital).

Diagnoses of psychiatric cases in primary and secondary care		
	Primary care	Secondary care
Psychoses	5%	25%
Depression	26%	25%
Other neuroses	36%	10%
Substance abuse	3%	6%
Personality disorders	1%	10%
Organic	2%	14%
Other, e.g. adjustment	27%	10%

The perceived need for psychotherapy is very much a reflection of the GP's recognition rate of psychiatric illness, psychosocial problems or plain unhappiness in the community. Burach and Carpenter (1983) showed that most psychosocial problems were not identified at the initial consultation, but that good consultation skills and a willingness to look 'under all stones' improved the detection rate considerably.

At least one in three of the general population experiences an episode of depression at some point during their lives. Depression is diagnosed more frequently in women, especially those with young children and poor social supports. It is also common in those who are physically ill, which may be missed by GPs and specialists alike. Depression may also be missed when symptoms are atypical, as in some ethnic groups where somatic presentations are common. It is also less likely to be considered when it is chronic and taken to be part of the patient's normal presentation.

Paykel and Priest (1992) wrote a consensus statement on the recognition and management of depression in general practice. They estimated that the prevalence of major depression in the general population was about 5% of which half were diagnosed by their GPs as suffering from depression. Only about one-third of those depressions detected by a GP were given any psychotherapeutic or pharmacological treatment. Part of the reason for this may be the high natural remission rate (40–50%) of neurotic disorders. Only a tenth of those diagnosed as suffering from depression are referred to a psychiatrist, of whom one-third will be admitted to hospital.

Selection of patients for treatment must take into account the severity and chronicity of a patient's problem, and the level of training and skill of the GP who will carry out the treatment. Several diagnostic groups are unlikely to benefit, or be sufficiently contained in primary care. This includes those with longstanding self-harming behaviours, chronic obsessional or phobic symptoms, serious suicidal risks or chronic substance dependencies. Those with severe personality disorders may be too difficult, as may be those with chronic addictions. Patients with psychotic or suicidal tendencies may be best served by the local psychiatric services.

Self-selection sometimes occurs when a patient is resistant to accepting a referral for more specialized help but still comes to the GP. This uncomfortable situation, which is characteristic of the 'heartsink' patient, can be helped by adequate supervision and liaison.

Which therapist and why?

There is an uneven distribution of mental health professionals working in general practice settings and they tend to cluster together in larger training practices which do not necessarily have the greatest need. Only one in thirty practices in a 1993 British survey had a psychotherapist working on site, whereas a third had community psychiatric nurses. One in six GP practices had a counsellor attached, one in nine had a clinical psychologist and only one in twelve had a psychiatrist working on site.

There has been a global trend in moving psychiatric services out of the hospital into the community. This has been accompanied by a wide range of therapies provided by a variety of therapists. The huge variations between different countries, and an international perspective, are clearly described in the final chapter of Bennet and Freeman's *Community Psychiatry* (1991).

Liaison between psychotherapist and GP

Alexis Brook, a psychiatrist, and Jane Temperley, a social worker, both from the Tavistock Clinic in London, reported on the contribution of a psychotherapist to general practice in a 1976 paper published in the *Journal of the Royal College of General Practitioners*. Their experiment was to send out into practices a social worker, a psychologist or a psychiatrist who also had a training in psychotherapy. Rather than seeking to offload patients from the GP, their aim was to cooperate and share the workload. This was to reduce the amount of splitting and dissociation that can occur between professionals.

In some cases, the psychotherapist saw patients for assessment or brief therapy. In others there was more consultative and advisory work and in some, there was total collaboration with joint interviews taking place. After working through sometimes unrealistically high expectations, a level of mutual respect was achieved and the levels of general psychiatric referral were seen to fall. In all this, they were aided by weekly meetings at the Tavistock Clinic. This gave them an opportunity to present new cases, discuss existing ones and deal with other issues such as the inter-professional rivalry that was exposed.

Brook and Temperley demonstrated that, by seconding a psychotherapist to a general practice, patients with emotional problems received earlier help. The therapist was also able to see some patients who would not have accepted referral to a psychiatric clinic or outside agency. In addition, the therapist provided practice staff with help and consultation, which directly benefited the patients.

Wilson and Wilson (1985) noted the natural affinity between psychiatry and primary care in Oxford general practices. However, they stressed the need for attention to the dynamics within the working relationships. They found that the referral process itself was sometimes as complex as the issues presented by the patient, carrying with it some of the GP's own personal agenda. For example. there may have been a breakdown in the relationship between GP and patient, or a patient who presented with a problem too painfully close to that of the GP, which resulted in unresolved counter-transference problems. There may also be hopes of a magical cure for someone with longstanding or intractable problems. GPs may find the criteria regarding referrals to a psychotherapist very vague, in contrast to the clear-cut guidelines provided by mainstream psychiatry for patients with frank mental illness. It is therefore helpful if a therapist can give the GP guidelines for referral.

If the GP and the liaison psychotherapist form a close working relationship there may also be unexpected attachment and dependency which comes to light when the therapist leaves. This raises the question of a GP's own personal need for support, interpretation and understanding in a demanding job which leaves little time for such considerations.

Studies of the relative merits of a treatment from a psychotherapist or from the GP have given mixed results. Some show no significant difference while others show a reduction in prescription of psychotropics, and in general psychiatric referral.

There will be patients who continue to struggle despite everyone's best efforts. A typical example is that of a frequently attending middle-aged man or woman who presents with numerous somatic complaints and feelings of anxiety and depression. In the notes are countless consultations and prescriptions, none of which has made any lasting difference. Collective frustration labels this a classic 'thick-file', 'heartsink' patient of which every GP has a few. Then some major external trauma occurs, such as a bereavement or serious physical illness, and many of the neurotic symptoms abate. There is now a tangible problem around which to organize all the previous complaints. The perseverance, support and loyalty of the GP may be more important than any particular form of treatment offered by anybody.

This example also illustrates one of the difficulties faced by a psychotherapist working in general practice. The therapist will inevitably be referred many people with chronic neurotic complaints, and those with 'problems of daily living'. It may not be clear who is the best person to help – someone in the family, a priest, a friend or a health professional? Often the very absence of other supports leads to a process of self-selection and the subsequent medicalization of the problem. The GP is a captive audience, and what determines the referral to a psychotherapist may be the limits of the GP's capacity for containment, or simply a shortage of time and energy.

Training and supervision

Training in Balint's techniques is available in a variety of workshops, seminars and Balint groups, and also in psychotherapy courses tailored to the needs of GPs. Trainee GPs are taught something of his work during preparation for their qualifying examinations. Considerable time is spent in studying the process of the consultation using video recordings of consultations for discussion and feedback. This is described fully by Pendleton et al. (1984).

Exposure to general practice for psychotherapists and psychiatrists is encouraged in some training programmes, which include an attachment to a GP practice as part of the training.

There is a need for regular supervision and this may be part of the role of a liaison psychotherapist or some other therapist experienced in the specific technique the GP is using. Consideration should also be given to the GP's own need for analysis which may be personally beneficial as well as helpful in averting some of the pitfalls of working in the psychological domain.

Therapeutic setting

One of the prerequisites of therapy is a secure, stable setting. In general practice, many things conspire against this. A crucial issue is that of confidentiality, if the GP conducting the therapy is also responsible for the care of the rest of the family and others in the community. This may have advantages, in allowing vicarious contact to be maintained through family members, giving the GP an added feel of the situation, which is an opportunity not afforded to an outside therapist. However, this may be a less comfortable position when a hostile spouse assumes that the GP is taking the side of their partner, and wants to know what the partner is saying. There may likewise be concerns that the GP will leak information, perhaps inadvertently, when he or she meets a family member who is also a social acquaintance. Concerns also arise in regard to the security of information in the case notes – which are potentially available to any of the practice staff including nurses, receptionists, administrators, managers, domestic staff and other doctors. This may lead a GP therapist to keep a separate set of notes, or no notes at all.

Some therapists working in general practice settings have the experience of being shunted about from one room to another, depending upon which partner is away. Soundproofing may be inadequate and GPs are subject to constant interruptions by bleeps, telephones and surreptitious notes under the door. Firm boundaries must be set to make therapy time secure. If this cannot be done then it is doubtful whether the GP should attempt this sort of work.

Therapists may prefer prospective patients to be given their name and number by the GP so that the patients can make independent contact. Therapy works best when actively sought out by patients, rather than prescribed and arranged for them.

Problems in therapy

Perhaps the most common error is in the inappropriate selection of patients. This is usually a product of inexperience. Whilst the training offered by brief intensive courses on psychotherapy may be tempting to many GPs, they may also prove inadequate without further experience under specialist supervision.

Occasionally delay in referral, or not considering referral soon enough, may lead to serious disturbance or even disaster, such as suicide. Although there is always uncertainty about how preventable such events are, they will always cause uncertainty and anxiety to referrers who are responsible for their treatment. This uncertainty can only be mitigated by careful consideration of risks and options beforehand, and peer review, audit and support afterwards.

GP therapists can get out of their depth, and this is where adequate supervision is important. Transference and countertransference may become a problem and a successfully completed personal analysis may be of great value. Over-involved relationships between GPs or therapists and their clients are not uncommon and have serious therapeutic, ethical and legal implications.

Confidentiality has been mentioned, and it can be a serious difficulty a GP faces when seeing other members of a patient's family while privy to confidential information about them, such as the presence of sexual abuse.

Evaluation of therapy

The value of treatment

A busy GP may feel under pressure to prescribe, rather than talk and engage in psychological treatment. Catalan and colleagues (1984) looked at the effects of non-prescribing of anxiolytics in general practice. Half of the patients in the observed group with a minor affective disorder were prescribed anxiolytics while the other half were given counselling alone. Both groups showed similar improvement at subsequent psychological and social assessments. It was shown that there was no increased demand on the doctor's time in the counselled group. Withholding an anxiolytic did not prolong psychological distress nor did it lead to increased consumption of other substances such as alcohol. It was also found that patients did not necessarily expect a prescription as a treatment for their condition.

Many GPs fear that if they search too hard for evidence of mental illness, they will only find more than they have time or energy to address. Andrews and Brodaty (1980) looked at this issue by following a cohort of 1500 consecutive GP attenders over six months. They found that only 5% of new consultations required active psychological intervention. In terms of cost-effectiveness the benefits in the longer term are considerable, with prevention of the consequences of unattended psychological morbidity for the good of the individual, the family and society.

As they gain more financial and managerial autonomy, GPs have been able to exercise choices about psychotherapy and counselling services for their patients, who in turn have expressed increasing demand for such services. One of the consequences is a trend for GPs to buy in counsellors in addition to existing local mental health services. Evaluation of their effectiveness is at an early stage, but the demand for such services is clearly rising.

Cost-effectiveness

In today's finance-driven health economy, the cost-effectiveness of all forms of psychotherapy has become a pertinent issue. There have been enough difficulties in setting up good controlled trials to show efficacy let alone whether or not it pays for itself. But even if psychotherapy services were 'rationalized' or just marginalized to the private sector, the needs would remain unmet – and the GP would still be faced with the same problems.

Cost offset is a major question. Namely, does psychotherapy lead to a decrease in the use of medical and other services, and an enhanced degree of well-being in the home and workplace, which together equate to a gross economic benefit? Some estimate that a 20% reduction in utilization of primary medical services may result from psychotherapeutic intervention. Similarly, in short-term behavioural psychotherapy, major cost benefits have been calculated in terms of reduced use of health services and increased time spent being productive at work, particularly if patients remained well for two years or more. Therapeutic work with sufferers of irritable bowel syndrome and chronic functional dyspepsia has demonstrated marked improvement: there could be substantial savings on physical investigations and treatments if appropriate patients' numerous physical and psychosomatic conditions could be identified earlier and appropriate psychological intervention offered.

Although behaviour therapy and cognitive behaviour therapy have stood up well to cost–benefit analyses, there is as yet no clear-cut evidence available to the GP in deciding which brief dynamic therapies a health service should offer. The role of long-term therapies remains equally unclear. At the end of the day patients, as consumers, may play an increasingly important role in determining the future face of psychotherapy services in general practice.

Further reading

Balint, M. (1957) *The Doctor, His Patient and the Illness.* London: Pitman.
Balint, E. and Norell, J.S. (eds) (1973) *Six Minutes for the Patient: Interactions in General Practice Consultation.* London: Tavistock.
Gask, L. and McGrath, G. (1989) Psychotherapy and general practice. *British Journal of Psychiatry,* **154**, 445–453.
Pendleton, D., Schofield, T., Tate, P. and Havelock, P. (1984) *The Consultation: an Approach to Learning and Teaching.* Oxford: Oxford University Press.
Pullen, I., Wilkinson, G., Wright A. *et al.* (eds) (1994) *Psychiatry and General Practice Today.* London: Royal College of Psychiatrists and Royal College of General Practitioners.
Shepherd, M., Cooper, B., Brown, A.C. *et al.* (1966) *Psychiatric Illness in General Practice* Oxford: Oxford University Press. Second edition, 1981.

Bibliography

Andrews, G. and Brodaty, H. (1980) General practitioner as psychotherapist. *Medical Journal of Australia,* **2**, 655–659.
Balint, M. (1957) *The Doctor, His Patient and the Illness.* London: Pitman.
Balint, E. (1974) A portrait of Michael Balint: the development of his ideas on the use of the drug 'doctor'. *International Journal of Psychiatry in Medicine,* **5**, 211–222.
Balint, E. and Norell, J.S. (eds) (1973) *Six Minutes for the Patient: Interactions in General Practice Consultation.* London: Tavistock.
Bennet, D.H. and Freeman, H.L. (1991) *Community Psychiatry.* Edinburgh: Churchill Livingstone.
Brook, A. and Temperley, J. (1976) The contribution of a psychotherapist to general practice. *Journal of the Royal College of General Practitioners,* **26**, 86–94.
Burach, R.C. and Carpenter, R.R. (1983) The predictive value of the presenting complaint. *Journal of Family Practice,* **16**, 749–754.
Catalan, J., Gath, D.H., Edmonds, G. *et al.* (1984) The effects of non-prescribing of anxiolytics in general practice. *British Journal of Psychiatry,* **144**, 593–602.
Egan, G. (1986) *The Skilled Helper,* 3rd edn. Pacific Grove, CA: Brooks–Cole.
Huxley, P.J. *et al.* (1979) The prediction of the course of minor psychiatric disorders. *British Journal of Psychiatry,* **135**, 535–543.
Mynors-Wallis, L.M., Gath, D.H., Lloyd-Thomas, A.R. *et al.* (1995) Randomised controlled trial comparing problem solving treatment with amitriptyline and placebo for major depression in primary care. *British Medical Journal,* **310**, 441–445.
Paykel, E.S. and Priest, R.G. (1992) Recognition and management of depression in general practice: consensus statement. *British Medical Journal,* **305**, 1198–1202.
Pemberton, J. (1949) Illness in general practice. *British Medical Journal,* **i**, 306.

Pendleton, D., Schofield, T., Tate, P. and Havelock, P. (1984) *The Consultation: an Approach to Learning and Teaching*. Oxford: Oxford University Press.

Salinsky, J. and Curtis-Jenkins, G. (1994) Counselling in general practice. *British Journal of General Practice,* **44,** 194–195.

Shepherd, M., Cooper, B., Brown, A.C. *et al.* (1966) *Psychiatric Illness in General Practice.* Oxford: Oxford University Press. Second edition, 1981.

Teasdale, J.D., Fennell, M.J.V., Hibbert, G.A. and Amies, P.L. (1984) Cognitive therapy for major depressive disorder in primary care. *British Journal of Psychiatry,* **144,** 400–406.

Wilson, S. and Wilson, K. (1985) Close encounters in general practice: experiences of a psychotherapy liaison team. *British Journal of Psychiatry,* **146,** 277–281.

19

Psychotherapy Research

*Jennifer Stein, Rex Haigh, Alice Levinson and
Samuel M. Stein*

> *The observer who is reasonably free to find what is to be observed, not having to
> guard too much (for personal reasons) against finding whatever is to be found, can
> choose from many different methods for objective study!*
>
> Winnicott, 1964

Introduction

Health care services are increasingly being asked to explain and justify their
existence. Psychotherapy departments are also under growing pressure to
quantitatively evaluate what they do and base clinical treatment choices
on evidence-based research. There is a trend within general psychotherapy
research which has aligned itself with humanistic traditions but this has
been largely confined to 'psychotherapy process research'. Psychotherapy
outcome research has been strongly dominated by the methods of the natural
sciences. Because of its reliance on the case history as a basis for its theorizing,
psychoanalysis has had great difficulty in fitting experimental research
paradigms.

Twenty years ago, Brown and Pedder (1979) commented that research in
psychotherapy was unlikely to be adequately tackled unless methods were
devised which match the complexity and subtlety of human beings and their
problems. Several authors have described psychotherapy research as being
complex, and there has been a recognition that compromises have to be
made. Gelder *et al.* (1988) concluded that psychotherapy research has been
most informative when applied to simple forms of treatment. While there
is a belief that 'adherence to scientific method can only be mechanistic and
limiting' (Bloch, 1982), there is a strong argument in favour of opening up
psychoanalysis to the wider scientific community and thereby helping to
break down what is often seen as an esoteric and inward-looking discipline.

The Review of Strategic Policy of NHS Psychotherapy Services in England
by the NHS Executive (1996) gives a clear message that psychotherapy, of
all types, will be required to face up to the current demand for evidence-
based practice. The point is made, however, that 'where the appropriate
control treatment research has not yet been undertaken, the absence of
evidence for efficacy is not evidence for ineffectiveness ... and clinically

effective care should not perish for lack of funding'. While the evaluation of psychoanalysis and psychotherapy remains a challenge for the future, the need is now growing and this pressure is likely to influence psychotherapy research in general.

The history of psychotherapy research

Freud located psychoanalysis firmly in the scientific domain. In 1926, he wrote, 'In psychoanalysis there has existed from the very first an inseparable bond with research.' Freud's observations of the structure of the human psyche and its processes were developed within this framework. For example, transference was initially seen as a block to this empirical observation and only later recognized as a tool for observing and understanding the unconscious. Freud's tradition of empiricism continued in Europe in the form of thinking about cases and reporting on them, and was seen as synonymous with research.

The work of Melanie Klein and Anna Freud extended analytic thinking to actual observations of children, and others became interested in groups, families and organizations. Clinics in Berlin and London in the late 1920s and early 1930s reported systematic studies of patients.

The most significant impetus to psychotherapeutic research was the highly critical paper by H.J. Eysenck (1952), in which he contended that psychotherapy of neurotic patients was no more effective than an absence of treatment. Clinicians such as Allen Bergen and David Malan demonstrated the inadequacy of Eysenck's studies and the arbitrary manner in which he designated levels of improvement (Bloch, 1982). Malan (1963, 1973) went on to research brief analytic psychotherapy at the Tavistock Clinic. In the United States Margaret Mahler (1975) undertook observational studies of children, and the Menninger Foundation study, started in 1954, was a large case series which produced important findings relevant to psychodynamic and psychoanalytic work.

Many clinical reviews have addressed the efficacy of psychoanalytic treatment for a diverse range of psychopathology (Freud, 1937; A. Freud, 1954; Tyson & Sandler, 1971; Schlessinger, 1984). Fonagy and Target (1994) have reported on 763 cases of child psychoanalysis and psychotherapy at the Anna Freud Centre. There have also been a small number of systematic studies with adult patients (Weber et al., 1985; Kantrowitz, 1987; Wallerstein, 1989). Bachrach et al. (1991) give a comprehensive review of studies of psychoanalytic work. In addition to psychoanalytic studies, Rogers and Dymond (1954) described investigations into client-centred therapy. Behavioural and cognitive behavioural work poses fewer problems for research than analytic and psychodynamic psychotherapy, and there is consequently a much larger body of research relating to these treatments.

Aims of psychotherapy research

- The role of psychotherapy research is to increase the understanding of mechanisms of change (Evans et al., 1996).

- Research should be of help in modifying and shaping the discipline (Levinson, 1997).
- Research enables psychoanalysis to scrutinize and refine itself in order to discard what is outmoded or unworkable, and to develop what is most valuable (Bateman and Holmes, 1995).
- Research can reassure clinicians that their work is effective.
- Research helps in the clarification of clinical concepts, and in generating new hypotheses for clinical work and future research.
- Research can give psychoanalysis a better public face, re-establishing itself through facts which are more readily understood by a larger number of people and thereby avoiding the charge of rigidity and ossification.
- Research into normal developmental processes might be of value in understanding clinical problems and inspire effective modes of intervention (Fonagy, 1993).

Methods of research in psychotherapy

Qualitative and quantitative methods

Pope and Britten (in Greenhalgh and Taylor, 1997) presented a paper to the BSA Medical Sociology Group Conference in 1993 entitled 'Barriers to Qualitativeness in the Medical Mind Set'. They described their collection of rejection letters from biomedical journals which revealed a striking ignorance of qualitative methodology on the part of the reviewers. They also maintained that 'the critical appraisal of qualitative research is a relatively under-developed science'.

Qualitative methods aim to make sense of or interpret phenomena in terms of the meanings people bring to them. This kind of research may define preliminary questions which can then be addressed in quantitative studies. Good qualitative research will use more than one research method to address a clinical problem, and it is both possible and useful to combine qualitative with quantitative methods. This is known as triangulation, and involves the use of independent analysis of the data by more than one researcher. A characteristic of qualitative research is that there is often participant observation, in other words the researcher also occupies a role or part in the setting in addition to observing. Greenhalgh and Taylor (1997) make the point that there is 'no way of abolishing, or fully controlling, observer bias in qualitative research. This is most obviously the case when participant observation is used; it is also true for other forms of data collection and data analysis.'

It has been claimed by several psychotherapy researchers that a conceptual dichotomy has been created between qualitative and quantitative research which is artificial. Qualitative research includes content analysis, discourse and conversational analysis, and narrative analysis. There is a growing interest in qualitative research, and the development of research methods which aim to make sense of or find meaning for clinical problems. This work has been aided by the increasingly sophisticated analysis of language and gesture, often using computer translations to operationalize video-taped material. The strength of qualitative research is that 'data collection methods . . . touch the core of what is going on rather than just skimming the surface' (Greenhalgh and Taylor, 1997). They go on to say 'by it's very nature, qualitative research is non-standard, unconfined, and dependent on the subjective experience of both the researcher and the researched . . . Doctors have traditionally placed high value on numerical data, which may in reality be misleading, reductionist and irrelevant to the real issues'.

Comparative and correlational methods

In the correlational approach, the researcher does not differentiate between independent and dependent variables. Rather, he measures the phenomena that interest him and notes how they relate to one another through a statistical process of correlation. No causal relationship can be assumed. The investigator simply seeks to clarify the associations between different phenomena (Bloch, 1982). Associations between variables revealed by observational methods allow the possibility of many different explanations for the association, and the comparisons are either comparative or correlational (Evans et al., 1996). If a research finding statistically links a large number of different factors then the correlation is said to be high, whereas if few factors are brought together statistically in a single explanation, then the correlation will be low. The greater the statistical correlation, the more reliable is the result and it can therefore be generalized to a larger section of the population. Group comparison studies provide data that can be generalized to similar populations and compared with other groups, but they do not provide information about the individual subjects (Levinson, 1997).

Descriptive method

Another type of research of process is purely descriptive, recording as accurately and reliably as possible what occurs in therapy. It simply describes a set of events. Psychotherapy espouses such non-numerical descriptive data, leaning very heavily on discussions of observational data from the treatment of individuals. Descriptive research serves a number of functions: to define the scope of the research area, to identify a range of questions that may then be explored further through comparative, correlational or true experimental methods, and to provide numerical parameters. Descriptive research has been given more validity through the use of meta-analysis, a statistical manoeuvre in which studies are pooled in order to provide 'increased precision over their descriptive estimates' (Evans et al., 1996).

Process methods

Psychotherapy research is often divided into outcome studies (looking at the research results of psychotherapy treatment) and process research (studying what goes on in the psychotherapy process itself). Some have argued that there is an arbitrary distinction between outcome and process research since psychotherapy process can be viewed as a collection of many small outcomes. However, process and outcome are inevitably brought together if one can identify factors in the therapy that promote or hinder its effectiveness and efficiency. From both a research and clinical perspective, it may then be appropriate to manipulate such factors in order to note the result (Bloch, 1982).

Process research uses a variety of methodologies to explore change in psychotherapy, and to facilitate our understanding of the therapeutic process and of the factors that are most effective in clinical work (Evans et al., 1996). Greenberg and Pinsoff (1986) wrote that 'process research is the study of the interaction between patient and therapist systems. The goal of process research is to identify the change processes in all of the behaviours and experiences within these systems. Process research covers all of the behaviours and experiences of the systems, within and outside of treatment sessions, which pertain to the process of change.'

The variables of process research are broadly distinguished input variables which are present before therapy and which include personality structure, personal history, history of mental illness and other individual characteristics. Process variables are also distinguished from other variables which may change during therapy. External variables include domestic circumstances, social support network and life events. These process variables are distinguished from outcome variables. Thorough process research provides the foundation for erecting hypotheses about outcome and is applicable to all forms of psychotherapy. It is most helpful in combination with outcome research and individual case analyses (Evans et al., 1996).

Outcome methods

Brown and Pedder (1979) described the assessment of outcome in psychotherapy as 'an important challenge'. Outcome studies require the following in order to be meaningful:

- Sufficient sample sizes to give statistical power
- A homogeneous sample
- Operationalized diagnostic criteria (e.g. DSM-IV or ICD-10)
- Standardized measures of known reliability and validity
- Multidimensional measures covering different levels of intrapsychic processes
- A prospective design measuring changes temporally before, during and after treatment as well as at follow-up
- Long-term follow-up to reflect the long-term nature of treatment and the potential for change to continue after treatment

An inherent problem of outcome research for psychoanalysis is that it is likely to measure relatively course-grained data, such as symptomatology, which does not adequately reflect the nature of change that psychoanalysis aims to bring about. Research using only psychiatric psychometric instruments will not do justice to the rich and complex nature of the mind's subjectivity and inter-subjectivity (Levinson, 1977).

An outcome project of psychoanalysis that takes into account these inherent challenges is being conducted at the Anna Freud Centre. It aims to measure change during and after psychoanalysis, multidimensionally, on a number of standardized measures including psychiatric diagnoses, symptomatology, the Adult Attachment Interview (AAI) (George *et al.*, 1985) and Reflective Self-Function (RSF) scale (Fonagy *et al.*, 1997). It includes the further dimension of the analysts' evaluations of change by a random monthly session reported verbatim, and 'The Anna Freud Centre Young Adult Weekly Rating Scale' (Gerber, 1997). It is constructed to measure major themes of the psychoanalytic relationship, including the manifest themes, the analyst's understanding of these, the nature of the transference, forms of resistance and the main theme of the analyst's interpretations. The project aims to use innovative methodology that is scientific – using procedures that are open to inspection and are replicable – but which investigates meaningful constructs of psychoanalysis.

Randomized control trials (RCT)

Psychotherapy research has its origins in the experimental tradition in which research seeks to test hypotheses by manipulation of variables, and extend comparison or correlational analysis beyond its observational forms (Evans *et al.*, 1996). The application of experimental design in psychotherapy, however, has not followed easily from clinical practice. This has perhaps been in part because of the tradition for experimental research findings to be based on the randomized control trial.

The randomized control trial is generally considered the gold standard for treatment evaluation research. The aim of the controlled study is to provide a level of certainty that a significant difference between groups is due to the intervention which has been given to one group in comparison to a matched group receiving no treatment. Randomization ensures that any potential differences that might affect the outcome are randomly distributed between both groups. It will not automatically produce equal groups, but the likelihood that the groups are equivalent increases as the sample size increases.

The control group has to be selected from patients who are not receiving treatment. This may introduce a distortion into the research as there may be a reason why treatment is being withheld. Brown and Pedder (1979) commented that 'Controlled double blind trials of drug treatments are simple because every pill is the same and control groups of patients can be given dummy pills without their realizing it, so giving a measure of the placebo effect. In psychoanalysis and psychotherapy neither the patient nor the therapist can be blind to the control treatment group.' Several writers have also made the point that it is not ethical to use randomization to select a control group in psychotherapy as this treatment has been shown to be of greater benefit than no treatment.

As there has not yet been any empirical research into the use of randomized control trials in psychoanalytic psychotherapy, it remains questionable whether the RCT is the best way of evaluating these treatments. Fonagy and Higgitt (1989) have reviewed this approach to psychotherapy research. Clarke, writing with both Cornish (1972) and Sinclair (1973), has described the difficulties that arise when conducting RCTs in educational therapeutic communities.

There are a number of serious problems with using the RCT in psychotherapy outcome research, especially in long-term psychodynamic psychotherapy:

- Psychoanalysis deals with a relatively small population of subjects and therefore the sample size is small.
- A small sample prevents adequate matching between groups and randomization across groups.
- Construction of an adequate control group is usually impossible. In addition to problems in matching psychopathology, there are ethical problems in withholding treatment or asking people to wait for treatment (waiting-list control design).
- Control groups are unlikely to participate in long-term follow-up, which is essential in psychotherapy research studies.
- Double blind trials in psychotherapy are impossible to construct.
- There is no evidence to support the idea that results from any one psychotherapy study can be generalized to another, or to individual treatments, since neither the sample nor the treatment can be precisely defined.
- Suitable measures for psychotherapy have yet to be identified. Measures designed primarily to demonstrate short-term treatment gains are not necessarily applicable to a study of longer-term gains such as personality change or quality of relationships. The measures may also lack reliability in addition to internal and external validity.

Single case studies

Single case and small sample designs can be of use in appropriate circumstances as they offer the opportunity for fine-grained investigation which is necessary to explore the rich and complex domain of subjectivity (Levinson, 1997). They are particularly useful in looking at the process of psychoanalytic psychotherapy where the focus is the complex interactional sequences between therapist and patient in order to explore the elaborate changes in the patient–therapist interaction. The individual case study has a long tradition in clinical psychotherapy, as clinicians have carefully observed their individual patients to note whether or how they changed in treatment (Bloch, 1982).

Single case and small sample designs have been considered unrigorous and unscientific by empirical researchers as they do not provide statistically analysable data. They have been criticized as 'a sophisticated creation in which the events of a clinical encounter are filtered, shaped, tidied up, reflected upon, romanticized, condensed and generally tailored to theoretical preconceptions, in a way that makes it highly unreliable as a source of information about what actually happens between analyst and patient' (Bateman and Holmes, 1995).

There are also problems of therapist bias and the lack of generalizability or repeatability. The generalization of findings from small samples can be improved and replication made possible by the use of operationalized diagnostic criteria at baseline and standardized measures of known reliability and validity. Some workers have modified the single case study in order to improve its objectivity and address the issue of therapist bias. Kernberg (1994) conducted a case study, audio-recording every session of a patient's treatment over a number of years, and demonstrated how changes in the transference can be measured by observing the nature of the patient's responses to the analyst's interpretations. Sandler (1995) has described a method of study with small numbers of subjects by using a research group to discuss the therapists' observed data in order to gain some objective view of the material. The method was found to be helpful in examining and clarifying some psychoanalytic concepts.

There is now a growing body of opinion which believes that a repeated measures design of single analytic treatments ($n = 1$) should become the standard for psychoanalytic psychotherapy research. Such studies provide the ground for ideas to emerge and hypotheses to be created which can then be tested clinically, and by further research with larger groups (Levinson, 1997). This work is currently under way using the Adult Attachment Interview (AAI) and the Reflective Self-Function Scale (RSF).

Clinical audit

A useful distinction between research, particularly routine clinical research, and audit is the direction of the end product. Audit of clinical work is now widespread within the NHS and much has been written about the construction of audit and the necessity for closure of audit loops. Audit is not required to produce information which is generalizable and therefore publishable as a comment on general psychotherapy practice. Audit is intended to inform individual clinical practice but, as with research, it will only do so in so far as the measures accurately reflect the questions being asked. Feldman (1992) has described how audit, rather than being anxiety-provoking, can be useful in focusing clinicians' interest and curiosity through careful scrutiny of clinical practice.

Audit can also be useful in describing and 'selling' the value of psychotherapy to those bodies who commission or provide it. The models that are employed for audit are often simple and based on concise and straightforward questions. Bearing in mind Gelder's comments on the need for simple issues to be addressed first in psychotherapy (Gelder *et al.*, 1988), potential researchers may be able to learn lessons from successful audit projects.

Cost effectiveness and cost-offset research studies

Several writers have drawn attention to the importance of making use of cost-offset studies to monitor outcome and efficacy. For example, the cost of one year's treatment in a specialist in-patient unit is comparable and frequently more expensive than five years of psychoanalysis. There are now a number of cost-offset studies for the evaluation of therapeutic community treatment, showing an overall cost reduction when the cost of the treatment is set against the reduction in the use of other resources (Menzies *et al.*, 1993). It has been argued that studies using health care consumption as a research measure have particular validity for patients with borderline personality disorders who may make excessive and chaotic use of general practitioners, casualty departments, psychiatric in-patient and out-patient units, social service facilities, probation services and other caregiving agencies (Haigh, 1998).

Problems in psychotherapy research

The nature of psychotherapy research

Freud, in 1933, said:

> At one time a complaint was made against psychoanalysis that it was not to be taken seriously as a treatment since it did not dare to issue any statistics of its successes. Since then, the Psychoanalytic Institute in Berlin ... has published a statement of its results during the first ten years. Its therapeutic successes give grounds neither for boasting nor for being ashamed. But statistics of that kind are generally uninstructive; the material worked upon is so heterogeneous that only very large numbers would show anything. It is wiser to examine one's own individual experience.

Ricoeur (1970) also advocated criteria of internal coherence and narrative plausibility as the basis for settling disputes. Research studies are now being developed which use methodology based on internal world descriptives. This type of investigative tool draws on existing psychoanalytic and psychodynamic theory in the way that cognitive therapy has incorporated its research outcome measures into the clinical method.

This work is as yet in its infancy but demonstrates how psychotherapy research is becoming more sophisticated, including the use of audio-visual recording and other research instruments. Fonagy (1993) described the need for a change in the direction in which psychotherapy research is moving since the 'almost unique emphasis on anecdotal clinical data ... left the epistemology of psychoanalysis and psychotherapy dependent on an outmoded epistemic paradigm: enumerative inductivism (i.e. generalizing from a number of examples). Enumerative inductivism, finding examples consistent with a proposition, is at most an educational device and not a method of scientific scrutiny ... The almost universal application of this epistemic tool in psychoanalytic writings has created a situation where, currently, psychoanalysis has no method of discarding ideas once they have been proposed and made to sound plausible.' Psychoanalysis as a 'hermeneutic' discipline, attempting to find external validation for its truths, is doomed to failure.

Methodology

Gelder, writing in 1988, said that 'until recently, psychotherapy research suffered from over ambitious attempts to investigate complex problems, although the available methods of assessment were only suited to simple issues' (Gelder *et al.*, 1988). While some of these criticisms have been overcome in cognitive behavioural therapy research, dynamic and psychoanalytic research are still struggling with these issues. Dynamic psychotherapy research is criticized for its poor methodology, particularly the small sample size and lack of operationalized diagnostic criteria. Many of the measures used in psychotherapy research are unstandardized, and the research design is uncontrolled and retrospective. There is also often insufficient follow-up.

Clinical problems

Bateman and Holmes (1995) draw attention to the traditional reluctance of analysts to subject themselves to scientific scrutiny, and the difficulty in operationalizing the theoretical concepts which are worked with in psychoanalytic psychotherapy. Several writers have drawn attention to the difficulty of introducing what amounts to a third party into the psychoanalytic or psychotherapeutic relationship. This intrudes upon what is usually a highly personal and private encounter; in more analytic terms it introduces an oedipal dynamic which has both conscious and unconscious reverberations. There is also no objective way of monitoring information which passes between a patient and his therapist at unconscious levels, and the personal qualities of the therapist enter into the equation (Evans *et al.*, 1996). Problems are compounded by the hidden selection processes which may operate before a patient is accepted for psychotherapy (Gelder *et al.*, 1988). In addition to this, therapists who belong to the same theoretical school may in practice have widely differing clinical styles (Bloch, 1982).

Ambivalence

For many practising psychoanalysts and psychotherapists the preoccupations of contemporary science seem largely irrelevant to their day to day experience (Bateman and Holmes, 1995). This is particularly true of those working in private practice who have fewer of the institutional pressures to provide evidence for the efficacy of their work. Some practitioners have challenged the appropriateness of psychotherapy as a subject for scientific study (Bloch, 1982), and others have felt that psychotherapy is more comparable to an educational process than to a medical model (Brown and Pedder, 1979). It is often maintained that the inner world with which psychoanalysis is concerned can only be reached by introspection, and is therefore inherently unresearchable (Steiner, 1996). Research that is remote from clinical practice is likely to be viewed as irrelevant by many clinicians as statistical significance may not reflect clinical significance. Measures of clinical relevance therefore need to be incorporated (Levinson, 1997).

Analytic psychotherapy in particular has a chequered history in terms of its image and acceptability, which often has had little to do with its proven efficacy (Steiner, 1985). It is possible therefore that the resistance to psychotherapy provision sometimes originates in the unconscious minds of those who influence its delivery. Practitioners themselves must also bear some responsibility for the way in which they are perceived, and research may be influential in changing this.

Advances in psychotherapy research

Dynamic psychotherapy

Although it has now been widely accepted that psychological treatments are an effective alternative in many different psychological and psychiatric disorders, the evidence for this from research studies has not been satisfactorily incorporated into the body of knowledge. One reason for this is the problems psychotherapy has in devising suitable research methods, and of collecting data.

In a recent report to the National Health Service (NHS), Roth and Fonagy (1996) looked at dynamic psychotherapy but concluded that this had been insufficiently researched. They made the point that absence of evidence for the effectiveness of psychodynamic therapy should not be taken as evidence of ineffectiveness. Uncontrolled studies and case studies have demonstrated the effectiveness of psychodynamic psychotherapy, particularly when there has been a high level of skill in the therapist. It was felt that an essential aspect of treatment evaluation would be the development of outcome measures that capture the type of changes these therapies aim to produce. Short-term symptomatic relief, whilst of value, is not a sufficient measure of improvement, and they suggested that reliable measures of changes in core interpersonal conflicts, general functioning and quality of life would be important.

Other workers in psychodynamic psychotherapy have pointed to research studies, for example the work on expressed emotion, which have clearly defined psychological antecedents to psychiatric problems, and the benefits of psychological treatments in such situations; nevertheless the evidence has not been able to be integrated into routine clinical practice. There have been several studies (Luborsky et al., 1988) which have shown that treatment gains in dynamic psychotherapy are maintained at long-term follow-up whereas a recent review by Fonagy (1993) suggested that the gains of brief therapy were not always maintained. Despite these findings, it is clear that the policy-makers are choosing to substantially ignore this data, and are either supporting short-term psychotherapy on financial and resource grounds, or are choosing not to fund psychological treatments at all.

Linehan (1997) has developed a model which can be applied to dynamic, cognitive and behavioural therapy research. She describes the passage of psychotherapeutic techniques through a three-stage process: development, validation and dissemination. Development starts with the generation of ideas, moves on to the standardization of therapies and finishes with pilot tests of efficacy. The validation stage includes thorough testing of efficacy, investigation of mechanisms of action, and determination of utility. Dissemination is accomplished through service development, programme evaluation and formal effectiveness studies.

Cognitive behaviour therapy

Cognitive therapy was originally developed to treat depression in the 1970s, and its methodology has been specifically developed in order to fulfil the necessary requirements for an evidence based approach. A meta-analysis by Dobson (1989) suggested that cognitive therapy is more effective than either no treatment or non-specific treatment, and at least as effective as alternative and pharmacological intervention in the treatment of unipolar depression. Follow-up studies have also suggested that cognitive therapy reduces the risk of relapse by 50% as compared to pharmacotherapy. These kinds of studies have been related to evaluative or service research, whereas the work by people such as Clark and Teasdale (1982) has been more exploratory and theoretical. Their work has linked memory retrieval with changes in mood, and they have described a bias in autobiographical memory in depressed people who tend to remember negative events in their life more quickly than positive events. Williams (1997) suggests that in depression there is an over-general retrieval of events and that this leads to difficulties in generating alternative solutions, and problem-solving. He suggests that the prophylactic effect of cognitive behaviour therapy may be due to patients learning to 'de-centre' from their troubling negative thoughts and prevent further deterioration of their mood.

Barlow and Hoffman (1997) give a full description of the efficacy and dissemination of these treatments. They thought that the recent report to the National Health Service (NHS) by Roth and Fonagy (1996) 'underscored the effectiveness of a number of psychological interventions, particularly of cognitive behaviour therapy and interpersonal psychotherapy (IPT)'. There is a large body of evidence on the effectiveness of cognitive and behavioural interventions in a wide range of psychiatric disorders, and in most instances these treatments are better than no treatment and as good or better than effective drug treatment. Barlow and Hoffman (1997) suggest that when out-patient treatment is considered, pharmacological approaches are often recommended by policy-makers, and psychological approaches are excluded. This bias seems to be related to public relations, accessibility and dissemination.

Shapiro and Firth (1987) compared prescriptive (cognitive behavioural) with exploratory (relationship-oriented) psychotherapy in a cross-over design with each client seeing the same therapist throughout. This was a very short therapy of only sixteen sessions in total and the results favoured prescriptive therapy although this difference was of moderate extent. This study illustrates some of the problems encountered in researching psychotherapy using a methodology perhaps more suited to a drug trial.

Specific areas of research

Naturalistic studies

A naturalistic study that has been performed is the Menninger Project (Wallerstein, 1986). It is a prospective study spanning twenty-five years, incorporating measures at assessment, during treatment and at outcome. The sample included 42 cases of severe personality disturbance, 22 who received psychoanalysis and 20 psychotherapy. As is frequently the case for naturalistic studies, the treatment conditions varied so that by the end of the study only six of the psychoanalytic sample had traditional psychoanalysis, the others having a modified psychoanalytic treatment, making the results less clear. In this study there was no evidence that psychoanalysis was more effective than supportive therapy in that patient group. In a final report on this project by Kernberg (1973) it was concluded that the outcome of therapy was highly dependent upon patient variables such as initial ego strength and initial level of anxiety. Manning (1989) has also developed a sophisticated naturalistic methodology, and has conducted a similar study involving six therapeutic communities in Australia.

Attachment research

There have been various reports of statistically significant positive correlations between negative childhood experience and adult psychopathology. The observation history repeats itself, and that there exists an intergenerational concordance in relationship patterns has been borne out by epidemiological research. Attachment research has demonstrated that there are marked continuities in children's security of attachment, maintained probably by the stable quality of the parent/child relationship. Parents' interviews concerning their own childhood have been shown to predict their children's attachment pattern even before the infant is born (Fonagy et al., 1991a). There are a number of simple indicators of family stress and deprivation which have been reported in a number of studies dramatically to increase the probability of poor attachment and adverse childhood development. These indicators (Fonagy et al., 1993) included:

- Single parent families
- Residing separately
- Overcrowding
- Paternal unemployment
- Chronic or acute life-threatening illness of father or mother
- Parental criminality
- Psychiatric illness of the parents
- Major illness in childhood
- Prolonged separation from parents before the age of eleven
- Boarding school before the age of eleven.

The Adult Attachment Interview (AAI) is one intrapsychic measure that has been devised to examine subjects' internal working models of attachment (George et al., 1985). Based on Bowlby's attachment theory it has been shown to have reliability (Main et al., 1985; Fonagy et al., 1991a) and validity, and has therefore opened a gateway for psychoanalytic and psychotherapy research. It is an audio-recorded interview consisting of a series of open questions followed by probes, that enquires into the subject's childhood attachment experiences. It is transcribed verbatim and rated on a number of scales, including experiences and states of mind. It has been found that the way a person is able to talk about their experiences – the coherency of their narrative – determines their attachment status, rather than the historic facts of their experiences. This is thought to be because coherency of narrative is a reflection of the subject's psychic organization and ability to think autonomously about their experiences.

There are three main categories of attachment, secure-autonomous, insecure-dismissive and insecure-preoccupied, in addition to which a fourth – unresolved to trauma or loss – can be given. Early findings suggest that the dismissive category may make a better response to psychotherapy than the entangled-preoccupied group (Fonagy et al., 1996). Reflective self-function (RSF) is a measure developed by Fonagy and colleagues (Fonagy et al., 1991b, 1997) of a person's capacity to think about their own mental state and the mental states of others. It is an attachment-related capacity and the Reflective Self-Function Scale is therefore applied to AAI transcripts. It has been shown to be the most powerful predictor of adult attachment security and, transgenerationally, of the infant's attachment to its parent

(Fonagy *et al.*, 1991a). RSF is one part of the capacity for psychoanalytic thinking and insight, and its operationalization in the form of the RSF Scale is therefore a valuable instrument for psychoanalytic research.

Exposure based therapy

Three recent surveys in the United States (Barlow and Hoffman, 1997) reported that a large percentage of phobic individuals in three major cities received counselling, hospitalization or medication, but only 15–38% were being treated with exposure based procedures. This is despite an agreement by psychotherapists from all theoretical persuasions that exposure based treatment is a desirable part of effective treatment in such disorders. Marks (1987), working at the Institute of Psychiatry in London, reported that over half of all sufferers of anxiety disorders (including Obsessive Compulsive Disorder) identified in community studies in both the United States and Germany had not sought treatment for their problem and remained untreated primarily because there are not enough therapists.

The patient/therapist relationship

Research has, until recently, looked at psychotherapy in a rather crude way, often ignoring the differences between therapists and between patients. Bloch (1982) said that 'patients may share certain common features but their differences may be crucial in influencing their outcome'. Bateman and Holmes (1995) drew attention to the differential contribution of common factors and specific interventions in any psychotherapy. They went on to say that the therapist/patient relationship appears to be a crucial factor in producing good outcome. Roth and Fonagy (1996) reported that good matching of an individual patient to the form of therapy, and the therapist's skill at developing and maintaining a working alliance, are probably at least as important as the specific effects of therapeutic technique for whatever particular diagnosis. Other studies have shown that treatment outcome is correlated with therapist's competency and protocol adherence (Crits-Christoph *et al.*, 1991), however despite this a number of writers have pointed out that the prevailing attitude in many mental health settings is that anyone who is capable of forming a good relationship with the patient can practise psychotherapy. This is clearly an area that needs more research.

Physical symptoms and psychological functioning

Both cognitive behaviour therapy and analytic therapy has looked at the close links between physical symptoms and psychological functioning. Patients with panic disorder often ascribe physical symptoms of anxiety to an impending heart attack. This was described by Freud (1895) and recently confirmed by others (Gelder, 1997). Whereas behaviour therapy attends to an understanding or decatastrophization of physical symptoms through behavioural learning, the cognitive component of therapy seeks to reassure, educate and retrain a thinking style. Work described by Gelder in the 1980s and currently being prepared by Clark and Salkovskis in relation to the development of hyperventilation in panic, clearly makes the case for the effectiveness of both behavioural and cognitive interventions. Moran and Fonagy (1987) have described analytic work with a diabetic patient, and used physical markers, in that case blood sugar levels, in order to monitor progress of the treatment. Guthrie described randomized control trials of conversational model psychotherapy in the treatment of irritable bowel syndrome (IBS) (Guthrie, 1991; Guthrie *et al.*, 1993). Other studies by these workers have looked at the relationship between marital therapy and IBS.

Summary

From this general review of results of research studies, the following may be concluded:
- Cognitive behavioural therapy is now well supported by research studies which have been accepted as part of an evidence based approach to psychological treatments.
- Despite this, the implementation of treatment following from such research studies is not yet widespread.
- Dynamic psychotherapy and psychoanalysis has not been sufficiently well researched using the paradigms of evidence based medicine.
- There have been several studies that have demonstrated the effectiveness of longer-term psychotherapy.
- The gains of brief therapy are not always maintained at long-term follow-up.
- Despite these findings neither research nor clinical practice of psychotherapy are being adequately funded and supported.

Routine clinical research

Many clinicians and researchers now believe that one way to address the need to satisfy both the policy-makers and providers of services, and the professionals working within psychotherapy, is to introduce a core battery of measures which are routinely administered. There is currently a project in progress, funded by the Mental Health Foundation, which aims to implement such a core battery approach. This type of approach may both facilitate a wider examination of psychotherapy and encourage individual clinicians to research their own practice.

The disadvantages of such a routine procedure might be the loss of a more creative research approach, and the shifting emphasis from flexible individual thinking to an adherence to established norms in clinical practice. While the latter will undoubtedly suit the overstretched clinically oriented therapist, there remains the question of where the creativity lies in the practice of psychotherapy. To some extent this brings us back to the dilemma of where psychotherapy locates itself. This has been addressed by Hobson (1988), who argues for the preservation of subjectively-based research saying that 'there are certain things about relationships that can only be understood from within relationships'.

The adoption of routine clinical measures in psychotherapy practice would bring analytic and dynamic psychotherapy into line with cognitive behavioural therapy. This would undoubtedly ease discussions with those who commission services and may help to restore the analytic therapies to a more secure and influential position within medicine and the NHS (Barlow and Hoffman, 1997). However, this may not be a panacea for the provision of psychotherapy, nor sufficient to secure evidence based service development.

As with other areas of psychiatry, the availability of psychotherapy is likely to be influenced by consumer opinion. We are fortunate therefore that, at the current time, commissioners and providers of mental health services are attentive to patient opinion and choice. It would seem important therefore to include this component of psychotherapy research into routine clinical measures.

Setting up psychotherapy research projects

The evaluation of psychoanalysis remains a challenge for the future. Crammer and Freeman (1985) define the research attitude as 'one of being wide awake in the course of everyday clinical work and of asking questions instead of taking things for granted. There is a satisfaction in solving problems, making discoveries, perhaps finding a new treatment or a new hypothesis which can be tested.'

The essential factor for research is the quality of the methodological design, including careful consideration of statistical power where appropriate, as this will enhance the meaning of the results whether or not they attain statistical significance. The specific goal of any research project will depend on the questions being asked by it and must take account of ethical issues.

When planning a research project, it is important to bear in mind that:
• Research is hard work, requires discipline and is time-consuming.
• Often the beginner becomes disillusioned.
• It is useful to persuade a colleague to collaborate at an early stage.

Conclusion

Bateman and Holmes (1995) have suggested that Freud's insistence that psychoanalysis be accepted as a science remains a legitimate contemporary hope and possibility. The very nature of psychotherapy gives the required culture of enquiry a central place; the same curiosity that makes psychotherapists strive towards understanding their patients also makes them strive towards understanding the nature of the process in which they are engaged.

In this spirit of not taking things for granted, psychotherapy research not only asks questions about the process of psychotherapy but also challenges and scrutinizes the paradigms of research itself – as a comprehensive understanding is not possible without consideration of the context in which research takes place.

Further reading

Bergin, E.A. and Garfield, S.L. (1994) *Handbook of Psychotherapy and Behaviour Change*. New York: John Wiley.

Clark, D.M. and Fairburn, C. (1997) *Science and Practice of Cognitive Behaviour Therapy*. Oxford: Oxford University Press.

Freeman, C. and Tyrer, P. (1989) *Research Methods in Psychiatry: A Beginner's Guide*. London: Gaskell.

Greenhalgh, T. and Taylor, R. (1997) Papers that go beyond numbers (qualitative research). *British Medical Journal*, **315**, 740–743.

Malan, D. (1963) *A Study of Brief Psychotherapy*. New York: Plenum Press.

Roth, A. and Fonagy, P. (1996) *What Works for Whom? A Critical Review of Psychotherapy Research*. New York: Guilford Press.

Bibliography

Bachrach, H.M., Galatzer-Levy, R., Skolnikoff, A. and Waldron, S. (1991) On the efficacy of psychoanalysis. *Journal of the American Psychoanalytic Association*, **39**, 871–916.

Barlow, D.H. and Hoffman, S.G. (1997) Efficacy and discrimination of psychological treatments. In: D.M. Clark and C. Fairburn (eds), *Science and Practice of Cognitive Behaviour Therapy*. Oxford: Oxford University Press, pp. 95–118.

Bateman, A. and Holmes, J. (1995) *Introduction to Psychoanalysis*. London: Routledge.

Bloch, S. (1982) *What is Psychotherapy?* Oxford: Oxford University Press.

Brown, D. and Pedder, J. (1979) *Introduction to Psychotherapy. An Outline of Psychodynamic Principles and Practice*. London: Tavistock.

Clark, D.M. and Teasdale, J.D. (1982) Diurnal variation in clinical depression and accessibility of memories of positive and negative experiences. *Journal of Abnormal Psychology*, **91**, 87–95.

Clarke, R.V.G. and Cornish, D.B. (1972) *The Controlled Trial in Institutional Research*. London: HMSO.

Clarke, R.V.G. and Sinclair, I. (1973) *Towards More Effective Treatment Evaluation*. Strasbourg: Council of Europe.

Crammer, J.L. and Freeman, C.P. (1985) *Hints on Research*. London: Royal College of Psychiatrists Research Committee.

Crits-Christoph, P., Baranackie, K., Kurcias, J.S. *et al.* (1991) Meta-analysis of therapist effects in psychotherapy outcome studies. *Psychotherapy Research*, **1**, 81–91.

Dobson, K.S. (1989) A meta-analysis of the efficacy of cognitive therapy for depression. *Journal of Counselling and Clinical Psychology*, **57**, 414–417.

Evans, C., Carlyle, J. and Dolan, B. (1996) *Research: An Overview*. In: C. Cordess and M. Cox (eds), *Forensic Psychotherapy: Crime, Psychodynamics and the Offender Patient*. London: Jessica Kingsley, pp. 509–542.

Eysenck, H.J. (1952) The effects of psychotherapy: an evaluation. *Journal of Consulting Psychology*, **16**, 319–324.

Feldman, M.M. (1992) Audit in psychotherapy: the concept of Kaizen. *Psychiatric Bulletin*, **16**, 334–336.

Fonagy, P. (1993) Psychoanalytic and empirical approaches to developmental psychopathology: can they be usefully integrated? *Journal of the Royal Society of Medicine*, **86**, 577.

Fonagy, P. and Higgitt, A. (1989) Evaluating the performance of Departments of Psychotherapy. *Psychoanalytic Psychotherapy*, **4**, 121–153.

Fonagy, P. and Target, M. (1994) The efficacy of psychoanalysis for children with discipline disorders. *Journal of the American Academy for Child and Adolescent Psychiatry*, **33**, 44–55.

Fonagy, P. and Target, M. (1996) Playing with reality I: Theory of mind and the normal development of psychic reality. *International Journal of Psychoanalysis*, **77**, 217–223.

Fonagy, P., Leigh, T., Steele, M. *et al.* (1996) The relationship of attachment states, psychiatric classification, and response to psychotherapy. *Journal of Consulting and Clinical Psychology*, **64**, 1–10.

Fonagy, P., Steele, M., Moran, G. *et al.* (1991b) The capacity for understanding mental states: the reflective self in parent and child and its significance for security of attachment. *Infant Mental Health Journal*, **13**, 200–217.

Fonagy, P., Steele, M. and Steele, H. (1991a) Maternal representations of attachment during pregnancy predict the organisation of infant–mother attachment at one year of age. *Child Development*, **62**, 880–893.

Fonagy, P., Steele, M., Steele, H. and Target, M. (1997) *Reflective Functioning Manual: Version 4.1. For Application to Adult Attachment Interviews.* London: University College London, Psychoanalysis Unit.

Freud, A. (1954) The widening scope of indications for psychoanalysis: discussion. *Journal of the American Psychoanalytical Association*, **2**, 607–620.

Freud, S. (1895) Studies in hysteria. In: *Standard Edition of the Complete Psychological Works of Sigmund Freud*, vol. 2. London: Hogarth Press.

Freud, S. (1926) Inhibitions, symptoms and anxiety. In: *Standard Edition of the Complete Psychological Works of Sigmund Freud*, vol. 20. London: Hogarth Press.

Freud, S. (1933) New introductory lectures on psycho-analysis. In: *Standard Edition of the Complete Psychological Works of Sigmund Freud*, vol. 22. London: Hogarth Press.

Freud, S. (1937) Analysis terminable and interminable. In: *Standard Edition of the Complete Psychological Works of Sigmund Freud*, vol. 22. London: Hogarth Press.

Gelder, M., Gath, D. and Mayou, R. (1988) *Oxford Textbook of Psychiatry.* Oxford: Oxford University Press.

Gelder, M. (1997) The scientific foundations of cognitive therapy. In: D.M. Clark and C. Fairburn, *Science and Practice of Cognitive Behaviour Therapy.* Oxford: Oxford University Press, pp. 27–46.

George, G., Kaplan, N. and Malan, M. (1985) The Adult and Attachment Interview. Unpublished manuscript. Berkeley, CA: University of California Press.

Gerber, A. (1997) The Anna Freud Centre Young Adult Weekly Rating Scale. Unpublished PhD in progress. London: Anna Freud Centre.

Greenberg, L. and Pinsoff, W. (1986) *The Psychotherapeutic Process.* New York: Guilford Press.

Greenhalgh, T. and Taylor, R. (1997) Papers that go beyond numbers (qualitative research). *British Medical Journal*, **315**, 740–743.

Guthrie, E. (1991) Brief psychotherapy with patients with refractory irritable bowel syndrome. *British Journal of Psychotherapy*, **8**, 175–188.

Guthrie, E., Creed, F., Dawson, D. and Tomenson, B. (1993) A randomised controlled trial of psychotherapy in patients with refractory irritable bowel syndrome. *British Journal of Psychiatry*, **163**, 315–321.

Haigh, R. (1998) Economics of attachment disorders. *British Journal of Psychiatry*, **172**, 448–449.

Hobson, R.P. (1988) *Psychotherapy and Research – Are They Compatible?* London: Tavistock Papers, No.126.

Kantrowitz, J. (1987) Suitability for psychoanalysis. In: *The Yearbook of Psychoanalysis and Psychotherapy.* New York: Guilford Press, pp. 403–415.

Kernberg, O. (1973) Summary and conclusions of 'Psychotherapy and Psychoanalysis: A Final Report of the Menninger Foundation's Psychotherapy Research Project'. *International Journal of Psychiatry*, **11**, 62–77.

Kernberg, O. (1994) *Identity Diffusion and Structural Change.* Research Findings Presented to the Fourth International Psychoanalytic Association Conference on Psychoanalytic Research. London: March 1994.

Levinson, A. (1997) Research. In: E. Welldon and C. van Velsen (eds), *A Practical Guide to Forensic Psychotherapy.* London: Jessica Kingsley. 261–269.

Linehan, M. (1997) *Treatment Development, Validation and Dissemination: Thoughts from the Trenches.* Keynote Address at Society for Psychotherapy Research (UK) Annual Conference, Ravenscar, Yorkshire, 24 March 1997.

Luborsky, L., Crits-Cristoph, P., Mintz, J. and Auerbach, A. (1988) *Who Will Benefit From Psychotherapy? Predicting Therapeutic Outcomes.* New York: Basic Books.

Mahler, M.S. (1975) *The Psychological Birth of the Human Infant: Symbiosis and Individuation.* New York: Basic Books.

Main, M., Kaplan, N. and Cassidy, J. (1985) Security in Infancy, Childhood and Adulthood. A Move to the Level of Representation. In: I. Bretherton and E. Waters (eds), *Growing Points of Attachment Theory and Research.* Monographs of the Society for Research in Child Development, **50**, 60–104.

Malan, D. (1963) *A Study of Brief Psychotherapy.* New York: Plenum Press.

Malan, D. (1973) The outcome problem in psychotherapy research. *Archives of General Psychiatry*, **29**, 719–729.

Manning, N. (1989) *The Therapeutic Community Movement: Charisma and Routinization.* London: Routledge.

Marks, I. (1987) *Fears, Phobias and Rituals.* Oxford: Oxford University Press.

Menzies, D., Dolan, B. and Norton, K. (1993) Are short term savings worth long-term costs? Funding psychotherapeutic in-patient treatment of personality disorders. *Psychiatric Bulletin*, **17**, 517–521.

Moran, G. and Fonagy, P. (1987) Psychoanalysis and diabetic control: a single case study. *British Journal of Medical Psychology*, **60**, 357–372.

NHS Executive (1996) *NHS Psychotherapy Services in England: A Review of Strategic Policy.* Wetherby: Department of Health.

Rogers, C. and Dymond, R.F. (1954) *Psychotherapy and Personality Change.* Chicago: University of Chicago Press.

Roth, A. and Fonagy, P. (1996) *What Works for Whom? A Critical Review of Psychotherapy Research.* New York: Guilford Press.

Ricoeur, U.P. (1970) *Freud and Philosophy. An Essay on Interpretation.* New York: Yale University Press.

Sandler, J. (1995) *Research Without Numbers: An Approach to Conceptual Research in Psychoanalysis.* Presented to the British Psycho-Analytical Society, London, 5 July 1995.

Schlessinger, N. (1984) On analysability. In: J. Gedo and G. Pollock (eds), *Psychoanalysis: The Vital Issues.* Madison, CT: International Universities Press, pp. 249–274.

Shapiro, D. and Firth, J. (1987) Prescriptive v. exploratory psychotherapy. *British Journal of Psychiatry*, **151**, 790–799.

Steiner, J. (1985) Psychotherapy under attack. *Lancet*, **i**, 266–267.

Steiner, J. (1996) The aim of psychoanalysis in theory and practice. *International Journal of Psychoanalysis*, **77**, 1073–1083.

Tyson, A. and Sandler, J. (1971) Problems in the selection of patients for psychoanalysis: comments on the application of concepts of 'indications', 'suitability' and 'analyzability'. *British Journal of Medical Psychology*, **44**, 211–218.

Wallerstein, R.S. (1986) *Forty-Two Lives in Treatment: A Study of Psychoanalysis and Psychotherapy.* New York: Guilford Press.

Wallerstein, R.S. (1989) The Psychotherapy Research Project of the Menninger Foundation: an overview. *Journal of Consulting and Clinical Psychology*, **57**, 195–205.

Weber, J., Bachrach, H. and Solomon, M. (1985) Factors associated with the outcome of psychoanalysis: report of the Columbia Psychoanalytic Centre Research Project. *International Review of Psychoanalysis*, **12**, 127–141.

Williams, J.M.G. (1997) Depression. In: D.M. Clark and C. Fairburn (eds), *Science and Practice of Cognitive Behaviour Therapy.* Oxford: Oxford University Press, pp. 259–284.

Winnicott, D.W. (1964) *The Child, the Family and the Outside World.* London: Penguin.

Index